Emerging Advancements for Virtual and Augmented Reality in Healthcare

Luis Pinto Coelho
Polytechnic of Porto, Portugal

Ricardo Queirós
Polytechnic of Porto, Portugal

Sara Seabra Reis
Polytechnic of Porto, Portugal

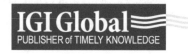

A volume in the Advances in Medical Technologies and Clinical Practice (AMTCP) Book Series

Published in the United States of America by
　　IGI Global
　　Medical Information Science Reference (an imprint of IGI Global)
　　701 E. Chocolate Avenue
　　Hershey PA, USA 17033
　　Tel: 717-533-8845
　　Fax: 717-533-8661
　　E-mail: cust@igi-global.com
　　Web site: http://www.igi-global.com

Library of Congress Cataloging-in-Publication Data

Names: Coelho, Luis, 1977- editor. | Queiros, Ricardo, 1975- editor. |
　　Reis, Sara, 1981- editor.
Title: Emerging advancements for virtual and augmented reality in
　　healthcare / Luis Coelho, Ricardo Queirós, and Sara Reis, editor.
Description: Hershey, PA : Medical Information Science Reference, [2022] |
　　Includes bibliographical references and index. | Summary: "The goal of
　　this book is to show how to put Virtual Reality in action by linking
　　academic and informatics researchers with professionals who use and need
　　VR in their day-a-day work, with a special focus on healthcare
　　professionals and related areas for the purpose of exchanging the
　　knowledge, information and technology from the international communities
　　in the area of VR, AR and XR"-- Provided by publisher.
Identifiers: LCCN 2021038631 (print) | LCCN 2021038632 (ebook) | ISBN
　　9781799883715 (hardcover) | ISBN 9781799883722 (ebook)
Subjects: MESH: Virtual Reality | Augmented Reality | Therapeutics |
　　Education, Medical
Classification: LCC R859.7.A78 (print) | LCC R859.7.A78 (ebook) | NLM W
　　26.55.V6 | DDC 610.285--dc23
LC record available at https://lccn.loc.gov/2021038631
LC ebook record available at https://lccn.loc.gov/2021038632

This book is published in the IGI Global book series Advances in Medical Technologies and Clinical Practice (AMTCP) (ISSN: 2327-9354; eISSN: 2327-9370)

British Cataloguing in Publication Data
A Cataloguing in Publication record for this book is available from the British Library.

For electronic access to this publication, please contact: eresources@igi-global.com.

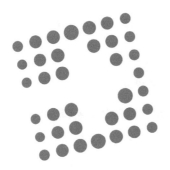

Advances in Medical Technologies and Clinical Practice (AMTCP) Book Series

Srikanta Patnaik
SOA University, India
Priti Das
S.C.B. Medical College, India

ISSN:2327-9354
EISSN:2327-9370

MISSION

Medical technological innovation continues to provide avenues of research for faster and safer diagnosis and treatments for patients. Practitioners must stay up to date with these latest advancements to provide the best care for nursing and clinical practices.

The **Advances in Medical Technologies and Clinical Practice (AMTCP) Book Series** brings together the most recent research on the latest technology used in areas of nursing informatics, clinical technology, biomedicine, diagnostic technologies, and more. Researchers, students, and practitioners in this field will benefit from this fundamental coverage on the use of technology in clinical practices.

COVERAGE

- Biometrics
- Biomechanics
- E-Health
- Clinical Nutrition
- Diagnostic Technologies
- Clinical Studies
- Nursing Informatics
- Clinical High-Performance Computing
- Clinical Data Mining
- Biomedical Applications

IGI Global is currently accepting manuscripts for publication within this series. To submit a proposal for a volume in this series, please contact our Acquisition Editors at Acquisitions@igi-global.com or visit: http://www.igi-global.com/publish/.

Titles in this Series

For a list of additional titles in this series, please visit: http://www.igi-global.com/book-series/advances-medical-technologies-clinical-practice/73682

Assistive Technologies for Assessment and Recovery of Neurological Impairments
Fabrizio Stasolla (University Giustino Fortunato of Benevento, Italy)
Medical Information Science Reference • © 2022 • 396pp • H/C (ISBN: 9781799874300) • US $295.00

Ethical Implications of Reshaping Healthcare With Emerging Technologies
Thomas Heinrich Musiolik (Berlin University of the Arts, Germany) and Alexiei Dingli (University of Malta, Malta)
Medical Information Science Reference • © 2022 • 242pp • H/C (ISBN: 9781799878889) • US $295.00

Innovative Approaches for Nanobiotechnology in Healthcare Systems
Touseef Amna (Albaha University, Saudi Arabia) and M. Shamshi Hassan (Albaha University, Saudi Arabia)
Medical Information Science Reference • © 2022 • 424pp • H/C (ISBN: 9781799882510) • US $395.00

Machine Learning and Data Analytics for Predicting, Managing, and Monitoring Disease
Manikant Roy (Lovely Professional University, India) and Lovi Raj Gupta (Lovely Professional University, India)
Medical Information Science Reference • © 2021 • 241pp • H/C (ISBN: 9781799871880) • US $395.00

Advancing the Investigation and Treatment of Sleep Disorders Using AI
M. Rajesh Kumar (Vellore Institute of Technology, Vellore, India) Ranjeet Kumar (Vellore Institute of Technology, Chennai, India) and D. Vaithiyanathan (National Institute of Technology, Delhi, India)
Medical Information Science Reference • © 2021 • 290pp • H/C (ISBN: 9781799880189) • US $345.00

Machine Learning in Cancer Research With Applications in Colon Cancer and Big Data Analysis
Zhongyu Lu (University of Huddersfield, UK) Qiang Xu (University of Huddersfield, UK) Murad Al-Rajab (University of Huddersfield, UK & Abu Dhabi University, UAE) and Lamogha Chiazor (University of Huddersfield, UK)
Medical Information Science Reference • © 2021 • 263pp • H/C (ISBN: 9781799873167) • US $345.00

Handbook of Research on Nano-Strategies for Combatting Antimicrobial Resistance and Cancer
Muthupandian Saravanan (Mekelle University, Ethiopia & Saveetha Dental College, Saveetha Institute of Medical and Technical Sciences (SIMATS), India) Venkatraman Gopinath (University of Malaya, Malaysia) and Karthik Deekonda (Monash University, Malaysia)
Medical Information Science Reference • © 2021 • 559pp • H/C (ISBN: 9781799850496) • US $375.00

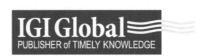

701 East Chocolate Avenue, Hershey, PA 17033, USA
Tel: 717-533-8845 x100 • Fax: 717-533-8661
E-Mail: cust@igi-global.com • www.igi-global.com

Table of Contents

Section 2
Education and Training

Section 3
Physical Intervention

Detailed Table of Contents

Section 1
Preventive Healthcare and Awareness

Chapter 1
Virtual Reality in Healthcare: A Survey
    Dorota Kamińska, Lodz University of Technology, Poland
    Grzegorz Zwolińsksi, Lodz University of Technology, Poland
    Anna Laska-Leśniewicz, Lodz University of Technology, Poland
    Luis Pinto Coelho, Polytechnic of Porto, Portugal

Over the past few years, the rapid development of virtual reality has led to the technology finding its way into the professional sector in addition to the gaming market. It plays a particularly important role in medical applications by providing a virtual environment to enable therapy, rehabilitation, and serving as an educational platform. The chapter provides an overview of the applications of virtual reality in medicine about some of the most important areas. Both scenario development and application validation methods are presented, as well as their impact on the end user. Finally, the technological potential and future development of VR applications used for improving medical service delivery are summarized and briefly discussed.

Chapter 2
Virtual and Augmented Reality Awareness Tools for Universal Design: Towards Active
Preventive Healthcare
    Luis Coelho, Polytechnic of Porto, Portugal
    Idalina Freitas, Polytechnic of Porto, Portugal
    Dorota Urszula Kaminska, Lodz University of Technology, Poland
    Ricardo Queirós, School of Media Arts and Design, Polytechnic of Porto, Portugal
    Anna Laska-Lesniewicz, Lodz University of Technology, Poland
    Grzegorz Zwolinski, Lodz University of Technology, Poland
    Rui Raposo, Universidade de Aveiro, Portugal
    Mário Vairinhos, Universidade de Aveiro, Portugal
    Elisabeth Pereira, Universidade de Aveiro, Portugal
    Eric Haamer, University of Tartu, Estonia

Gholamreza Anbarjafari, University of Tartu, Estonia

This chapter will be focused on contributing to the increase of universal design competencies of future engineers, educators, and designers through the use of mixed reality technologies, closing the gap between theory and field application of principles, towards a more inclusive world and promoting health and wellbeing for all. The experience of a situation where limitations arise in relation to what is taken for granted is an important experience that leads to a personal knowledge of the difficulties. By the use of simulators, especially virtual (VR) and mixed reality (MR) technologies, it is possible to create such experiences. Training based on MR can prepare future and current professionals for up-to-date requirements of the labor market. In addition, it can ensure that the standards such as barrier-free concepts, broader accessibility, adaptive and assistive technology will be familiar to trainees.

Section 2
Education and Training

Chapter 3

Sonia Rodriguez Cano, Facultad de Educación, Universidad de Burgos, Spain
Vanesa Delgado-Benito, Facultad de Educación, Universidad de Burgos, Spain
Vitor Gonçalves, CIEB, Instituto Politécnico de Bragança, Portugal

Educational technology is contributing towards diversity awareness as it allows you to create more personalized and student-centered learning situations. This chapter addresses specific learning difficulties (SpLD) and, specifically, dyslexia, since it is one of the most prevalent challenges in the educational field. Information and communication technologies allow direct intervention with students who have special educational needs as an alternative to traditional resources, which is much more motivating. In this sense, as an example, various projects and applications are presented that allow working on this type of difficulties with students. This chapter highlights the virtual reality and augmented reality software carried out in the context of the European Erasmus + FORDYSVAR project, of which the authors are part.

Chapter 4

Catherine Hayes, University of Sunderland, UK

This chapter provides an insight into the theoretical perspectives which form the foundation of extended reality (XR) and its emergence in practice as a fundamental part of medical and healthcare curricula. Issues such as the authenticity of learning, the validity and reliability of XR within processes of assessment, and the theoretical underpinnings of pedagogical approaches in health professions pedagogy are illuminated. Also considered are the implications of XR within the context of non-patient-based learning and the delineation of cognitive, affective, and psychomotor domains of learning in relation to patient outcomes at the front line of care in applied practice. The COVID-19 pandemic, which has impacted all global higher education institutional (HEI) learning since March 2020, is also considered in the context of moves to ensure that medical and healthcare education can continue, albeit via hybrid models of learning as opposed to traditional pedagogical approaches, which have remained little altered over the last century.

Chapter 5

Virtual simulation is a learning tool that employs specific hardware and software technology for simulation-based provider training within a digital domain. Extended reality or XR software includes virtual reality (VR), augmented reality (AR), and mixed reality (MR) programs that represent a rapidly growing area within the field of virtual simulation. This training may provide either provider- or patient-centered learning modules, with dedicated hardware and software centered on skill-based, 3D modeling or case-based learning. Demand for these learning programs in healthcare education was fueled by the remote learning needs of the COVID-19 pandemic. In addition to this growing demand, there is a significant role for many virtual simulation software programs within the traditional classroom and lecture hall. This is a previously untapped resource for simulation education. The flipped classroom model provides an opportune framework for the incorporation of immersive, virtual simulation learning programs within spaces previously limited to the more passive, podium-based lecture.

Chapter 6

The advancement of virtual reality (VR) technology for educational instruction and curricular (re)design have become highly attractive and newly demanding areas of both the technology and healthcare industries. However, the quickly evolving field is still learning about each of the associated VR technologies, whether they are evidence-based, and how they are validated to decrease cognitive load and in turn increase student/learner comprehension. Likewise, the instructional (re)design of the content that the student/learner is exposed to in VR, and whether it is immersive, and promotes memorable content and experiences can influence their learning outcomes. Here the Revinax® Handbook content library that is displayed in an immersive virtual reality application in first-person point-of-view (IVRA-FPV) is contrasted with third-person point-of-view (IVRA-TPV) through VR headsets to an individual, and computer displays to many individuals along with augmented reality (AR) are evaluated as emerging advancements in the field of VR and AR.

Section 3
Physical Intervention

This chapter seeks to explore from the reflexivity approach the current state of virtual and augmented technologies in various surgical procedures, analyzing the most relevant technological progress as well as the latest practical applications that have been developed. Bibliographic, documentary, and descriptive were the methodologies of research; the information was collected from various scientific articles from indexed journals and websites, using keywords such as "virtual reality," "augmented reality," and "surgical procedure" in search engines. Furthermore, technological progress in various branches that include surgery is explored in this chapter, which is focused on the research and technology application of virtual and augmented reality as well as the challenges.

Chapter 8

Ranjit Barua, CHST, Indian Institute of Engineering Science and Technology, Shibpur, India
Surajit Das, R. G. Kar Medical College and Hospital, India

Present signs of development in virtual and augmented reality have offered an important amount of inventive outfits into the customer market. Virtual reality (VR) technology has now affected the optimistic features of treatment. Surgeries in especially urology are constantly emerging, and the virtual reality model has become an important supplement in urologist teaching and training lists. This chapter provides a summary of the significance and varieties of virtual reality methods, their present applications in the area of urology (surgery), and upcoming implications.

Chapter 9

Anmol Bagaria, CynoDent, India
Sonal Mahilkar, Maitri College of Dentistry and Research Centre, India
Subash C. Sonkar, Multidisciplinary Research Unit, Maulana Azad Medical College,
*   University of Delhi, New Delhi, India*

The skill of visual reality has matured, and VR and AR are increasingly being used in educational and surgical settings. The development of virtual reality technologies allows users to mix medical knowledge, medical data, and graphical data. It can provide more precise information, allowing users to increase their safety and reduce their risk. Virtual reality (VR) or augmented reality (AR) simulators that provide direct feedback and objective evaluation could be a useful tool in dental education in the future. Not only has it been applied to education, but it has also been created in therapeutic therapy. The authors believe that in the future VR and AR training and teaching will be extended and used in every aspect of dentistry, enabling students to develop their abilities on their own. In comparison to augmented reality, virtual reality offers a far more immersive experience. It would establish a trusting relationship between patients and doctors based on the experience of the dentists and the use of different hardware and software.

Section 4
Mental Intervention

Chapter 10
Charles V. Trappey, National Yang Ming Chiao Tung University, Taiwan
Amy J. C. Trappey, National Tsing Hua University, Taiwan
C. M. Chang, Chang Gung Memorial Hospital, Taiwan
M. C. Tsai, Taoyuan General Hospital, Taiwan
Routine R. T. Kuo, National Tsing Hua University, Taiwan
Aislyn P. C. Lin, National Tsing Hua University, Taiwan

Anxiety disorders are diagnosed when people become overreactive, disassociated, and feel emotionally unable to control feelings to the extent that their daily lifes are affected. Driving phobia is one of the widespread anxiety disorders in modern society, which cause problematic disruptions of a patient's daily activities. Exposure therapy is an approach gaining popularity for treating patients with stress disorders. Virtual reality (VR) technology allows people to interact with objects and stimuli in an immersive way. The VR for phobic therapy using indirect exposure, which can be safely discontinued or lowed in terms of intensity, is the area of research with literature published and patents granted. This research focuses on reviewing virtual reality exposure therapy (VRET) literature and patents. The chapter also presents the research and development of a novel driving phobia VRET system with the detailed experiments to demonstrate the design, development, implementation, enhancement, and verification of VRET.

Chapter 11
Jagrika Bajaj, Touchkin eServices Private Limited., India
Aparna Sahu, Turiyan Psyneuronics Private Limited., India

The advancements in immersive technologies have impacted various sectors, with mental healthcare being one of them. The subsequent interaction between immersive technologies, particularly virtual reality and mental health, has created interesting effects that call for a closer look. This chapter intends to provide a comprehensive picture of mental health conditions, namely anxiety and related disorders, post-traumatic stress disorder, and major depressive disorder, as tackled by VR-based therapy. The focus is on its effectiveness and how the results compare to the traditional modes of treatment in terms of efficacy. The impact of user experience towards this approach of intervention and the importance of ethical consideration when VR intersects with the field of mental health are addressed.

Chapter 12
Aparna Sahu, Turiyan Psyneuronics Private Limited, India
Jagrika Bajaj, Touchkin eServices Private Limited, India

The merging of immersive technologies and cognition has been around for a while. However, it is only in the last decade or so that immersive technologies' contributions in the areas of cognitive assessments and interventions have gathered recognition. This chapter covers findings from published research in cognition-based assessments and interventions using the immersive technologies of virtual reality (VR) and augmented reality (AR). The role of immersive technologies in cognition is critically evaluated to inform all its stakeholders about its potential for use in the future.

Section 5
Trends

Virtual reality (VR) is defined as a simulation of the real world using computer graphics. The basic components of a VR application or program are interaction and immersion. Human-computer interaction is achieved through multiple sensory channels that allow individuals to explore virtual environments through senses. Immersion is considered the degree to which the individual feels engrossed or enveloped within the virtual environment. Scope of virtual reality is quite wide and varied, including technology, industry, education, and health. In the health sector, it has a significant role in assessment as well as intervention. Specific to human behavior and cognition, virtual reality's (VR) application is for cognitive assessment and rehabilitation. VR offers the potential to develop human testing and training environments that allow for the precise control of complex stimulus presentations in which human cognitive and functional performance can be accurately assessed and rehabilitated.

Chapter 14

The visual field (VF) examination is a useful clinical tool for monitoring a variety of ocular diseases. Despite its wide utility in eye clinics, the test as currently conducted is subject to an array of issues that interfere in obtaining accurate results. Visual field exams of patients suffering from additional ocular conditions are often unreliable due to interference between the comorbid diseases. To improve upon these shortcomings, virtual reality (VR) and deep learning are being explored as potential solutions. Virtual reality has been incorporated into novel visual field exams to provide a portable, 3D exam experience. Deep learning, a specialization of machine learning, has been used in conjunction with VR, such as in the iGlaucoma application, to limit subjective bias occurring from patients' eye movements. This chapter seeks to analyze and critique how VR and deep learning can augment the visual field experience by improving accuracy, reducing subjective bias, and ultimately, providing clinicians with a greater capacity to enhance patient outcomes.

Preface

INTRODUCTION

In the last few years, devices that are increasingly capable of offering an immersive experience close to reality have emerged. Goggles, gloves, suits and other devices are able to work in conjunction to stimulate the user's senses while monitoring his reaction, creating a technological closed loop where the human is the central system. As the cost of devices drops and their size decreases, interest and application possibilities increase. In the health area, there is an enormous potential for VR and AR development, as this technology allows, on the one hand, the perception and execution of operations or processes at a distance, decoupling realities, and on the other hand, it offers the possibility of simulation for training purposes, whenever there are contexts of risk to the patient or to the health professional. The application possibilities and their impact are transversal to all areas of health, and fields such as education, training, surgery, pain management, physical rehabilitation, stroke rehabilitation, phobia therapy or telemedicine are the focus of a lot of attention.

To obtain natural immersive experiences, where the virtual world is not distinguished from the real world, there are still many technical challenges. In addition to the supporting hardware, the development of a virtual reality encompasses a wide range of areas: idealization of scenarios and actors, 3D modeling of scenarios and actors, modeling of laws of physics and rules of interaction between objects, navigation and interaction between humans and virtual world, integration of artificial intelligence in virtual environments, among others. Additionally, the use of virtual reality devices and immersion in virtual environments still requires some improvements as complaints of headaches or nausea are still common. Both causes and consequences must be investigated to offer the best user experience

Virtual Reality (VR) is the use of computer technology to construct an environment that is simulated. VR places the user inside and in the center of the experience, unlike conventional user interfaces. Users are immersed and able to connect with 3D environments instead of seeing a screen in front of them. The computer has the role to provide the experiences of the user in this artificial environment by simulating as many senses as possible, such as sight, hearing, touch, and smell. In Augmented Reality (AR) we have an enhanced version of the real physical world that is achieved through the use of digital visual elements, sound, or other sensory stimuli delivered via technology. It can be seen as VR imposed into real life.

In both VR and AR, the experience is composed of a virtual or extended world, an immersion technology, sensory feedback, and interactivity. These elements use a multitude of technologies that must work together and presented to the user seamlessly integrated and synchronized.

GOALS

The book *Emerging Advancements for Virtual and Augmented Reality in Healthcare* is dedicated to applications, new technologies and emerging trends in the fields of virtual reality and augmented reality in the healthcare realm. This comprises, by definition, the prevention, diagnosis, treatment, recovery, or cure of disease, illness, injury, and other physical and mental impairments in people, either as an active form or in a passive action, towards or by promoting such outcomes. In terms of scope, it is intended to cover technical areas as well as areas of applied intervention. In a technological perspective, it is expected to cover hardware and software technologies while encompassing all components of the virtual experience.

A potential reader should be able to understand how Virtual Reality can be put in action by linking academic and informatics researchers with professionals who use and need VR in their day-a-day work, with a special focus on healthcare professionals and related areas. Within this scope, it is intended to disseminate and exchange the knowledge, information and technology provided by the international communities in the areas of VR, AR and XR throughout the beginning of 21st century.

Another important goal is to synthesize trends, best practices, methodologies, languages, and tools which are used to implement VR. To shape the future of VR, new paradigms and technologies should be discussed, not forgetting aspects related to regulation and certification of VR technologies, especially in the healthcare area. These last topics are crucial for the standardization of VR.

This book will present important achievements and will show how to use VR technologies in a full range of settings able to provide decision support anywhere and anytime using this new approach. The mission of this book is promoting the cross-fertilization of knowledge across professional and geographical boundaries, catalyzing the users engaging in several areas like education, healthcare, industry, among others.

This book will be submitted to be indexed in Scopus, which will increase their visibility and interest to the community.

The target audience comprises professionals and researchers working in the field of VR/AR for healthcare. This encompasses a wide range of professionals, from health professions (doctors, nurses, audiologists, psychologists, occupational therapists, etc.) to engineers, designers, story tellers and others that must work together to build VR and AR technology.

DESCRIPTION AND ORGANIZATION OF THE BOOK

The book contains contributions from academia and from industry, and all world regions are represented in terms of authorship. This diversity ensures to provide a global vision of the topic from many different perspectives. All fifteen chapters help to understand the present and shape the future of VR/AR in healthcare. For accomplishing it, the book is divided into five sections: I. Preventive Healthcare and Awareness; II. Education and Training; III. Physical Intervention; IV Mental Intervention; and V. Trends.

The first section, "Preventive Healthcare and Awareness," presents some studies conducted through theory and surveys on the use of VR/AR in healthcare. Then, the chapters of the second section, "Education and Training," show some innovative strategies for using mixed reality in healthcare education. The third section, "Physical Intervention," presents some strategies and approaches for the use of these technologies with people with disability and for advanced treatments in specific areas. The next section, "Mental Intervention," exposes some approaches to address issues on the treatment of mental health such as stress disorders. The last section, "Trends," explores new techniques (like deep learning) to foster the use of VR/AR in complex healthcare challenges.

The first section of this book, entitled "Preventive Healthcare and Awareness," has two chapters. This first chapter, entitled "Virtual Reality in Healthcare: A Survey," provides an overview of some of the most important applications of virtual reality in medicine. Methods for scenario development and application validation, as well as their impact on the end user, are presented. Finally, the technological potential and future development of virtual reality (VR) applications for improving medical service delivery are summarized and briefly discussed. The second chapter, entitled "Virtual and Augmented Reality Awareness Tools for Universal Design: Towards Active Preventive Healthcare," is focused on contributing to the increase of Universal Design competencies of future engineers, educators, and designers through the use of mixed reality technologies, closing the gap between theory and field application of principles, towards a more inclusive world and promoting health and well-being for all. The authors also present results of a survey about the use of VR/AR as a learning technology and an example application.

The second section of this book, covering the areas of "Education and Training," is constituted by four chapters. The first, entitled "Educational Technology Based on Virtual and Augmented Reality for Students With Learning Disabilities: Specific Projects and Applications," addresses Specific Learning Difficulties (DEA) and, specifically, dyslexia, since it is one of the most prevalent difficulties in the educational field. The authors show that Educational Technology can contribute as a motivational boost to direct intervention with students who have special educational needs as an alternative in relation to more traditional resources. As an example, various projects and applications are described. The following chapter, "A Pedagogical Paradigm Shift: Prospective Epistemologies of Extended Reality (XR) in Health Professions Education," explores the key epistemologies or ways of knowing, from a theoretical perspective, that can be used to ensure the necessary authenticity level to highlight the pedagogical shifts in the application of learning theory which now characterize responsive curriculum design and adaptation to accommodate XR in practice. The next chapter, with the title "Virtual Simulation: A Flipped Classroom Teaching Tool for Healthcare Education," seeks to offer readers a detailed description of the variety of virtual simulation programs within healthcare education as well as their crucial role within the traditional classroom and lecture hall within the flipped classroom model. The flipped classroom model provides a suitable framework for integrating immersive, virtual simulation learning programs within spaces previously limited to the more traditional, passive, podium-based lecture. Still, in this section, in "Building an Extended Reality Pedagogical Continuum: The Use of 180° First Person Point-of-View Video to Upskill, Reskill, and Support Learning Technical Procedures From VR-to-Computer and Mobile Displays-to-AR," the Revinax® content library that is displayed in an Immersive Virtual Reality Application in first-person point-of-view (IVRA-FPV) is contrasted with third-person point-of-view (IVRA-TPV) through VR headsets to an individual and computer displays to many individuals along with Augmented Reality are evaluated as emerging advancements in the field of VR and AR.

The third section of this book is aimed towards the "Physical Intervention" area, being comprised of three chapters. In "Application of Virtual/Augmented Reality in Surgical Procedures: Bibliographic Revision of Recent Advances," the authors seek to explore from the reflexivity approach the current state of virtual and augmented technologies in various surgical procedures, analyzing the most relevant technological progresses, as well as the latest practical applications that have been developed. Additionally, the technological progress in various branches that include surgery is explored, focusing in the research and technological application of virtual and augmented reality, as well as the current challenges to massify the use of these tools in the future. Then, an application area is explored in "Improvements of

Virtual and Augmented Reality for Advanced Treatments in Urology". Here the authors present how VR and AR had a revolutionary role on the area and how these technologies can benefit the several stages of urology treatments. Another application area is explored in "Emerging Advancement for Augmented Reality (AR) and Virtual Reality (VR) in Dentistry," where the authors explore novel approaches to the use of VR and AR in dentistry.

The fourth section of this book is focused on "Mental Intervention" and has three chapters. The first chapter, entitled "Virtual Reality Exposure Therapy and Physiological Data Analysis for Immersive Treatment of Stress Disorders," provides a review of Virtual Reality Exposure Therapy (VRET) literature and patents, and also presents the research and development of a novel driving phobia VRET system, with detailed experiments to demonstrate the design, development, implementation, enhancement, and verification of VRET. The following chapter, "Evidence-Based Virtual Reality Use for Mental Health Conditions," presents an approach to the use of virtual reality therapy for psychiatric disorders. Considering the characteristics of anxiety related disorders, posttraumatic stress disorder and major depressive disorder, the possibilities, findings, and advantages of using virtual reality therapy are presented. Also, ethical considerations are made in the context of the use of this technique in mental disorders. To close the section, we can find in "Evidence-Based Immersive Technology Use in Cognitive Assessments and Cognition-Based Interventions," psychometrics requirements for cognitive tests are covered. The use of immersive technologies for cognition-based assessments and interventions is presented. A critical evaluation of the use of these techniques is also made.

The fifth and final section of this book, entitled "Trends," tries to anticipate the future by providing a vision of what can be done and what challenges need to be overpassed. In the first of the two chapters, "The Future of Virtual Reality and Deep Learning in Visual Field Testing," the authors will further explain the issues with the current visual field test and how virtual reality and deep learning have the potential to augment the exam to allow for a more accurate portrayal of a patient's visual field to improve patient care. The next and final chapter, "Application of Virtual Reality in Cognitive Rehabilitation: A Road Ahead," is focused in an area of major importance in modern world. The author, after providing a thorough overview of the cognitive rehabilitation area, exposes outcomes, limitations, future plans, and implications of VR and AR technology in such field.

CONCLUSION

This book has a transversal and convergent impact because it addresses the use of VR/AR applied to several areas in the healthcare realm. The included chapters bring ideas of how to use VR/AR in particular healthcare domains, providing the required specificities, but also by creating bridges with other areas and applications. The practical examples can clarify and motivate the researchers to conduct their works in applied VR/AR. The book can help to prove that the application of VR/AR mechanisms can help to solve many issues and that this technology has a promising future.

We hope that this book can be a vital contribution in the area and help engage the community of VR/AR by bringing new researchers and professionals of this topic to the challenging and demanding domain of healthcare.

Acknowledgment

First of all, we thank all the authors, reviewers and the editorial board who have contributed to this book's success. Then, a particular thanks to IGI and their editorial team for the help provided during the editing process.

Section 1
Preventive Healthcare and Awareness

Chapter 1
Virtual Reality in Healthcare:
A Survey

Dorota Kamińska
Lodz University of Technology, Poland

Grzegorz Zwolińsksi
Lodz University of Technology, Poland

Anna Laska-Leśniewicz
Lodz University of Technology, Poland

Luis Pinto Coelho
iD https://orcid.org/0000-0002-5673-7306
Polytechnic of Porto, Portugal

ABSTRACT

Over the past few years, the rapid development of virtual reality has led to the technology finding its way into the professional sector in addition to the gaming market. It plays a particularly important role in medical applications by providing a virtual environment to enable therapy, rehabilitation, and serving as an educational platform. The chapter provides an overview of the applications of virtual reality in medicine about some of the most important areas. Both scenario development and application validation methods are presented, as well as their impact on the end user. Finally, the technological potential and future development of VR applications used for improving medical service delivery are summarized and briefly discussed.

PREAMBLE

Over the past few years, the rapid development of virtual reality has led to the technology finding its way into the professional sector in addition to the gaming market. It plays a particularly important role in medical applications by providing a virtual environment to enable therapy, rehabilitation and serving

DOI: 10.4018/978-1-7998-8371-5.ch001

as an educational platform. The following chapter provides an overview of the applications of virtual reality in medicine about some of the most important areas. Both scenario development and application validation methods are presented, as well as their impact on the end user. Finally, the technological potential and future development of VR applications used for improving medical service delivery are summarized and briefly discussed.

INTRODUCTION

It is well known that the use of modern technologies in the medical industry helps to improve the quality of services provided. The cooperation of these two fields is constantly developing, and researchers are looking for more and more advanced solutions to improve the work of medics, but above all to increase the quality of treatment of diseases and disorders. In recent years, virtual reality (VR), by providing an interactive computer-generated environment, has found its way into various medical fields. VR simulates the physical presence of the user in an artificially generated world and allows them to interact with this environment. The use of VR in medicine is an area of great opportunity, as evidenced by clinical studies and experienced physicians (Riva, 2003). For example, VR can serve as a training environment that helps healthcare professionals improve their skills through hands-on learning. The key strength of such solutions is the ability to include even very rare clinical cases in scenarios and the total lack of consequences for wrong decisions and actions undertaken. Although the field is completely new, there are already several such applications that have been shown to have a significant impact on improving both medical education and patient treatment and therapy.

The term virtual reality refers to a computer simulation representing an environment in which one can move and interact with virtual space, events, objects, and people (avatars). The virtual environment is usually three-dimensional and often replicates the real world in terms of appearance and physical phenomena occurring in it. Typically, VR applications can be divided into three groups based on the degree of immersion into applications using: VR displays (e.g., stereoscopic (Alfalah et al., 2018), large-format (Hsieh et al., 2017), virtual caves (Flaconer et al., 2016)), augmented reality (AR) and virtual reality helmets.

The first type is a partially or semi-immersive VR environment (Lee et al., 2008). It is usually projected onto a wall or monitor using special goggles used to view 3D objects. Interaction with the virtual world is based on simple input devices such as keyboard, mouse, joystick, or touch screen. Augmented reality is based on combining the real world with the virtual world, thus superimposing 3D graphics in real time, e.g., using translucent glasses. Such applications are very often used in medical imaging - specialists have access to visualization of the structure or function of the patient's internal organs.

Figure 1. Types of virtual reality used in medical applications.
From left - stereoscopic screen (Alfalah et al., 2018), AR for learning anatomy, VR headset for depression treatment

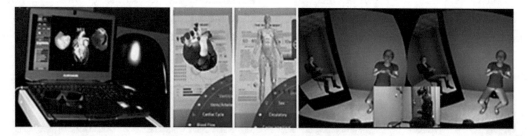

The creation of the first Oculus Rift prototype (2010) marked the beginning of the strong development of head-mounted display (HMD) virtual reality helmets. At the current level of technology development, most VR applications are based on HMDs, with players such as Sony, HTC, Facebook, and Google competing to produce them. Their main aim is to create cheaper yet more powerful hardware, which is essential for the popularization of VR (Gutierrez et al., 2017). The simplest VR platform has been developed by Google. It includes simple, cheap, foldable cardboard frames in which a smartphone is placed (many popular smart phone models can be used). More complex, and therefore more expensive solutions, such as Oculus Rift or HTC Vive, require complex hardware infrastructure so they are rather used in laboratories and specially adapted rooms. These types of VR platforms do not require additional hardware for interaction, as they come standard with headsets and controllers with a built-in set of sensors.

One of the major challenges for VR technology is to provide deeper immersion. Special external sensors such as Kinect (Kurillo et al., 2014) or the MYO Gesture control band (Sathiyanarayanan et al., 2016), sensory gloves (Lin et al., 2018) or dedicated suits (Kunze et al., 2017) can be used to solve this problem. For example, motor rehabilitation applications very often use EMG electromyographic signals. Typically used in the rehabilitation of post-stroke patients, they show both high effectiveness and comfort in use (Yang et al., 2017). Another example is an application in which the authors evaluate the effectiveness of combining an immersive VR game with stationary cycling as a health physical activity (Kim et al., 2018). More advanced and precise systems often use so-called tailor-made solutions, i.e., customized for a specific application. Secodont, for example, is a pre-clinical dental training based on a VR application that has been combined with haptic technology to simulate realistic rough textures (Wang et al., 2016). Another example is an app for training people with autism spectrum disorders. The application scenario involves the selection and manipulation of tangible objects and locomotion, using HMDs and large-format screens (Bozgeyikli et al., 2018). A selection of examples is shown in figure 2.

Figure 2. Selected examples of technologies that increase the level of immersion.
From left: MYO Gesture control band (Sathiyanarayanan et al., 2016), virtual exercise bike platform (Kim et al., 2018), Si-modont (Wang et al., 2016).

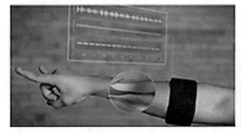 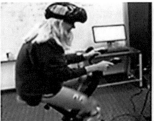 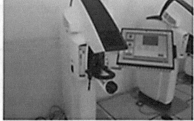

Another challenge of VR technology is still the relatively expensive and inconvenient hardware and the limited options available to use it. This is slowly beginning to change, but while devices have been developed that have become affordable, easy to use and enable amazing effects, the shortcomings of the available technology still mean that the glory days of VR and AR have not yet begun. However, all indications are that fifth-generation mobile technology will change a lot!

5G mobile networks can provide a reduction in the cost of mobile communications and, more importantly, a huge amount of data transfer without delay. For example, it is possible to control robots, from anywhere, and 5G technology will make this fully accurate and seamless, eliminating any potential technical errors almost to zero (Rao et al., 2018). Another example is the automotive industry, which is investing heavily in VR and 3D visualization technologies to improve product design, by virtually creating, examining, and testing them (Lawson et al., 2015). The deployment of 5G networks and use in virtual technologies is undoubtedly a step in the right direction.

Educational Applications

One of the most important applications of virtual reality are training and educational applications. Solutions of this type also work well for medical training. Thanks to simulators reflecting the human body, young doctors can gain experience, experiment, and learn from their mistakes without risking the health and lives of patients. One of the most interesting examples is the Physical Heart Model, an application that presents the three-dimensional structure of the human heart (Alfalah et al., 2018). The virtual heart is set in space and the user can freely manipulate it by rotating it at different angles, analyzing cross-sections and relations between its parts. The application was tested at the Faculty of Medicine at the University of Jordan, and its effectiveness was compared with learning on a traditional physical model. The test results indicated the superiority of the virtual model. A similar approach was presented by the authors of an application aimed at learning the anatomy of the canine skeletal system (Seo et al., 2017). The virtual environment allows interaction with individual bones, their identification, and the construction of the animal skeleton in 3D.

The virtual environment can simulate situations that medical personnel must deal with daily. Life Support, for example, is an application designed to train the performance of advanced resuscitation (Vankipuram et al., 2014). The scenario consists of a series of timed, team-based tasks, providing guidance on clinical interventions during cardiac arrest and respiratory failure. Another example is an application that prepares nurses for the nursing profession. The virtual environment replicates a hospital ward full of patients with dementia, their family members, and medical staff. The user experiences real-life scenarios and learns about the responsibilities and activities required of staff who care for patients (Elliman et al., 2016). A similar goal is pursued by the application, which supports learning how to prepare hands for a surgical procedure, which is key to preventing infections (Harrison et al., 2017).

A more advanced device is Simodont (Wang et al., 2016), a virtual simulation that prepares dental students to create a dental crown. Interestingly, the simulator can differentiate between students and residents based on both the time it takes to make a crown and their skills. Because it replicates realistic clinical situations, it is a much better learning environment than a phantom or plastic mannequin. VRmagic (Radia et al., 2018), is also an advanced surgical simulator that provides a realistic environment for acquiring psychomotor skills and developing microsurgical spatial awareness. The skills thus acquired are applied by novice eye surgeons during real cataract and vitreoretinal surgeries. This type of training allows young doctors to become familiar with techniques of moving in the patient's eye space, thus minimizing the stress accompanying the procedure in the real life of an operating theatre. Screenshots of VR applications used for educational purposes are presented in figure 3.

Figure 3. Screenshots of VR applications used for educational purposes.
From left: Life Support (Vankipuram et al., 2014), learning the anatomy of the dog's skeletal system (Seo et al., 2017), Physical Heart Model (Alfalah et al., 2018), Simodont (Wang et al., 2016)

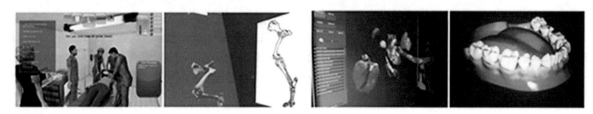

Motor Rehabilitation

The use of VR for motor rehabilitation has long been a focus of research, and the increasing popularity of hardware and software has led to growing interest in the use of such solutions in both clinical and home settings (Powell et al., 2017). One of the most important groups of recipients of such applications are post-stroke patients with mobility problems. An example is the upper limb rehabilitation system, which offers a range of interactive exercises using feedback. Ten people with upper limb paresis due to stroke were recruited for the pilot study. Patients participated in ten sessions (two sessions per week). Clinical studies have shown that virtual training is beneficial for motor function recovery (a mean improvement of 5.3\% was observed) even in the chronic stage. At this point, studies are being conducted on a larger sample size to confirm the effectiveness of the therapy (Perez-Marcos et al., 2017). A similar approach was used in an application for hand motor rehabilitation. The app uses a flexible orthosis to help perform hand exercises via a virtual interface (Cartagena et al., 2017).

Another example is the use of VR as a motor skills training tool in the rehabilitation of balance and gait disorders. Most studies are conducted on neurological patients such as patients diagnosed with Parkinson's disease, multiple sclerosis, after acute and chronic stroke, traumatic brain injury or cerebral palsy. More than ninety different studies confirm that the use of VR improves balance and gait in all the cohorts, especially when combined with conventional rehabilitation (Porras et al., 2018).

A typical application of VR is also to prepare the patient for life after amputation. After surgery, the patient must not only undergo expensive rehabilitation treatment, but also wait several months before receiving a properly fitted prosthesis (Sharma et al., 2018). An example of this type of application is a virtual training environment in which hand amputation patients can train independently, interacting with holographic objects using Microsoft HoloLens goggles, while receiving tactile and proprioceptive sensations. This type of environment can also be used in motor therapy after leg amputation (Winkler et al., 2016).

Figure 4. VR applications used for physical rehabilitation.
From left: upper limb rehabilitation (Perez-Marcos et al., 2017), motor skills training too (Porras et al., 2018), preparing the patient for life after amputation (Winkler et al., 2016), Face to Face (Breedon et al., 2016)

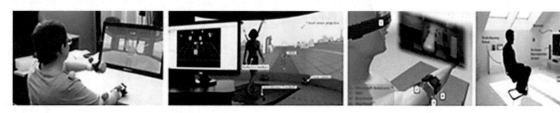

Very interesting research is being done in the use of VR for training facial muscles. An example is the Face-to-Face (Breedon et al., 2016) system, which aims to treat facial muscle spasticity caused by stroke. The patient's task is to perform exercises presented by a virtual therapist on the screen. The system records and simultaneously provides feedback using a face recognition algorithm captured by a Kinect sensor. Clinical studies indicate that the system is more effective than exercises performed in front of a mirror. Face to Face encourages the patient to exercise, but more importantly records their progress. Another example is a system that supports facial recovery using functional electrical stimulation after facial transplantation (Topçu et all, 2018).

Psychological Therapy

Virtual reality also helps in professional psychotherapy, especially in cognitive behavioral therapy. For example, it can be used for the treatment of patients with anxiety disorders and phobias, post-traumatic stress disorder, addictions and other disorders that negatively affect the patient's daily life. One of the most common types of phobias is social phobia, affecting approximately 7-9\% of the population. Numerous studies indicate that virtual reality applications based on cognitive behavioral therapy together with the use of biological feedback are an effective way to improve this type of disorder. The most common scenarios for such applications are based on creating an anxiety-provoking environment for the user, e.g., public speaking or job interview for non-generalized phobia, and social contact or everyday social interaction in hospitals, offices, etc. for generalized phobia (Reyna et al., 2018). Similar applications can be used to treat acrophobia (Krijn et al., 2004), arachnophobia (Shiban et al., 2013), claustrophobia (Botella et al., 2000), aerodromophobia (Braga et al., 2017) and many others (Maples-Keller et al., 2017).

VR technology is very often used to treat post-traumatic stress disorder (PTSD). Its effectiveness in this area is confirmed by numerous studies because it has been used for over twenty years, and the first clinical trials were conducted on American soldiers fighting in Vietnam. The scenario of such applications takes the treated soldiers to the virtual world of warfare (e.g., inside a Huey helicopter). The therapist stimulates the patient with audio-visual experiences tailored to their individual trauma. Therapies of this type are still used successfully, only the technology and the scenarios used have changed (Rizzo et al., 2016). One of the most important applications is DeepVR, an underwater world in which the control is by breath and thus contributes to stress reduction: with each inhalation, the user swims upwards, and with each exhalation, downwards. The app can also be used for relaxation and is extremely popular with young patients in cancer wards and hospices. Another interesting approach is presented in (Kamińska et al., 2020), where the authors integrated VR with the bilateral stimulation used in EMDR as a tool to relieve stress.

The potential benefits of using VR as a tool to support behavioral therapy for children and adults with autism spectrum disorder (ASD) are increasingly evident in the literature. An example is a VR application that enhances the social adaptability of children with ASD (Ip et al., 2018). The app consists of six unique learning scenarios, such as controlling emotions and relaxation, simulating different social situations, facilitating consolidation and generalization. Another example is the job interview simulator, which is designed to help autistic people find a job (Arter et al., 2018). VR applications used for psychological rehabilitation are presented in figure 5.

Figure 5. VR applications used for psychological rehabilitation.
From the left, therapy for: aerodromophobia (Braga et al., 2017), PTSD (Rizzo et al., 2016), ASD (Ip et al., 2018).

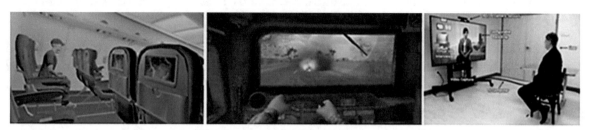

SUMMARY AND DIRECTIONS FOR FURTHER DEVELOPMENT

The examples provided prove that VR has great potential in supporting healthcare operations. By providing an immersive environment that stimulates different senses, medical care becomes more enjoyable for both patient and employee. Although it is a new method, there are already many implementations on the market for medical purposes. Nevertheless, the market is not yet saturated with them. We observe their constant development both in technological areas (use of more sensors, elements enabling interaction with more senses) and for use in medical areas not yet supported by VR technology. Some areas of medicine such as neurology, ophthalmology or telemedicine require deeper analysis.

One of the key problems that needs to be addressed soon is the lack of visual realism, as well as the reality of dynamics and interaction. It can be deduced that the techniques used to generate and display graphics are quite limited. It is worth mentioning that the psycho-visual design of the human brain allows the detection of even small unrealistic details, which can easily break the immersion and distract the patient and involve the need to repeat the exercise.

The high cost of VR equipment limits mass usage, so the technology remains available only to a narrow audience for the time being. Tools that provide advanced VR experiences cost between $400 and $600, plus the equipment has high technological requirements. There are also products available on the market that use mobile phones, such as Samsung Gear VR or Google Cardboard. Unfortunately, the possibilities of these solutions are significantly limited. This is a pity, because the possibility of training outside a specialist institution could contribute to more effective therapy, faster results, and thus less expenditure on health care.

It is also important to be aware of the side effects that VR brings with it. Studies show that excessive use of HMDs can cause anxiety, stress, isolation, addiction, and affect mood changes. Furthermore, simulated movements can cause feelings of disorientation and nausea. Therefore, before starting therapy or treatment, it is advisable to successively prepare the patient for the virtual environment, as well as to use motion sickness medication if necessary.

REFERENCES

Alfalah, S., Falah, J., Alfalah, T., Elfalah, M., Muhaidat, N., & Falah, O. (2018). A Comparative Study Between a Virtual Reality Heart Anatomy System and Traditional Medical Teaching Modalities. *Virtual Reality (Waltham Cross).*

Botella, C., Baños, R. M., Villa, H., Perpiñá, C., & García-Palacios, A. (2000). Virtual Reality in the Treatment of Claustrophobic Fear: A Controlled, Multiple-baseline Design. *Behaviour Research and Therapy*, *31*(3), 583–595. doi:10.1016/S0005-7894(00)80032-5

Bozgeyikli, E., Alqasemi, R., Raij, A., Katkoori, S., & Dubeyet, R. (2018). Virtual Reality Interaction Techniques for Individuals with Autism Spectrum Disorder. In *International Conference on Universal Access in Human-Computer Interaction*. Springer. 10.1007/978-3-319-92052-8_6

Braga, R., Camello, L., Costa, V., Raposo, A., Rodrigues, H., & Ventura, P. (2017). Virtual Reality as a Support Tool for the Treatment of Flying Phobia: A Pilot Study. *19th Symposium on Virtual and Augmented Reality (SVR)*. 10.1109/SVR.2017.17

Breedon, P., Logan, P., Pearce, D., Edmans, J., Childs, B., & O'Brien, R. (2016). Face to Face: An Interactive Facial Exercise System for Stroke Patients with Facial Weakness. *11th International Conference on Disability, Virtual Reality&Associated Technologies*.

Cartagena, P. D., Naranjo, J. E., Garcia, C. A., Beltran, C., Castro, M., & Garcia, M. V. (2018). *Virtual Reality-Based System for Hand Rehabilitation Using an Orthosis, w: Augmented Reality, Virtual Reality, and Computer Graphics*. AVR. doi:10.1007/978-3-319-95282-6_8

Elliman, J., Loizou, M., & Loizides, F. (2016). Virtual Reality Simulation Training for Student Nurse Education. *8th International Conference on Games and Virtual Worlds for Serious Applications*.

Falconer, C. J., Rovira, A., King, J. A., Gilbert, P., Antley, A., Fearon, P., Ralph, N., Slater, M., & Brewin, C. R. (2016). Embodying Self-compassion within Virtual Reality and its Effects on Patients with Depression. *BJPsych Open*, *2*, 74–80.

Górski, Buń, Wichniarek, Zawadzki, & Hamrol. (n.d.). Effective Design of Educational Virtual Reality Applications for Medicine using Knowledge-Engineering Techniques. Eurasia Journal of Mathematics, Science and Technology Education, 13(2), 395–416.

Gutierrez, J. M., Anorbe-Dıaz, C., & Gonzalez-Marrero, A. (2017). Virtual Technologies Trends in Education. *Eurasia Journal of Mathematics, Science and Technology Education*, *13*(2), 469–486.

Harrison, B., Oehmen, R., Robertson, A., Robertson, B., De Cruz, P., Khan, R., & Fick, D. (2017). Through the Eye of the Master: The Use of Virtual Reality in the Teaching of Surgical Hand Preparation. *5th International Conference on Serious Games and Applications for Health*.

Hsieh, M. C., & Lee, J. J. (2017). Preliminary Study of VR and AR Applications in Medical and Healthcare Education. *Journal of Nursing and Health Studies*, *3*(1), 1.

Kamińska, D., Smółka, K., Zwoliński, G., Wiak, S., Merecz-Kot, D., & Anbarjafari, G. (2020). Stress reduction using bilateral stimulation in virtual reality. *IEEE Access: Practical Innovations, Open Solutions*, *8*, 200351–200366.

Kim, G., & Biocca, F. (2018). Immersion in Virtual Reality Can Increase Exercise Motivation and Physical Performance. *International Conference on Virtual, Augmented and Mixed Reality*, 94–102.

Krijn, M., Emmelkamp, P. M., Biemond, R., de Wilde de Ligny, C., Schuemie, M. J., & van der Mast, C. (2004). Treatment of Acrophobia in Virtual Reality: The Role of Immersion and Presence. *Behaviour Research and Therapy, 42*, 229–239.

Kunze, K., Minamizawa, K., Lukosch, S., Inami, M., & Rekimoto, J. (2017). Superhuman Sports: Applying Human Augmentation to Physical Exercise. *IEEE Pervasive Computing*, (2), 14–17.

Kurillo, G., Han, J., Nicorici, A., & Bajcsy, R. (2014). *Tele-MFAsT: Kinect-Based Tele-Medicine Tool for Remote Motion and Function Assessment.* MMVR.

Lawson, G., Salanitri, D., & Waterfield, B. (2015, August). Vr processes in the automotive industry. In *International Conference on Human-Computer Interaction* (pp. 208-217). Springer.

Lee, L., & Wong, K. W. (2008). *A Review of Using Virtual Reality for Learning, Transactions on Edutainment* (Vol. 5080). Lecture Notes in Computer Science. Springer.

Lin, B.-S., Lee, I.-J., Yang, S.-Y., Lo, Y.-C., Lee, J., & Chen, J.-L. (2018). Design of an Inertial-Sensor-Based Data Glove for Hand Function Evaluation. *Sensors (Basel), 18*(5), 15–45.

Maples-Keller, J. L., Bunnell, B. E., Kim, S.-J., & Rothbaum, B. O. (2017). The Use of Virtual Reality Technology in the Treatment of Anxiety and Other Psychiatric Disorders. *Harvard Review of Psychiatry, 25*(3), 103–113.

Perez-Marcos, D., Chevalley, O., Schmidlin, T., Garipelli, G., Serino, A., Vuadens, P., Tadi, T., Blanke, O., & Millán, J. R. (2017). Increasing Upper Limb Training Intensity in Chronic Stroke Using Embodied Virtual Reality: A Pilot Study. *Journal of Neuroengineering and Rehabilitation, 14*(119).

Porras, D. C., Siemonsma, P., Inzelberg, R., Zeilig, G., & Plotnik, M. (2018). Advantages of Virtual Reality in the Rehabilitation of Balance and Gait: Systematic Review. *Neurology, 29*(90), 1017–1025.

Powell, W., Rizzo, A., Sharkey, P., & Merrick, J. (2017). Innovations and Challenges in the Use of Virtual Reality Technologies for Rehabilitation. *Journal of Alternative Medical Research, 10*.

Radia, M., Arunakirinathan, M., & Sibley, D. (2018). A Guide to Eyes: Ophthalmic Simulators. *The Bulletin of the Royal College of Surgeons of England, 100*(4), 169–171.

Rao, S. K., & Prasad, R. (2018). Impact of 5G technologies on industry 4.0. *Wireless Personal Communications, 100*(1), 145–159.

Reyna, D., Caraza, R., Gonzalez-Knoell, M., Ayala, A., Martinez, P., Loredo, A., Rosas, R., & Reyes, P. (2018). Virtual Reality for Social Phobia Treatment. *Smart Technology, 213*, 165–177.

Riva, G. (2017). Applications of Virtual Environments in Medicine. *Methods of Information in Medicine, 42*(5), 524–534.

Rizzo, A., & Talbot, T. (2016). *Virtual Reality Standardized Patients for Clinical Training, w: The Digital Patient.* John Wiley&Sons, Inc.

Sathiyanarayanan, M., & Rajan, S. (2016). MYO Armband for Physiotherapy Healthcare: A Case Study Using Gesture Recognition Application. *8th International Conference on Communication Systems and Networks (COMSNETS)*.

Seo, J. H., Smith, B. M., Cook, M., Malone, E., Pine, M., Leal, S., Bai, Z., Suh, J., & Anatomy Builder, V. R. (2017). Applying a Constructive Learning Method in the Virtual Reality Canine Skeletal System. *International Conference on Applied Human Factors and Ergonomics*, 245–252.

Sharma, Hunt, Maheshwari, Osborn, Levay, Kaliki, Soares, & Thakork. (2018). A Mixed-Reality Training Environment for Upper Limb Prosthesis Control. *Conf. IEEE Biomed. Circuits Syst. (BioCAS)*.

Shiban, Y., Pauli, P., & Mühlberger, A. (2013). Effect of Multiple Context Exposure on Renewal in Spider Phobia. *Behaviour Research and Therapy*, *51*, 68–74.

Topçu, Ç., Uysal, H., Özkan, Ö., Özkan, Ö., Polat, Ö., Bedeloğlu, M., Akgül, A., Naz Döğer, E., Sever, R., & Çolak, Ö. H. (2018). Recovery of Facial Expressions Using Functional Electrical Stimulation After Full-face Transplantation. *Journal of Neuroengineering and Rehabilitation*, *15*(15).

Vankipuram, A., Khanal, P., Ashby, A., Vankipuram, M., Gupta, A., Drumm Gurnee, D., Josey, K., & Smith, M. (2014). Design and Development of a Virtual Reality Simulator for Advanced Cardiac Life Support Training. *IEEE Journal of Biomedical and Health Informatics*, *18*(4), 1478–1484.

Wang, F., Liu, Y., Tian, M., Zhang, Y., Zhang, S., & Chen, J. (2016). Application of a 3d Haptic Virtual Reality Simulation System for Dental Crown Preparation Training. *8th International Conference on Information Technology in Medicine and Education (ITME)*, 424–427.

Winkler, S. L., Kairalla, J. A., Cooper, R., Gaunaurd, I., Schlesinger, M., Krueger, A., & Ludwig, A. (2016). Comparison of Functional Benefits of Self-management Training for Amputees Under Virtual World and E-learning Conditions. *11th International Conference on Disability, Virtual Reality & Associated Technologies*.

Yang, X., Yeh, S.-C., Niu, J., Gong, Y., & Yang, G. (2017). Hand Rehabilitation Using Virtual Reality and Electromyography Signals. *5th International Conference on Enterprise Systems*.

Chapter 2
Virtual and Augmented Reality Awareness Tools for Universal Design:
Towards Active Preventive Healthcare

Luis Coelho
https://orcid.org/0000-0002-5673-7306
Polytechnic of Porto, Portugal

Idalina Freitas
Polytechnic of Porto, Portugal

Dorota Urszula Kaminska
Lodz University of Technology, Poland

Ricardo Queirós
https://orcid.org/0000-0002-1985-6285
School of Media Arts and Design, Polytechnic of Porto, Portugal

Anna Laska-Lesniewicz
Lodz University of Technology, Poland

Grzegorz Zwolinski
Lodz University of Technology, Poland

Rui Raposo
https://orcid.org/0000-0002-5275-6200
Universidade de Aveiro, Portugal

Mário Vairinhos
Universidade de Aveiro, Portugal

Elisabeth Pereira
Universidade de Aveiro, Portugal

Eric Haamer
University of Tartu, Estonia

Gholamreza Anbarjafari
University of Tartu, Estonia

ABSTRACT

This chapter will be focused on contributing to the increase of universal design competencies of future engineers, educators, and designers through the use of mixed reality technologies, closing the gap between theory and field application of principles, towards a more inclusive world and promoting health and wellbeing for all. The experience of a situation where limitations arise in relation to what is taken for granted is an important experience that leads to a personal knowledge of the difficulties. By the use of simulators, especially virtual (VR) and mixed reality (MR) technologies, it is possible to create such experiences. Training based on MR can prepare future and current professionals for up-to-date requirements of the labor market. In addition, it can ensure that the standards such as barrier-free concepts, broader accessibility, adaptive and assistive technology will be familiar to trainees.

DOI: 10.4018/978-1-7998-8371-5.ch002

PREAMBLE

This chapter will be focused on contributing to the increase of Universal Design competencies of future engineers, educators and designers through the use of mixed reality technologies, closing the gap between theory and field application of principles, towards a more inclusive world and promoting health and wellbeing for all.

LIVING WITH DISABILITY

According to the World Report on Disability (WHO, 2011) about 15% of the world's population is living with some kind of disability, of whom 2-4 per cent experience relevant difficulties in functioning. In the US, for example, about 61 million adults live with a disability (CDC, 2021). Children are also affected worldwide, with 93 million children – or 1 in 20 of those aged 14 or younger – live with a moderate or severe disability of some form (UNICEF, 2013). In countries with life expectancies over 70 years, individuals spend around 8 years, or 11.5 per cent of their life span, on average, living with disabilities (Disabled World, 2021). These numbers are dramatically increasing in the last decades, due to demographic trends and increases in chronic health conditions, among other causes, leading to an important public health problem that must be tackled.

Disability can encompass an extremely diverse range of conditions, often classified under six types: mobility (serious difficulty walking or climbing stairs; 13.7%), cognition (serious difficulty concentrating, remembering, or making decisions; 10.8%), independent living (difficulty doing errands alone; 6.8%), hearing (serious difficulty hearing; 5.9%), vision (serious difficulty seeing; 4.6%), and self-care (difficulty dressing or bathing; 3.6%) (Okoro, 2018). We can also distinguish between permanent disability and short-term disability (usually lasting for less than 6 months), which can be due to pregnancies (25%), musculoskeletal disorders affecting the back and spine, knees, hips, shoulders, and other parts of the body (20%), digestive disorders, such as hernias and gastritis (7.8%), mental health issues including depression and anxiety (7.7%), and injuries such as fractures, sprains, and strains of muscles and ligaments (7.5%) (Integrated Benefits Institute, 2017).

While some health conditions associated with disability do not directly impact health, most of them result in poor health and extensive healthcare needs. In fact, adults with disabilities are more likely to have obesity, suffer from depression, smoke, have hear diseases and have diabetes (CDC, 2021). Additionally, people with disabilities often encounter a multitude of barriers when they attempt to manage healthcare issues. Difficulties on accessibility, high-costs, limited availability of services, physical barriers, inadequate skills, or insufficient knowledge of health workers are some of the reported challenges.

Disabilities can also impact education and employment. Ninety per cent of children with disabilities in developing countries do not attend school (UNESCO, 2016). In higher education, students with disabilities remain under-represented, although their number is also increasing. Concerning employment, an estimated 386 million of the world's working-age people have some kind of disability (ILO, 2007). Unemployment among the persons with disabilities is as high as 80 per cent in some countries, more than quadruple of people without disabilities. Often employers assume that persons with disabilities are unable to work or to be productive.

UNIVERSAL DESIGN

Trying to mitigate some of the challenges disabled people face, the concept of Universal Design (Mace et al., 1991) have been gaining special importance, especially in the last decade. It has been defined as "…simply a way of designing a building or facility at little or no extra cost so it is both attractive and functional for all people disabled or not.". Universal design is not a specific field of design practice but rather an approach to design and engineering, a mental reference, a mindset leading to the idea that objects, environments, systems, or services should be planned and idealized as equally accessible and experienced by all persons or at least by the largest number of individuals possible. This attitude has also been explored in accessible design, usable design, barrier-free design, and inclusive design, all adjacent concepts that, despite their normative differences and distinct implications, provide similar ethical guidelines and propose compatible development frameworks.

When the main principles of universal design are applied, products and environments meet people's needs and encompass a wide range of features. Disability is just one of the many characteristics that an individual can have. A group of architects, product designers, engineers and researchers defined seven universal design principles (Burgstahler, 2009): equitable use, flexibility in use, simple and intuitive use, easy to understand information, error tolerance, low physical effort, dimensioning and space for approximation and use.

1. The first principle, equitable use, is a design that is useful and has the potential to be marketed to people with diverse abilities. It is essential to provide the same means of use for all people whenever possible and thus avoid segregating or stigmatizing any user as it appeals to everyone.
2. Regarding flexibility in use, this refers to design that has a wide range of individual preferences and abilities. It must allow the choice of methods of use and be adaptable to the user's pace.
3. Simple and intuitive use consists in the ease of understanding the information, regardless of the user's experience, their language skills or the user's level of concentration. It is necessary to organize information according to its importance and that is consistent with the user's expectations and intuition.
4. In the principle of easily perceptible information, the design communicates the necessary information effectively, regardless of environmental conditions or sensory abilities. It is important to provide an adequate contrast between essential information and its surroundings.
5. Error tolerance is when the design minimizes the risks and adverse consequences of accidental or unintended actions. It discourages unconscious action in tasks that require vigilance and fail-safe features, for example the "undo" feature in software programs that allows the user to correct a mistake without being penalized.
6. The low-effort principle is implemented when a design that be used efficiently and comfortably and with minimal fatigue.
7. Size and space are provided for approach, reach, manipulation and use, regardless of the user's body size, configuration or mobility. Provides a clear line of sight to elements important to any user sitting or standing. Makes the reach of all components comfortable for any user who is either sitting, standing or other compatible positions.

Both people with disabilities (PWD), permanent or temporary, and people with age-related impairments are strongly affected by the built environment in terms of their mobility and safety. A mismatch between the built environment and functional ability can cause problems of safety and independence for those populations (Pynoos et al., 2003). Universal design seeks to reduce functional and mobility difficulties not just for those with disabilities but to everyone. The Disability Act 2005 defines that universal design should be applied so that the results of the development to the greatest extent, in the most independent and natural manner possible, in the widest possible range of situations and without the need for adaptation, modification, assistive devices or specialized solutions, by any persons of any age or size or having any physical, sensory, mental health or intellectual ability or disability. Hence, universal design principles, when correctly applied during design and engineering stages, may help people with challenging conditions to increase physical activity, foster socialization, and enhance access to community resources, thereby positively affecting wellness and promoting health, directly and indirectly (HAPI, 2015). The applications of these general principles can encompass areas such as education, information technologies, industry, among others.

VIRTUAL AND AUGMENTED REALITY AS AN AWARENESS TOOLS

Despite the good intentions of universal design principles its application is often neglected, either due to the lack of knowledge, due to the need of a rapid market response or, in most cases, because there is insufficient awareness and training. These last aspects are essential, as a complement to theoretical knowledge, to raise awareness to the challenges experienced by people with disabilities.

Virtual Worlds and Virtual Products

The "ultimate display" was a concept developed by Ivan Sutherland, in 1965, presented at the International Federation for Information Processing (IFIP). Its goal was to imitate reality to the point where the user couldn't discern the difference between virtual and real life. It featured a simple virtual world, viewed through a head-mounted display (HMD), and a realistic augmented 3D environment with tactile input, allowing users to interact with virtual objects in a realistic manner. This was the dawn of virtual reality (VR) as we know it today, integrating essential pillars that were only defined later (Sherman et al., 2003): a) A virtual world. An imaginary space, independent from the real world, built from computer generated graphics, and where rules and interactions are defined by its creator; b) Immersion. When the participant is engaged in an activity in a virtual world to the extent that his or her mind are isolated from the real space in which he or she is present; c) Sensory feedback, giving the participants the ability to observe the results of their actions; and d) Interactivity, where the users' actions, such as viewpoint motion control, selection, or manipulation lead to changes in the virtual world (Muhanna, 2015). To ensure a complete and satisfying virtual reality experience, several components must operate integrated and completely synchronized. In figure 1 we can observe a generic model of a virtual reality system. On the left we find input devices that collect information from the user. These can be specific controllers for the purpose of interacting with the VR system, wearable devices but also a myriad of other devices that can collect useful information for a better integration of the user with the VR system. It is also necessary to have a tracking system to capture bode movement, body pose, eye tracking or others. All this information is then acquired, integrated and processed by a computation unit. The main element is the simulation engine, where algorithms are used to decide what should happen every time instant, using current or previous information. As a complement, an artificial intelligence module can also be used. These have underlying sophisticated mathematical models that can detect specific patterns and allow you to create personalized experiences, considering one or several variables and the relationships between them. As a complement, an artificial intelligence module can also be used. These have underlying sophisticated mathematical models that can detect specific patterns and allow you to create personalized experiences, considering one or several variables and the relationships between them. The several outputs are then generated and presented to the user. Any delay in one of the systems, either by inappropriate software or hardware, will result in a desynchronization of the stimulus modalities, leading the user to realize that the virtual environment where he is immersed does not behave as expected. The quality of the various elements and the guarantee of their absolute time synchronization are critical to creating and maintaining a good sense of immersion. Inadequate synchronization (among other VR related issues) can the cause of dizziness, nausea or even headaches, sweating, feeling tired, eye strain and a general lack of balance (Chang et al., 2020). The selection and generation of audio and image contents should also follow preference guidelines, based on psychologic preference scales, to create a more engaging experience (Coelho et al., 2011; Ibarra et al., 2017)

Figure 1. Basic components of a virtual reality system

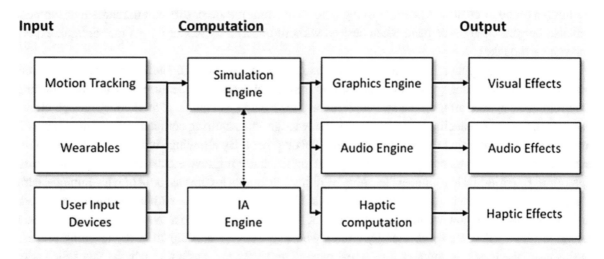

VR has continued to evolve with technologies, such as graphical processing, display technologies, and input systems, becoming more powerful, with higher quality and with lower cost. In the next years it is expected that full sensorial experiences will be available and additional stimuli, involving simulating touch, taste and smell, and sensations such as hot or cold, using new hardware technology and improved algorithms, will make VR more and more natural. At the same time, input devices and wearable sensor will be able to capture a wider set of data and at higher rates, leading to a near symbiotic experience. Artificial intelligence will be able to predict behaviors and create usage profiles for providing personalized worlds and improving user experience.

Inside an immersive universe, a VR experience entirely isolates the user from the outside world. As a result, the user can be transported into both simulated and speculative situations. This concept has also evolved, and technological advance has also made it possible to broaden the scope of virtual reality, leading to the creation of new concepts. In Augmented Reality (AR) systems, virtual contents are superimposed on the real-world to provide an enhanced experience (Furht, 2011). This happens in real time as the user interacts with the system, with elements of the environment or other real-world items being acquired and processed in 3D using computer vision techniques (Schmalstieg and Hollerer, 2016). In this approach, augmented reality can be utilized to improve real-world engagement and learning, such as better elucidating ideas and concepts. In Mixed Reality, different technologies are combined, and work in collaboration, to provide a Reality–Virtuality Continuum. A real and virtual world can be explored, as well as their elements, without a noticeable technological frontier (Speicher et al., 2019). The term Extended Reality (XR) is used is a hypernym for all technologies that extend or replace human perception of reality, encompassing VR, AR and MR. The X can represent any computer-assisted modifications of reality.

These technologies have enormous potential and, besides the typical daily life situations, they can be particularly interesting for simulating specific contexts. Dangerous environments, situations or procedures, for example, can be simulated in a VR world and explored without the inherent risks (e.g. entering a volcano or performing a heart surgery). High-cost situations or equipments can be computer generated and experienced or used many times without significant cost (e.g. traveling to a distant place or using expensive equipments). Impossible contexts can also be experienced by the user (e.g. traveling through the human blood circulation system or living in ancient Rome); Rare or difficult to recreate phenomena can also be generated on-demand when desired without uncertainty (e.g. seeing a rare animal, experience an earthquake).

The number of application areas continues to grow and we can find successful projects in areas such as automotive industry, healthcare, retail, tourism, real estate, architecture, learning and training, entertainment, sports, arts, events and conferences, well-being, socializing, marketing, among others. For the purpose of enhancing skills, improving knowledge and acquiring competences we are especially interested in the areas that can support personal development. By allowing students to study in an immersive, experiencing manner, virtual reality can significantly improve education and student success outcomes. Experiential learning, or "learning by doing," accounts for the vast bulk of what humans learn. Virtual reality provides a way for students to obtain hands-on experience without doing the real work/task. This is not only how we learn the majority of the time, but it is also a modality with great mental retention rates. VR can also be used by a tutor who may actively participate in the teaching process. In this case, the lesson is conducted by a real person, and VR serves as a tool which makes the lesson more interesting (Kamińska et al., 2019). VR is highly effective because it is emotional and impactful, misleading your brain because the human senses are being stimulated in a near natural way. VR experiences can affect how individuals think about themselves and how they see others in ways that any other media can't. VR is also being used in the learning and development business to improve soft skills, such as shared decision-making, or to evoke emotional intelligence abilities such as empathy and compassion. Additionally, VR has the potential to help people develop empathy. Because empathy requires "placing oneself in another's shoes," there is no better medium than virtual reality to do this. Empathy allows people to understand each other and their situations on a more personal level, making virtual reality the ideal instrument for promoting causes.

Figure 2. How VR/AR models can be generated and experienced by users during a development process.

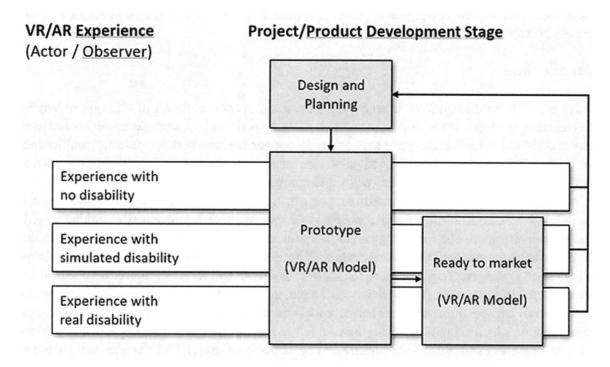

Using VR as a disability awareness tool allows the user to participate in the virtual experience in several different ways. In Figure 2 we can observe, on the right, the main stages of a project or product development process. Immediately after the design and planning, a VR/AR model of the prototype can be created as a first step towards the final, market-ready product. From this very early stage, where corrections or refinements are more effective and with less economic impact, the VR prototype can be experienced as an actor or as an observer (Larsson et al., 2001), left of the figure. When the VR user has a good awareness towards the obstacles that a person with a disability may face, then the virtual reality experience can be used to explore those particular aspects, checking if the principles of universal design are met. On the other hand, when there is a lack of disability awareness, then the VR user can experience one or more simulated disabilities. Experiencing virtual difficulties, which during the immersive experience are real, will allow the development of a particular sensitivity for future cases for the situations encountered. In addition, the VR experience can also be lived as an observer, requiring the virtual presence of other users (avatars of real persons or computer agents with algorithm-based behaviors). Observing a situation is a very impacting experience that can also help to raise awareness. In all cases, it is important to actively search for difficulties that may arise and effectively mitigate their effects by designing better products or environments.

By speeding up the process while also enhancing quality and usability, virtual reality opens up new opportunities in the realm of product development. Simulation, skills training, and communication with distant teams or third parties (e.g. users, experts, and associations) are three of the most important applications that provide great chances for product development in general. Additionally, users can test the use of the products before they exist, on site or remotely, which can lead to improved usability and better ergonomic design, leading to an overall enhanced user experience. By using VR, users and stakeholders can influence the features of a project or product idea and the layout plans (e.g. for a factory, a hospital, or a city) (Ottosson, 2002).

Gamification

The expression "gamification" has recently emerged as a way of defining the use of video game elements in nongaming systems with the purpose of improving User Experience (UX) and user engagement (Deterding et al., 2011) or, in a broader perspective, more focused on the process development, "gamification" can be seen as the process of making activities more game-like (Werbach, 2014). Gamification can be used to improve motivation for learning and skill improvement.

A reward-based strategy is often used to support extrinsic motivation and most gamification systems use points, levels, leader boards, awards, or badges to engage students in an interactive learning content. The most significant risk of this strategy is that, once the incentive is removed, there is a possibility that the behavior may cease until the student finds another reason to support its motivation. Reward based gamification is adequate as an approach for short term-change and its effect in user engagement has been reported (Hagger et al., 2020). On the other hand, in is important to develop intrinsic motivation, when the user engages in an activity or behavior for its inherent satisfaction. Fostering internal rewards helps to build a stimulating and satisfying drive for intrinsic motivation, which is independent of external controls. Intrinsic motivation can be undermined by extrinsic rewards, although some components of extrinsic cues can assist learners track their progress via a learning exercise without overriding intrinsic motivation (Ryan and Deci, 2005).

Nevertheless, gamification strategies must be used with caution, always bearing in mind the essential bioethical principles. Effects like addiction, undesired competition, and off-task behavior can also be found as undesired secondary effects of the gamification process (Andrade et al., 2016). These conducts can be detrimental and raise questions that must be addressed, not only to define limits to what can be asked to the gamification recipient but also to define control strategies that monitor unwanted behaviors and allow to detect design flaws or promote mitigating actions (Coelho and Reis, 2021).

To build a VR experience for learning with gamification it is possible to either embed game elements into an environment that has been designed with educational purposes or to integrate specific contents with pedagogical motivation into a game, the so called serious games (Lameras et al., 2017; Swacha et al., 2019). The objectives of educational games (Serious Games) are more focused on educational/ professional training purposes than on entertainment, and, therefore, they have become more popular and have an impact in several areas (Susi et al., 2007). As an example, "World Without Oil" is a game created to draw attention and create solutions for a possible global extinction of oil in the near future. The feedback from both players and creators was reflected in significant learning and knowledge about the domains that are presented (Bonsignore et al., 2012). Recent studies have revealed that, in the area of medicine, more precisely in advanced life support, a game called "EMSAVE" was developed, whose objective is to promote knowledge and skills associated with life support. There were also 40 tests with 38 multiple choice questions before and after playing. The results of these tests showed an increase in correct answers between the pre-test and post-test results (Buttussi et al., 2013).

VR/AR AS ASSISTIVE TECHNOLOGIES: A SURVEY

Education has a vital role to play in developing the knowledge, skills, attitudes and values that enable people to contribute to and benefit from an inclusive and sustainable future (OECD, 2018). To understand how disabilities impact young students, a survey has been conducted by the authors and some of the findings are presented in Figure 3. The study population was composed by a group of 62 university students, all of them with some kind of disability, with ages between 18 and 25 and a balanced gender distribution. The students attend different institutions and different degrees.

Figure 3. Survey results based on an university student population

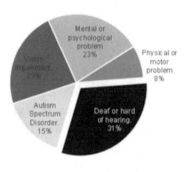

a)   Type of disability

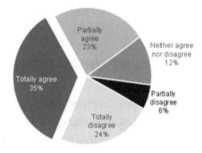

b)   My disability has a negative impact on
my activities

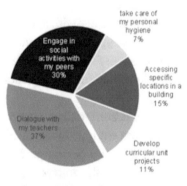

c)   I could need help on...

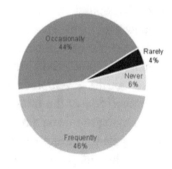

d)   VR could help me

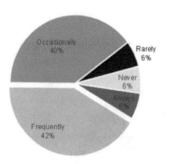

e)   AR could help me

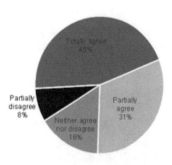

f)   I am motivated to use VR/AR

In Fig. 3a and 3b we can observe that hearing problems represent that hearing, vision and mental impairments are the most prevalent and most students report that this is negatively impacting their performance. Fig. 3c shows that social activities, to interact with teachers or even to integrate with colleagues, are those where the negative impact of having impairment is most felt. This may indicate that, in addition to the direct impacts, the existence of some type of disability also has serious indirect impacts that cover various aspects of the individual's daily life. In Figs. 3d and 3e, students report that VR and AR can be a useful technology as an assistive technology, boosting their academic performance while helping their life at the university. Finally, in Fig 3f, most student declare a positive or very positive attitude towards the use of VR and AR.

Despite the small study population we believe that the results obtained in this survey can be extrapolated to many other academic populations. The most important facts to retain are the existing motivation for the use of AR and VR and the perception that these technologies can play a positive role in a student's daily life, impacting direct and indirect aspects.

AN APPLICATION OF VR/AR FOR AWARENESS

To raise awareness about users that navigate spaces using a wheelchair, a VR game has been developed. It consists of two different environments, each with two different levels of navigation difficulty. The user can browse these spaces for exploratory purposes only or can participate in a gamified experience. The developed game aims to take the player to explore different areas of the virtual environments to collect tokens that are worth points, passing through areas with particular characteristics, especially included because they present potential difficulty when navigated in a wheelchair.

The proportion of the population using wheelchairs increases dramatically with age, but the increase is much more pronounced for manual than for electric wheelchairs. In all age groups, manual wheelchairs dominate compared to electric ones, the rate of use of manual wheelchairs among the elderly (2.76%) is almost 8 times compared to motorized ones (0.35%). Taking this into account, a 3D model of a manual wheelchair was chosen for the development of the project.

Regarding the composition of the house (as seen of Figure 4), it comprises a single floor with a kitchen, a bathroom, a living room and a bedroom. These divisions are equipped with furniture, decoration and electrical equipment to exactly simulate the daily activities that a person performs. To make the house more challenging, its geometric shape is identical to a rectangular trapeze and not the usual rectangular shape.

Figure 4. House floor plan for the developed VR environment.
On the left the simplified scenario, on the right, a more challenging scenario. The tokens that must be collected, in the gamified experience, are shown in light blue.

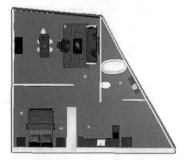 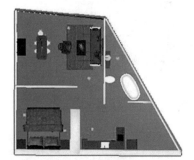

Additionally, another space was developed, with public characteristics and where it could be possible to include additional participants. A classroom was chosen as the ideal situation, a context where different challenges may arise for people with special needs. Again, two different versions were developed, with different levels of navigation difficulty, as seen in Figure 5. The access to the room can be made trough a ramp and the space between furniture varies. The location of the reward tokens was carefully chosen in order to force the user to explore specific locations.

Figure 5. Floor plan for a public space (classroom) for the developed VR environment.
On the left the simplified scenario, on the right, a more challenging scenario. The tokens that must be collected, in the gamified experience, are shown in light blue.

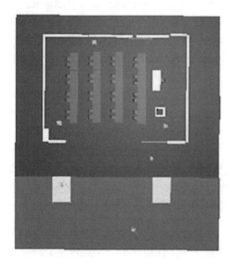 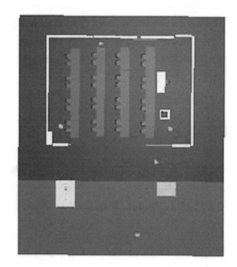

The game was tested by 10 persons (due to COVID-19 restrictions) and a small survey was conducted. Of the people surveyed, 80% had never experienced virtual reality equipment before. Of course, some of them had some knowledge about how the equipment works, even though they had not experienced it directly. Among all participants, there was not one wheelchair user, but 40% had already been using a wheelchair.

Then, you were asked to sort the scenarios (1 to 4) in relation to the level of difficulty. Comparing the versions of each virtual environment, the more challenging versions were always considered more difficult than the first version, as expected. Overall, most individuals considered the home scenario (easy version) to be the easiest and the school (challenging version) to be the most difficult.

From the observations taken during the simulations, it was found that users in the virtual home environment, in both versions, had greater difficulty in the living room due to the large amount of furniture and decoration. In relation to the school, the greatest difficulty was found on the ramps, especially on the steeper ramp in the second version.

All the players were able to collect all the tokens in the environments, despite some reported difficulties. This may indicate that additional tokens can be placed in the environment and more other locations can be chosen to create a more challenging and engaging game.

Overall, the players were quite satisfied with the experience and reported that this game has been useful to raise their awareness towards disabilities.

FINAL REMARKS

The experience of a situation where limitations arise in relation to what is taken for granted is an important experience that leads to a personal knowledge of the difficulties. By the use of simulators, especially virtual (VR) and mixed reality (MR) technologies, it is possible to create such experiences. MR applications along with a haptic and multisensory interfaces can enhance competences of future engineers and designers such as understanding what makes an environment completely tenable and functional for individuals, regardless of age, disability or other factors. Training based on MR can prepare future and current professionals for up-to-date requirements of the labor market. In addition, it can ensure that the standards such as barrier-free concepts, broader accessibility, adaptive and assistive technology will be familiar to trainees.

REFERENCES

Andrade, F. R. H., Mizoguchi, R., & Isotani, S. (2016). The Bright and Dark Sides of Gamification. In A. Micarelli, J. Stamper, & K. Panourgia (Eds.), *Intelligent Tutoring Systems* (pp. 176–186). Lecture Notes in Computer Science. Springer International Publishing. doi:10.1007/978-3-319-39583-8_17

Bonsignore, E., Kraus, K., Visconti, A., Hansen, D., Fraistat, A., & Druin, A. (2012). Game design for promoting counterfactual thinking. In *Proceedings of the SIGCHI Conference on Human Factors in Computing Systems, CHI '12*. Association for Computing Machinery. 10.1145/2207676.2208357

Burgstahler, S. (2009). *Universal Design: Process, Principles, and Applications, DO-IT*. DO-IT.

Buttussi, F., Pellis, T., Cabas Vidani, A., Pausler, D., Carchietti, E., & Chittaro, L. (2013). Evaluation of a 3D serious game for advanced life support retraining. *International Journal of Medical Informatics*, *82*(9), 798–809. doi:10.1016/j.ijmedinf.2013.05.007 PMID:23763908

CDC. (2021). *Disability Impacts All of Us (Disability and Health Data System)*. Center for Disease Control.

Chang, E., Kim, H. T., & Yoo, B. (2020). Virtual Reality Sickness: A Review of Causes and Measurements. *International Journal of Human-Computer Interaction*, *36*(17), 1658–1682. doi:10.1080/1044 7318.2020.1778351

Coelho, L., Braga, D., Dias, M., & García-Mateo, C. (2011). An Automatic Voice Pleasantness Classification System Based on Prosodic and Acoustic Patterns of Voice Preference. *Proc. of Interspeech*, 2460.

Coelho, L., & Reis, S. (2021). Ethical Issues of Gamification in Healthcare: The Need to be Involved. In *Handbook of Research on Solving Modern Healthcare Challenges With Gamification* (pp. 1–19). IGI Global. doi:10.4018/978-1-7998-7472-0.ch001

Deterding, S., Sicart, M., Nacke, L., O'Hara, K., & Dixon, D. (2011). Gamification. using game-design elements in non-gaming contexts. In *CHI '11 Extended Abstracts on Human Factors in Computing Systems, CHI EA '11* (pp. 2425–2428). Association for Computing Machinery. doi:10.1145/1979742.1979575

Disabled World. (2021). *Disability Statistics: Information.* Charts, Graphs and Tables.

Furht, B. (Ed.). (2011). *Handbook of Augmented Reality.* doi:10.1007/978-1-4614-0064-6

Hagger, M. S., Hankonen, N., Chatzisarantis, N. L. D., & Ryan, R. M. (2020). Changing Behavior Using Self-Determination Theory. In K. Hamilton, L. D. Cameron, M. S. Hagger, N. Hankonen, & T. Lintunen (Eds.), *The Handbook of Behavior Change, Cambridge Handbooks in Psychology* (pp. 104–119). Cambridge University Press. doi:10.1017/9781108677318.008

HAPI. (2015). Mobility, Universal Design, Health, and Place. Health and Place Initiative.

Ibarra, F. F., Kardan, O., Hunter, M. R., Kotabe, H. P., Meyer, F. A. C., & Berman, M. G. (2017). Image Feature Types and Their Predictions of Aesthetic Preference and Naturalness. *Frontiers in Psychology*, *8*, 632. doi:10.3389/fpsyg.2017.00632 PMID:28503158

ILO. (2007). *Disability in the World of Work: Factsheet.* International Labour Organization.

Integrated Benefits Institute. (2017). *Health and Productivity Benchmarking 2016.* Author.

Kamińska, D., Sapiński, T., Wiak, S., Tikk, T., Haamer, R. E., Avots, E., Helmi, A., Ozcinar, C., & Anbarjafari, G. (2019). Virtual Reality and Its Applications in Education: Survey. *Information (Basel)*, *10*(10), 318. doi:10.3390/info10100318

Lameras, P., Arnab, S., Dunwell, I., Stewart, C., Clarke, S., & Petridis, P. (2017). Essential features of serious games design in higher education: Linking learning attributes to game mechanics. *British Journal of Educational Technology*, *48*(4), 972–994. doi:10.1111/bjet.12467

Larsson, P., Västfjäll, D., & Kleiner, M. (2001). The actor-observer effect in virtual reality presentations. *Cyberpsychology & Behavior*, *4*(2), 239–246. doi:10.1089/109493101300117929 PMID:11710250

Mace, R., Hardie, G., & Plaice, J. (1991). Accessible environments: Toward universal design. In *Design Interventions: Toward a More Humane Architecture*. Van Nostrand Reinhold.

Muhanna, M.A. (2015). Virtual reality and the CAVE: Taxonomy, interaction challenges and research directions. *Journal of King Saud University - Computer and Information Sciences, 27*, 344–361. doi:10.1016/j.jksuci.2014.03.023

OECD. (2018). *The future of education and skills 2030.* OECD.

Okoro, C. A., Hollis, N. T. D., Cyrus, A. C., & Griffin-Blake, S. (2018). Prevalence of Disabilities and Health Care Access by Disability Status and Type Among Adults— United States. *MMWR. Morbidity and Mortality Weekly Report*, *67*(32), 882–887. Advance online publication. doi:10.15585/mmwr.mm6732a3 PMID:30114005

Ottosson, S. (2002). Virtual reality in the product development process. *Journal of Engineering Design*, *13*(2), 159–172. doi:10.1080/09544820210129823

Pynoos, J., Nishita, C., & Perelma, L. (2003). Advancements in the Home Modification Field. *Journal of Housing for the Elderly, 17*(1-2), 105–116. doi:10.1300/J081v17n01_08

Ryan, R., & Deci, E. (2005). Toward a Social Psychology of Assimilation: Self-Determination Theory in Cognitive Development and Education. doi:10.1017/CBO9781139152198.014

Schmalstieg, D., & Hollerer, T. (2016). Augmented Reality: Principles and Practice. Addison-Wesley Professional.

Sherman, W., Craig, A. B., Sherman, W. R., & Craig, A. B. (Eds.). (2003). *Understanding Virtual Reality: Interface, Application, and Design, The Morgan Kaufmann Series in Computer Graphics*. Morgan Kaufmann. doi:10.1016/B978-1-55860-353-0.50019-7

Speicher, M., Hall, B. D., & Nebeling, M. (2019). What is Mixed Reality? In *Proceedings of the 2019 CHI Conference on Human Factors in Computing Systems*. Association for Computing Machinery.

Susi, T., Johannesson, M., & Backlund, P. (2007). *Serious Games : An Overview*. Academic Press.

Swacha, J., Queirós, R., & Paiva, J. C. (2019). Towards a Framework for Gamified Programming Education. *2019 International Symposium on Educational Technology (ISET), 144–149.* 10.1109/ISET.2019.00038

UNESCO. (2016). *Global Education Monitoring Report: Education for People and Planet*. UNESCO.

UNICEF. (2013). *Children with Disabilities*. UNICEF.

Werbach, K. (2014). ReDefining Gamification: A Process Approach. In *Proceedings of the 9th International Conference on Persuasive Technology* - Volume 8462. Springer-Verlag. 10.1007/978-3-319-07127-5_23

WHO. (2011). *World report on disability 2011*. World Health Organization.

Section 2
Education and Training

Chapter 3
Educational Technology Based on Virtual and Augmented Reality for Students With Learning Disabilities:
Specific Projects and Applications

Sonia Rodriguez Cano
Facultad de Educación, Universidad de Burgos, Spain

Vanesa Delgado-Benito
Facultad de Educación, Universidad de Burgos, Spain

Vitor Gonçalves
(iD) https://orcid.org/0000-0002-0645-6776
CIEB, Instituto Politécnico de Bragança, Portugal

ABSTRACT

Educational technology is contributing towards diversity awareness as it allows you to create more personalized and student-centered learning situations. This chapter addresses specific learning difficulties (SpLD) and, specifically, dyslexia, since it is one of the most prevalent challenges in the educational field. Information and communication technologies allow direct intervention with students who have special educational needs as an alternative to traditional resources, which is much more motivating. In this sense, as an example, various projects and applications are presented that allow working on this type of difficulties with students. This chapter highlights the virtual reality and augmented reality software carried out in the context of the European Erasmus + FORDYSVAR project, of which the authors are part.

DOI: 10.4018/978-1-7998-8371-5.ch003

INTRODUCTION

At present, the incorporation of Information and Communication Technologies (ICT), the Instructional Design or design of Educational Technology (ET) and the development of software in the educational field contributes to educational intervention, offering playful and effective environments for the treatment of different disorders in children and adolescents, with the advantage of providing safe and controlled environments, generating motivation, providing a high level of interactivity, immediate feedback and contributing to the improvement of visual processing skills and short-term memory (Phipps, Sutherland & Seale, 2002; Kalyvioty & Mikropoulos, 2013).

The wealth of technology lies in the fact that it can present information through multimedia elements (audio, text, images or videos), having the possibility of storing and transferring it, combining the media or even carrying out transformations.

This is considerably beneficial for the attention of the individual needs of the students, contributing to the treatment of Specific Learning Difficulties such as dyslexia (Cuetos et al., 2012; Meyer, Rose & Gordon, 2014; Núñez & Santamaría, 2016).

In this line, research has been conducted using technological tools to facilitate intervention in specific disorders of learning to read and write (Cidrim, Braga & Madeiro, 2018; Cidrim & Madeiro, 2017; Kalyvioty & Mikropoulos, 2014; Saputra, Alfarozi & Nugroho, 2018; Skiada, Soroniati, Gardeli & Zissis, 2014; Suárez, Pérez, Vergara & Alférez, 2015; Williams, Jamali & Nicholas, 2006; Zikl et al. 2015).

Specifically, Virtual Reality (VR) and Augmented Reality (AR) are some of the emerging technologies, with an increasing trend in relation to their application in the educational field (Aznar Díaz, Romero-Rodríguez & Rodríguez-García, 2018).

In this sense, emerging technologies can facilitate constructivist learning, provide alternative forms of learning, enable collaboration between students beyond the physical space, increase motivation and interest, as well as the development of digital competence (Otero & Flores, 2011; Cuesta & Mañas, 2016).

The versatility it offers makes it adaptable to different contexts, one of them being learning disorders. Another of its potentials is that it is a safe and flexible tool and has high adherence rates (Mura et al., 2018).

Within the technological field, Virtual Reality and Augmented Reality can make important contributions to the treatment of Specific Learning Difficulties, since they offer more playful environments that can improve adherence to treatment as well as safe and controlled environments in which failure does not have negative consequences for the student. In addition, they provide immediate feedback and can have high levels of interactivity Kalyvioty and Mikropoulos (2013) together with the possibility of offering a multisensory approach (Broadhead et al., 2018), being considered one of the most promising treatment routes in this area since it allows more personalized and student-centered learning situations (Birsh, 2011).

This chapter addresses Specific Learning Difficulties (DEA) and, specifically, dyslexia, since it is one of the most prevalent difficulties in the educational field. In this regard, Educational Technology contributes to direct intervention with students who have special educational needs as an alternative to traditional resources, which is much more motivating.

As an example, we present various projects and applications that allow us to work on these types of difficulties with students.

BACKGROUND

Specific Learning Difficulties (SpLD)

The University of Cambridge defines Specific Learning Difficulty (SpLD) as a diagnosis in its own right, commonly used as an umbrella term to refer to one of the following diagnoses:

Dyslexia (an underlying language processing difficulty); Dyspraxia (a difficulty with motor co-ordination and visual perception and can hinder the efficiency with which the individual can plan and carry out motor tasks); Dyscalculia (primarily affects the ability to acquire arithmetical skills) and Dysgraphia (primarily affects handwriting).

Specific learning difficulty is considered to be the affectation of the cognitive processes involved in language, reading, writing and / or calculation, with relevant implications in the school environment.

In Spain, in Organic Law 8/2013, of December 9, for the improvement of educational quality (LOMCE), sections 1 and 2 of article 71 are worded as follows:

1. The educational Administrations will oversee obtaining the necessary means so that all students achieve their optimal intellectual, personal, emotional and social development, in the same way it must happen with the objectives proposed in general in this Law. The Administrations educational institutions will establish plans for priority centers to help those centers that enroll students in a socially disadvantageous situation.
2. It is the aim of the educational administrations to guarantee the necessary resources to students who require educational attention different from the ordinary ones due to special educational needs, specific learning difficulties, high abilities, ADHD, due to late incorporation into the educational system or other personal conditions or of school history, and achieve the objectives established in general.

In accordance with Organic Law 3/2020, of December 29, which modifies Organic Law 2/2006, of May 3, on Education (LOMLOE), in the area of attention to diversity, the need to individualize education in order to achieve the maximum personal, intellectual, social and emotional development of the students. The consideration of adaptations and adaptations for ACNEAE students in the post-mandatory stages will be opened.

The situation of legislation in Portugal regarding learning difficulties promotes development points similar to Spanish legislation:

According to article 3 of Decree-Law No. 54/2018, the principles of inclusive education are:

1. Universal education, the assumption that all children and students have the capacity for learning and educational development;
2. Equity, ensuring that all children and students have access to the support necessary to realize their potential for learning and development;
3. Inclusion, the right for all children and students to access and participate, fully and effectively, in the same educational contexts;
4. Personalization, educational planning centered on the student so that the measures are decided on a case-by-case basis according to their needs, potentials, interests and preferences, through a multi-level approach;

5.   Flexibility, flexible management of the curriculum, spaces and school days, for educational activities in its methods and time.

Dyslexia: Conceptual Approach

Taking into account the etymological origin of the word dyslexia, it comes from the Greek roots dys - which means difficulty - and lexia - which means reading, referring to difficulty in reading, a term coined at the end of 1880 (UNESCO, 2020).

According to the Diagnostic and Statistical Manual of Disorders (DSM-V), dyslexia is found in the subcategory of neurodevelopmental disorders called "Specific learning disorder" and refers to a pattern of learning difficulties characterized by problems with accurate or fluent word recognition, misspelling, and poor spelling skills (American Psychiatric Association, 2014).

Specifically, dyslexia is a learning disorder that is manifested by a difficulty in reading and writing, being its main signs or symptoms (De Marco, 2010):

- Difficulties in learning to read and write.
- Difficulties in reading speed.
- Difficulties in reading comprehension.
- Disruption in writing.
- Repeated omissions, substitutions, inversions, additions in their reading and writing.
- Handwriting problems.
- Spelling problems.
- Lack of attention, concentration and motivation.

Therefore, dyslexia can be defined as a specific reading and writing learning disorder that has a persistent and specific nature, its origin being derived from a neurodevelopmental disorder and characterized by the difficulties that the person has when recognizing certain words fluently and accurately as well as the ability to decode and spell due to a deficit in the phonological component of language and the field of reading being affected (Benítez-Burraco, 2010; Cidrim & Madeiro, 2017; National Institute of Neurological Disorder and Stroke, 2016).

People with dyslexia present a deficit in terms of phonological awareness, verbal memory and verbal processing speed that does not correspond to the stage of development in which the person is (Protopapas, 2019) and is prolonged in time, independent of good cognitive abilities and high performance of the person (Cuetos, Soriano & Rello, 2019).

They also have difficulties in differentiating sounds and words, memorizing, transforming isolated sounds into words, as well as remembering letters and their sound equivalents (Dymora & Niemiec, 2019). This is due to the fact that there is an alteration that affects the functionality of reading behavior that makes it impossible for the person to correctly and effectively extract written information and, therefore, influences their academic, personal and social adaptation (Cuetos et al., 2012).

Dyslexia affects 10% of the world's population and in four out of six people it causes failure in school. In Spain, it is calculated that the incidence in Primary and Secondary Education is between 5 and 10% of the student body (Artigas-Pallarés, 2009; Jiménez, Guzmán, Rodríguez & Artiles, 2009).

MAIN FOCUS OF THE CHAPTER

Educational Technology in Attention to Diversity

The emerging Information Society requires new skills at all levels, therefore, the educational field has multiple reasons to take advantage of the new possibilities provided by Educational Technology in order to promote this change towards a new, more personalized and focused educational paradigm centered in student learning.

Information and Communication Technologies allow us to develop certain key points that will allow us to see the student as a co-protagonist of their learning: increasing motivation when it comes to awakening interest in learning and understanding; allowing the immediacy of transmission and reception of information and providing a flexibility of pace and learning time (Sevillano and Rodríguez, 2013, p. 76).

The rapprochement that is being made between Information and Communication Technologies (ICT) and attention to diversity has reached very important levels (Correa & González, 2014). In this sense, it can be affirmed that the use of these tools facilitates the relationship of students with special educational needs with their environment, thus improving their quality of life in the personal, emotional, affective, work and professional spheres (Cabero, Córdoba & Fernández, 2007).

The evolution of Educational Technology, as well as its presence and implementation in schools, make it necessary to pose new challenges and lines of research since they offer a wide range of possibilities to work with people with special educational needs. In this regard, the use of audiovisual technological means provides great advantages to the educational needs of students (Cabero, 2002; Cabero, Córdoba & Fernández, 2007):

- help overcome the limitations that derive from the cognitive, sensory and motor disabilities of the students.
- favor the autonomy of the students since the tools can be adapted to the needs of each student in a personalized way.
- favor synchronous and asynchronous communication of students with the rest of their classmates and teachers.
- save time for the acquisition of skills and abilities in students.
- favor the diagnosis of students.
- support a multisensory communication and training model.
- promote individualized training for the student.
- facilitate the socio-labor insertion of students with specific difficulties.
- provide moments of leisure.
- promote the approach of the students to the scientific and cultural world, and to be up to date with the knowledge that is constantly being produced.
- favor the reduction of the sense of academic and personal failure.

The educator plays a fundamental role in the selection and use of the technology that he is going to use as an instrument for education and even more so if he must work with people with special educational needs. For this reason, in the selection and decision-making process, they must know the potential solutions offered by the different technologies and know which of them is the most appropriate to meet the special educational needs of their students (Hervás & Toledo, 2006, 2007).

On the other hand, when incorporating Educational Technology to serve students with special educational needs, we must not forget a series of important aspects such as (Cabero, Córdoba & Fernández, 2007):

- Its usage depends on the type of disability to which we are referring: visual, auditory, motor, cognitive...
- integration depends not only on the type of disability but also on its degree.
- perceive its use from the point of view of both hardware (physical component of computers: keyboards, monitors, printers...) and software (logical component: computer programs, browsers...).
- can find both the possibility of adapting conventional media, as well as the construction of specific ones.
- and that different professionals will come into play in their research and analysis, ranging from pedagogues, engineers, psychologists, designers, etc.

Specific Projects and Applications

In this section we will focus our attention on technological resources that allow educational intervention in students with Specific Learning Difficulties, specifically in students with Dyslexia.

FORDYSVAR

The European Project Erasmus + FORDYS-VAR (*Fostering inclusive learning for children with dyslexia in Europe by providing easy-to-use virtual and / or augmented reality tools and guidelines*) has been co-financed by the Erasmus + program of the European Union through the project 2018-1-ES01-KA201-050659.

FORDYS-VAR was awarded in 2018 by the Spanish Service for the Internationalization of Education (SEPIE) with a total funding of 367.544,00€ for the years 2018-2021.

It has a transnational focus and the coordination is carried out from the University of Burgos, being the Principal Investigator (PI) Professor Sonia Rodríguez Cano. In addition, the project consortium is made up of different European partners:

- Spain: University of Burgos, consulting firm K-Veloce and the IT development company AR-SOFT.
- Italy: Eugenio Medea Scientific Research Institute.
- Romania: Bucharest Dyslexia Association.

The FORDYS-VAR project addresses some of the horizontal priorities of Erasmus +, such as (FORDYS-VAR, 2020):

- Social inclusion, specifically, support for diversity and equal access to education for children with dyslexia.
- The use of ICT in educational settings to contribute to the access of students with dyslexia.
- And improve the skills of teachers, providing them with adequate tools to adapt their educational devices to schoolchildren with dyslexia.

Objectives

This project is included within the Strategic Partnerships Projects oriented to the field of school education (KA2), its main objective being to contribute to the educational inclusion of students with dyslexia, aged between 10 and 16 years, through the use of technology, specifically Virtual Reality (VR) and Augmented Reality (AR) to improve access, participation and learning achievements of students with this literacy disorder.

The purpose is to create a playful, fun and safe learning environment, thus achieving a greater commitment to treatment and improving their quality of life.

Consequently, it seeks to contribute to the improvement of quality standards in the educational field, promoting the academic success of boys and girls with dyslexia of school age and equal access and opportunities for all, increasing the skills and competencies of teachers and education professionals.

In summary, FORDYS-VAR pursues the following objectives:

- Contribute to the educational inclusion of children with Dyslexia using VR and AR.
- Generate adapted material and resources.
- Implement these resources in the classroom for their educational development.
- Provide tools to the teacher for the classroom.
- Disseminate results.
- Carry out transfer to other educational contexts.

Recipients

The target groups of the study are:

- Students with dyslexia, who will be the end users of the developed materials.
- Teachers and therapists, who will provide the formal and non-formal treatment.
- Families of boys and girls with dyslexia.

Expected Results

As a result, three intellectual products will be developed:

1. A toolkit

Including software to integrate VR and AR in educational and pedagogical settings for school-age children with dyslexia.

2. Electronic Book

With guidelines and good practices on dyslexia and the use of educational technology as well as the compilation of European regulations and the different approaches applied in the EU on dyslexia.

3. White Paper

For the establishment of educational policies for children with dyslexia.

All the intellectual products developed in the context of the European project will be freely available on its own website: https://fordysvar.eu

In the field of content localization and translation and in the context of the pandemic situation that we have been living, the Polytechnic Institute of Bragança has been invited to collaborate in the audio-visual translation of the applications produced within the scope of the project and to test it with a group of experts. A case study will be carried out in the first semester of 2021/2022.

Dissemination and Visibility

Communication, dissemination and visibility is undoubtedly one of the most important tasks in the development and implementation of European Erasmus + projects. This activity must be carried out from the beginning by all the partners involved, collecting evidence of the progress of the project and disseminating it both within and outside the beneficiary organization.

In the development and implementation of European Erasmus + projects, activities aimed at communication, dissemination and visibility of progress, development, implementation, as well as the results obtained during them, are particularly important in order to maximize their impact (Rodríguez, Delgado & Ausín, 2020).

By sharing the lessons learned, the results and conclusions of the projects, the aim is to raise awareness, maximize impact, engage stakeholders and target groups, share solutions and practical knowledge, influence practice and policies, and develop new ones. associations and contact networks.

The impact of an Erasmus + project is not only measured by the quality of the results obtained but also by the degree to which people outside the project know and use them.

Therefore, it can be deduced that reaching a large number of potential users through communication and dissemination tasks will help to achieve a higher return on investment from the European funds allocated to the projects.

In order to respond to communication and dissemination activities, it is important to determine what types of activities are appropriate to improve the education and training systems of the European Union. All this is described in detail in the project's Dissemination Plan, which tries to answer the questions: why, what, who, to whom, when, where and how the results obtained in the project will be disseminated, both during the funding period, as after this.

The project started in September 2018 and its duration is 36 months. At the present time, the dissemination plan is already being implemented through activities in the media (radio, press and television), institutional channels (University of Burgos, Medea Institute, Arsoft and Kveloce), various scientific events and congresses, international meetings, as well as various designated social networks.

Currently, it is essential to have a presence on Social Networks since, in recent times, they have gained relevance in the field of dissemination of projects (Rodríguez, Delgado, Ausín, Casado & Cuevas, 2020).

Social networks have become a powerful tool for communication, interaction and production of knowledge (Fain-holc, 2011). Based on the results of the latest study of the VII Wave of the Social Networks Observatory (The cocktail analysis, 2016), it is found that the penetration of social network users among regular Internet users has remained stable since 2011. In addition, 9 of each 10 regular Internet users have an active account on at least one social network (Facebook, Twitter, Google+, LinkedIn, Instagram, Pinterest).

Among the advantages of using Social Networks for dissemination we find the following:

- Increase knowledge about the subject of the project.
- They allow instant communication.
- They facilitate the sharing of knowledge and information.
- They contribute to the visibility of intellectual products.

From FORDYS-VAR we wanted to have a presence in four of the Social Networks, most used by the general population today:

- Twitter: @fordysvar [http://bit.ly/TW_fordysvar]
- Facebook: Fordysvar UBU [http://bit.ly/FB_fordysvar]
- Instagram: fordys_var [http://bit.ly/IG_fordysvar]
- YouTube: FORDYSVAR UBU [http://bit.ly/YT_fordysvar]

Programma DiTres

Rehasoft (2019a) is a company at the forefront of new educational technologies, with more than 15 years of experience that develops products that facilitate reading, writing, learning and communication for students with special educational needs who present Dyslexia, Dyscalculia or Attention Deficit Hyperactivity Disorder (ADHD).

In this regard, we will deal with the DiTres software whose specific programs are intended for students with Dysñexia.

DiTres (Rehasoft, 2019b) is a software package composed of three DiTex, DiDoc and DiLet programs, whose main idea is to make the computer read all the texts by incorporating a synthetic voice, applying multisensory learning. Listening to these texts, the person with Dyslexia can assume the content perfectly. This implies the opening of another sensory channel allowing to understand and assimilate any type of writing. This software is available in several languages and allows:

- Read any printed book / newspaper / magazine / text sheet (using the scanner), etc.
- Read any electronic document such as Word / Excel / PowerPoint documents, PDF documents, Web pages, email, etc.
- Listen to everything you write on the computer.
- Write faster using the word predictor.
- Eliminate spelling mistakes with ear-through auto-correction.

A demo of DiTres can be seen on Rehasoft's YouTube channel: https://www.youtube.com/watch?time_continue=8&v=OqXMbP1E9Qc&feature=emb_logo

DiTex

This program makes working with computers easier for people who have learning difficulties, speech problems, dyslexia or want to practice or follow a treatment to improve reading and writing. It is specially adapted to work with Microsoft Word and to read texts on the Internet. For this, it has an integrated voice that allows reading the texts on the computer screen in several languages. Its main options and functions are shown in Table 1.

Table 1. Characteristics of the DiTex program

DiTex	
Options	• Listen to the text that is written in Word, letter by letter, word by word or phrase by phrase. • Listen to a text in Word, a word, a line, a sentence, a paragraph or entire documents. • Listen to texts on the Internet or from other Windows programs. • Listen to texts, menus, icons while browsing the Internet.
Features	• Reading through the keyboard - listening to texts written on the computer. • Text reading - hear texts on the screen. • Read functions - hear menus, buttons, and dialog windows on the screen. • Reading texts on the Internet using the mouse or the function keys (F1 to F12) on the keyboard.
Display	
Demo link	http://www.rehasoft.com/descargas-demo/

Source: Rehasoft (2019c)

DiDoc

DiDoc is a program created to help people with reading problems. The program works with a scanner, once the desired document (a page, a book or a newspaper) has been scanned, the program reads the texts that appears on the computer screen, through a built-in voice that reads in different languages. Table 2 summarizes its main characteristics.

Table 2. Features of the DiDoc program

DiDoc	
Options	• Listen to the scanned document letter by letter. • Listen to the scanned document word for word. • Listen to the scanned document phrase by phrase. • Listen to an entire book or documents.
Features	• Reading of Books, Textbooks, Newspapers, Letters etc. • Scans in Black and White, Grayscale and Color. • Enlarge the letters of the text making it easier to read • Export the text of the scanned book to Word
Display	
Demo link	http://www.rehasoft.com/descargas-demo/

Source: Rehasoft (2019d)

DiLet

DiLet is a word predictor created to help people with Dyslexia to spell correctly. When you type one or more letters of a word, the program suggests a list of possible words. Also, in combination with DiTex you can hear the words. Another main feature is the creation of personalized word lists to better adapt the suggestions to the level of each student. Thanks to this, DiLet allows to carry out individualized work, combining the practice of writing to acquire more speed, with the improvement and increase of the vocabulary, which the user already has. Finally, Table 3 shows the main features of DiLet.

Table 3. Features of the DiLet program

DiLet	
Opciones	<ul><li>You can work with the suggestions offered by DiLet that come from a general dictionary included in the program.</li><li>Create a custom dictionary.</li><li>Dictionaries can be created with different levels of difficulty and on different topics. They can also be used in a pedagogical program for the student.</li><li>If the student has a very low vocabulary level, a personalized dictionary can be created with very few words, offering suggestions with only one letter. Thus the person can practice autonomously.</li><li>DiLet can read the suggestions through a synthetic voice in combination with DiTex.</li><li>By practicing with DiLet, people with dyslexia or other writing difficulties can improve and speed up writing, that is, write more, more correctly and faster.</li></ul>
Funtions	<ul><li>Examples of words according to the chosen dictionary.</li><li>Ability to create individual custom dictionaries.</li><li>Analysis of the development of vocabulary and the written word.</li><li>Reading of suggested words in combination with DiTex.</li></ul>
Visualización	
Demo link	http://www.rehasoft.com/descargas-demo/

Source: Rehasoft (2019c)

Table 4. Features of the Metaverse Studio

Metaverse Studio		
Options	•	Metaverse is a real-world gamification platform that annotates the physical world with interactive experiences.
	•	This program can be used to create virtual visits and other augmented reality environments.
	•	Metaverse can be used for all kinds of things including; gaming, scavenger hunts, loyalty programs, interactive storytelling, brand activations, retail gamification, fan coalescing, etc..
	•	Recommended for teachers to create and make content or activities available to students, but the creators have to acquire some ideas about dyslexia.
Funtions	•	Ability to create interactive stories, content presentations, augmented reality experiences, games, etc..
	•	Create user interaction interfaces.
	•	Create walls.
	•	Create polls.
Display		
Link	https://studio.gometa.io	

Source: Metaverse (2021)

ISSUES, CONTROVERSIES, PROBLEMS

In the coming years we will see a true educational revolution brought about using different emerging technologies that are emerging in the educational field, such as Augmented Reality, the Semantic Web or Virtual Reality. These can become a resource to face new educational challenges and given their flexibility and adaptability they can be incorporated in an appropriate way into the teaching-learning process, adapting this process to the times that each student needs with or without difficulties.

The motivation that a priori causes the use of these technologies, which stimulate and reinforce student learning by combining school content with playful environments and motor activity, encourages the acquisition of knowledge that becomes the central axis of the child's center of interest (Cano, Alonso, Benito & Villaverde, 2021).

Within the SpLD, dyslexia is one of the most common, and due to its close relationship with poor school performance, it has led to a multitude of researches. In addition, it is also known that as the child progresses through the different educational stages, the demand for literacy is greater, which implies a constant struggle towards academic success for students with dyslexia (Martínez, 2016).

SOLUTIONS AND RECOMMENDATIONS

Dyslexia is a Learning Difficulty with a prevalence of between 7 and 10%. Of this percentage, 90% will result in school failure.

The situation is aggravated by an educational system that is excessively based on reading and writing, both in content and in evaluation.

If the pandemic has taught us anything, it is that technologies will be part of the education of the future and that the better prepared and better uses we can give this technology, the better our education will be.

Children with dyslexia are a risk group, a risk that implies school failure, that implies low self-esteem, sometimes due to ignorance and other times because their circumstance goes unnoticed. They are children of normal intelligence, often branded as disorderly or rebellious bums. In short, they are a group that is still misunderstood by the school system, which often sets them apart and does not respond to their needs.

For this reason, research, training, innovation and the development of methodologies are necessary to help this, and other groups overcome their difficulties, from true inclusion, which means that the system adapts to the difficulties of the child and the response.

Dyslexia responds to speech therapy and psycho-pedagogical treatment, and it is committed to an early diagnosis and intervention, however, the treatments have little adherence because they are repetitive, demanding and sometimes not very motivating interventions. For this reason, the introduction of adapted and motivating technology is necessary and fundamental, which facilitates the educational inclusion of children diagnosed with this learning difficulty.

FUTURE RESEARCH DIRECTIONS

Currently, one of the most widely used instruments is ICT, which is integrated into the students' day-to-day life, which makes it a powerful tool. It is also a great help in creating interesting and motivating activities for students. For people with dyslexia, it is very useful since it can serve as support throughout their educational journey (Rodríguez-Cano, Delgado-Benito & Ausín-Villaverde, 2021).

For this reason, among others, the teaching staff must have as a task, almost obligatory, to frequently review and renew their educational practices. Lack of motivation in the classroom is one of the main impediments that teachers encounter, which can lead to future school failure. The use of ICT during their professional practice will undoubtedly be very beneficial in their performance and learning, as well as in the teaching process. Unlike the traditional system, ICTs immediately favor individualization since students are the ones in charge of working at their own pace with the computer. Likewise, it has been shown in different investigations that the computer-assisted instruction system is superior to the traditional system in different aspects, such as motivation, attention and cooperation, producing a very positive effect on the educational performance of people with some difficulty (Rodríguez, Jiménez, Díaz & González, 2011; Núñez & Santamarina, 2016).

DISCUSSION AND CONCLUSIONS

Educational Technology can contribute to generating spaces in which people with Specific Learning Difficulties such as Dyslexia can work through the difficulties they present, while also generating a personalized teaching place (Williams, Jamali & Nicholas, 2006). However, there are still few researches carried out in relation to this intervention (Broadhead, et al., 2018).

In this sense, we consider that the work carried out within the European Project Erasmus + *Fostering Inclusive Learning for children with Dyslexia in Europe by providing easy-touse Virtual and / or Augmented Reality tools and guidelines* can contribute to the advancement in the inclusion, treatment, and rehabilitation of the people with Dyslexia through AR and VR applications developed.

The three-dimensionality of these technologies makes it possible to bring knowledge, especially to those who have greater temporary or permanent difficulty, closer to their needs and interests, enhancing their level of competence, linked to perception, attention, memory, orientation, etc., and having a favorable impact in the understanding of language, in problem solving, the execution of tasks, among others, due to the high motivational component that the image provides. On the other hand, they can also be considered as teaching innovation tools that contribute to personalized education.

Currently, ICTs are conceived as an educational resource that favors the inclusion and integration of students. They have become powerful didactic tools that are integrated into the teaching-learning processes, achieving the acquisition of skills, competencies and strengthening the skills, performance and educational achievements of students (Román, Cardemil & Carrasco, 2011). In addition, they allow bringing content closer, increasing motivation, stimulating and reinforcing student learning, uniting school content and entertainment and inciting the acquisition of knowledge and generating curiosity (Pazmiño, Jácome, Santillán, & Freire, 2019).

The potential of these learning environments has also been recognized in the area of special educational needs (Stevens, 2004), coinciding with an increased interest in supporting the inclusion of people with learning difficulties such as dyslexia (Dyson, Farrell, Polat, Hutcheson & Gallanaugh, 2004).

However, and despite its advantages in terms of motivation and development of attention, some authors consider in their research that the difficulties that still generate the use of high-priced devices is a condition of inequality for students, no less important are the skills of teachers on applications or the use of devices whose difficulty has increased without schools have trained their professionals Marín,2014.

Virtual Reality is an incipient technology that lacks sufficient clinical studies at the moment to be able to demonstrate its long-term effects, which is why many manufacturers postpone its use to ages 12 and older.

Regarding the design of activities using technology, some authors state that the increase in information is difficult for students to sift through and this makes it difficult for them to pay attention and select the right materials and applications (Torres, Torres & Infante, 2015).

Our contribution in this field opens new possibilities for research and development of alternatives to work on dyslexia, however, we believe it is necessary to continue advancing in order to give scientific support to the use of these emerging technologies (VR and AR) in the diagnosis and dyslexia treatment.

ACKNOWLEDGMENT

Part of the content of this work has been co-financed by the Erasmus + program of the European Union through the project 2018-1-ES01-KA201-050659.

The support of the European Commission for the preparation of this publication does not imply acceptance of its contents, which is the sole responsibility of the authors. Therefore, the Commission is not responsible for the use that may be made of the information disclosed here.

This work has been supported by FCT – Fundação para a Ciência e Tecnologia within the Project Scope: UIDB/05777/2020.

REFERENCES

American Psychiatry Association. (2014). *Manual diagnóstico y estadístico de los trastornos mentales* (5th ed.). Editorial Médica Panamericana.

Artigas-Pallarés, J. (2009). Dislexia: enfermedad, trastorno o algo distinto. *Rev Neurol, 48*(2), 63-69.

Aznar Díaz, I., Romero-Rodríguez, J. M., & Rodríguez-García, A. M. (2018). La tecnología móvil de Realidad Virtual en educación: Una revisión del estado de la literatura científica en España. *EDMETIC. Revista de Educación Mediática y TIC, 7*(1), 256–274. doi:10.21071/edmetic.v7i1.10139

Benítez-Burraco, A. (2010). Neurobiología y neurogenética de la dislexia. *Neurologia (Barcelona, Spain), 25*(9), 563–581. doi:10.1016/j.nrl.2009.12.010 PMID:21093706

Birsh, J. R. (2011). Connecting research and practice. In J. R. Birsh (Ed.), *Multisensory teaching of basic language skills* (3rd ed., pp. 1–24). Paul H. Brookes Publishing.

Broadhead, M., Zad, D., MacKinnon, L., & Bacon, L. (2018). A multisensory 3D environment as intervention to aid reading in dyslexia: A proposed framework. *2018 10th International Conference on Virtual Worlds and Games for Serious Applications, VS-Games 2018 - Proceedings*, 1–4.

Cabero, J. (Ed.). (2000). *Nuevas tecnologías aplicadas a la educación*. Síntesis.

Cabero, J., & Fernández, J. (2007). *Las TIC para la igualdad*. Publidisa.

Cano, S. R., Alonso, P. S., Benito, V. D., & Villaverde, V. A. (2021). Evaluation of Motivational Learning Strategies for Children with Dyslexia: A FORDYSVAR Proposal for Education and Sustainable Innovation. *Sustainability, 13*(5), 2666. doi:10.3390u13052666

Cidrim, L., Braga, P., & Madeiro, F. (2018). Desembaralhando: A Mobile Application for Intervention in the Problem of Dyslexic Children Mirror Writing. *Revista CEFAC, 20*(1), 13–20. doi:10.1590/1982-0216201820111917

Cidrim, L., & Madeiro, F. (2017). Information and Communication Technology (ICT) applied to dyslexia: Literature review. *Revista CEFAC*, 19(1), 99- 108.Correa, M. R. & González, M. J. A. (2014). Las TIC al servicio de la inclusión educativa. *Digital Education Review*, (25), 108–126.

Cuetos, F., & Domínguez, A. (2012). *Neurología del lenguaje. Bases e implicaciones clínicas.* Editorial Médica Panamericana.

Cuetos, F., Soriano, M., & Rello, L. (2019). *Dislexia. Ni despiste, ni pereza: Todas las claves para entender el trastorno.* La Esfera de los Libros.

De Marco, M. (2010). Programas informáticos para trastornos de lectoescritura, Dislexia y/o TDAH. In *25 Años de Integración Escolar en España: Tecnología e Inclusión en el ámbito educativo, laboral y comunitario.* Consejería de Educación, Formación y Empleo.

Dymora, P., & Niemiec, K. (2019). Gamification as a supportive tool for school children with dyslexia. *Informatics (MDPI)*, 6(4), 48. doi:10.3390/informatics6040048

Dyson, A., Farrell, P., Polat, F., Hutcheson., G., & Gallanaugh, F. (2004). Inclusion and Pupil Achievement. London: Department for Education and Skills.

Hervás, C. & Toledo, P. (2007). Las tecnologías como apoyo a la diversidad del alumnado. In *Tecnología educativa* (pp. 233-248). Madrid: McGraw-Hill.

Jiménez, J. E., Guzmán, R., Rodríguez, C., & Artiles, C. (2009). Prevalencia de las dificultades específicas de aprendizaje: La dislexia en español. *Anales de Psicología*, 25, 78–85.

Kalyvioti, K., & Mikropoulos, T. A. (2013). A virtual reality test for the identification of memory strengths of dyslexic students in Higher Education. *Journal of Universal Computer Science*, 19(18), 2698–2721.

Kalyvioti, K., & Mikropoulos, T. A. (2014). Virtual Environments and Dyslexia: Review of literature. *Procedia Computer Science*, 27, 138–147. doi:10.1016/j.procs.2014.02.017

Marín, V. I. (2014). El uso del blog de aula como recurso complementario de la enseñanza presencial para el intercambio de información e interacción entre el profesorado y alumnado de primer año de química. *Educación en la Química*, 25, 183–189.

Martinez, E. (2016). *Dislexia en Adolescentes y Jóvenes Adultos: Caracterización Cognitiva y Afectivo-Motivacional.* http://hdl.handle.net/10550/56210

Metaverse. (2021). *Youtube Channel: Metaverse AR Platform.* https://www.youtube.com/channel/UCu-m7uPJBXug0HfqNi4AfQmQ

Meyer, A., Rose, D. H., & Gordon, D. (2014). *Universal design for learning: Theory and Practice.* CAST Professional Publishing.

Mura, G., Carta, M. G., Sancassiani, F., Machado, S., & Prosperini, L. (2018). Active exergames to improve cognitive functioning in neurological disabilities: A systematic review and meta-analysis. *European Journal of Physical and Rehabilitation Medicine*, 54(3), 450–462. doi:10.23736/S1973-9087.17.04680-9 PMID:29072042

National Institute of Neurological Disorder and Stroke. (2016). *Dyslexia Information Page.* http://bit.ly/2IoXY8H

Núñez, M. P., & Santamaría, M. (2016). Una propuesta de mejora de la dislexia a través del procesador de textos: "Adapro. *Revista Educativa Hekademos*, (19), 20–25.

Otero, A., & Flores, J. (2011). Realidad virtual: Un medio de comunicación de contenidos. Aplicación como herramienta educativa y factores de diseño e implantación en museos y espacios públicos. *Icono 14. Revista de Comunicación Audiovisual y Nuevas Tecnologías*, 9(2), 185–211.

Pazmiño, A., Jácome, J., Santillán, C., & Freire, M. (2019). El uso de las TIC para el aprendizaje de la programación. *Dominio de las Ciencias*, 5(1), 290–298. doi:10.23857/dc.v5i1.861

Phipps, L., Sutherland, A., & Seale, J. (Eds.). (2002). *Access All Areas: disability, technology and learning*. JISC TechDis Service and ALT.

Protopapas, A. (2019). Evolving Concepts of Dyslexia and Their Implications for Research and Remediation. *Frontiers in Psychology*, 10, 2873. doi:10.3389/fpsyg.2019.02873 PMID:31920890

Rehasoft. (2019a). *Dislexia, TDAH, Discalculia y Baja Visión*. https://www.rehasoft.com/

Rehasoft. (2019b). *DiTres*. https://www.rehasoft.com/dislexia/ditres/

Rehasoft. (2019c). *DiTex*. https://www.rehasoft.com/dislexia/ditex/

Rehasoft. (2019d). *DiDoc*. https://www.rehasoft.com/dislexia/didoc/

Rodríguez-Cano, S., Delgado-Benito, V., Ausín-Villaverde, V., & Martín, L. M. (2021). Design of a Virtual Reality software to promote the learning of students with Dyslexia. *Sustainability*, 13(15), 8425. doi:10.3390u13158425

Román, M., Cardemil, C., & Carrasco, A. (2011). Enfoque y metodología para evaluar la calidad del proceso pedagógico que incorpora TIC en el aula. *Revista Iberoaméricana de Evaluación Educativa*, 4(2), 9–35.

Saputra, M. R. U., Alfarozi, S. A. I., & Nugroho, K. A. (2018). LexiPal: Kinect- based application for dyslexia using multisensory approach and natural user interface. *International Journal of Computer Applications in Technology*, 57(4), 334. doi:10.1504/IJCAT.2018.10014728

Sevillano, M., & Rodríguez, R. (2013). Integración de tecnologías de la información y comunicación en educación infantil en Navarra. *Píxel-Bit. Revista de Medios y Educación*, 42, 75–87.

Skiada, R., Soroniati, E., Gardeli, A., & Zissis, D. (2014). EasyLexia: A mobile application for children with learning difficulties. *Procedia Computer Science*, 27(2), 218–228. doi:10.1016/j.procs.2014.02.025

Suárez, A. I., Pérez, C. Y., Vergara, M. M., & Alférez, V. H. (2015). Desarrollo de la lectoescritura mediante TIC y recursos educativos abiertos. *Apertura (Guadalajara, Jal.)*, 7(1), 38–49.

Torres, J. C., Torres, P. V., & Infante, M. A. (2015). Aprendizajemóvil:perspectivas.RUSC. *Universities and Knowledge Society Journal*, 12, 38–49. https://www.redalyc.org/articulo.oa?id=78033494005

UNESCO. (2020). *Embracing Dyslexia - Crossing the chasm and saving lives*. https://bit.ly/2Vzyey2

Williams, P., Jamali, H. R., & Nicholas, D. (2006). Using ICT with people with special education needs: What the literature tells us. *Aslib Proceedings*, 58(4), 330–345. doi:10.1108/00012530610687704

Zikl, P., Bartošová, I. K., Víšková, K. J., Havlíčková, K., Kučírková, A., Navrátilová, J., & Zetková, B. (2015). The possibilities of ICT use for compensation of difficulties with reading in pupils with dyslexia. *Procedia: Social and Behavioral Sciences*, *176*(1), 915–922. doi:10.1016/j.sbspro.2015.01.558

ADDITIONAL READING

Cano, S. R., Alonso, P. S., Benito, V. D., & Villaverde, V. A. (2021). Evaluation of Motivational Learning Strategies for Children with Dyslexia: A FORDYSVAR Proposal for Education and Sustainable Innovation. *Sustainability*, *13*(5), 2666. doi:10.3390u13052666

Cano, S. R., & Benito, V. D. (2020). Fordysvar: Realidad virtual y realidad aumentada en niños y niñas con dislexia. In *Libro de Actas del X Congreso Universitario Internacional sobre Contenidos, Investigación, Innovación y Docencia:(CUICIID 2020)* (p. 1141). Fórum Internacional de Comunicación y Relaciones Públicas (Fórum XXI).

García, S. A., Cano, S. R., Benito, V. D., & Villaverde, V. A. (2021). Material multimedia interactivo y de realidad aumentada para el conocimiento y la sensibilización de la dislexia en el aula. In *Desempeño docente y formación en competencia digital en la era SARS COV 2* (pp. 531–542). Dykinson.

Rodríguez, S., Ausín, V., Delgado, V., & Tuñón, M. (2020). Líneas de intervención para el diseño de toolkit en el proyecto FORDYSVAR. In *V Encontro International de Formação na Docência | Livro de Resumos*. Instituto Politécnico de Bragança.

Rodríguez-Cano, S., Delgado-Benito, V., Ausín-Villaverde, V., & Martín, L. M. (2021). Design of a Virtual Reality software to promote the learning of students with Dyslexia. *Sustainability*, *13*(15), 8425. doi:10.3390u13158425

KEY TERMS AND DEFINITIONS

Augmented Reality: It is the technology that allows virtual elements to be superimposed on elements of reality.

Dyslexia: Specific learning difficulty with neurobiological origin and characterized by a deficit in reading and writing skills.

Educational Inclusion: UNESCO defines inclusive education as the process of identifying and responding to the diversity of needs of all students.

Educational Technology: Set of knowledge, applications, and devices that allow the application of technological tools in the field of education.

Learning Difficulties: It refers to a heterogeneous group of disorders, manifested by significant difficulties in the acquisition and use of some linguistic, reading or calculation skills.

User-Centered Design: Is defined by the Usability Professionals Association (UPA) as a design approach whose process is driven by information about the people who go to make use of the product.

Virtual Reality: It is an environment of scenes and objects of real appearance that creates in the user the sensation of being immersed in it.

Chapter 4
A Pedagogical Paradigm Shift:
Prospective Epistemologies of Extended Reality in Health Professions Education

Catherine Hayes
University of Sunderland, UK

ABSTRACT

This chapter provides an insight into the theoretical perspectives which form the foundation of extended reality (XR) and its emergence in practice as a fundamental part of medical and healthcare curricula. Issues such as the authenticity of learning, the validity and reliability of XR within processes of assessment, and the theoretical underpinnings of pedagogical approaches in health professions pedagogy are illuminated. Also considered are the implications of XR within the context of non-patient-based learning and the delineation of cognitive, affective, and psychomotor domains of learning in relation to patient outcomes at the front line of care in applied practice. The COVID-19 pandemic, which has impacted all global higher education institutional (HEI) learning since March 2020, is also considered in the context of moves to ensure that medical and healthcare education can continue, albeit via hybrid models of learning as opposed to traditional pedagogical approaches, which have remained little altered over the last century.

INTRODUCTION

The justification of pedagogy in the context of Extended Reality (XR), which encompasses Virtual Reality (VR), Augmented Reality (AR) and Mixed/Hybrid Reality (MR) has become an ongoing source of complex ambiguity over the last decade, that the COVID-19 pandemic has only served to exacerbate (van der Niet and Bleakley, 2021). Ensuring the validity and reliability of XR experiences within health professions education remains central to the potential to rule out technologies as adjuncts to optimal pedagogic practice as an authentic means of providing insight and illumination of medical contexts, scenarios and disease processes (McGrath et al, 2018). For the purposes of this chapter there will be four fundamental operationally definitive terms of what the umbrella term XR actually encompasses, firstly

DOI: 10.4018/978-1-7998-8371-5.ch004

VR refers to the use of computer technology in the creation of simulated learning environments. Secondly, AR pertains to the addition of computerised content as an overlay to reality, which means that learners can actively interact both with real world and augmentations of it at the same time. Mixed or hybrid reality refers to the transection of virtual worlds and actual worlds, where physical and computerised objects can interact and exist concurrently. XR encompasses all of these and as a collective they have revolutionised health and medical training, particularly in relation to the practise of risk management and professional role identity in life and death situations, for example obstetric emergencies, as reported by Hayes, Hinshaw and Petrie (2018).

Training for the strategic management of risk in healthcare practice in situated contexts of healthcare provision has been a key focus in the use of XR in practice (Hilty et al, 2020). Not only does it involve rational aspects of cognitive knowledge or the purist demonstration of psychomotor skills and affective domain learning (Zulkilfli, 2019). It also encompasses the intuitive, tacit and largely intangible intellectual instincts that develop with sustained experiential learning (Humpherys, Bakir and Babb, 2021). One of the key issues has been the challenge of assessing the last of these, what XR has enabled is the benchmarking of perceived levels of interprofessional and multi-disciplinary teamwork, where intuitive knowledge can be used to measure risk, regardless of the level of the organisational hierarchy within which personnel are employed (Goh and Sandars, 2020; Hayes, Hinshaw and Petrie, 2018). This chapter will explore the key epistemologies or ways of knowing, from a theoretical perspective, that can be used to ensure the level of authenticity necessary to highlight the pedagogical shifts in the application of learning theory which now characterise responsive curriculum design and adaptation to accommodate XR in practice.

THE CURRENT CLIMATE OF HEALTH PROFESSIONS PEDAGOGY

The ongoing pandemic, which on July 8th, 2021 had reached 184 million confirmed cases and over 4 million fatalities, has not only changed the world of education in its current form, it has likely altered its mechanism of delivery for the foreseeable future (WHO International Data, 2021). In practice the pandemic has seen universities close, a switch to hybrid models of learning and education, a social science by definition, depleted in terms of its capacity to engage people in face to face meetings (Okoye et al, 2021). The plethora of academic articles surrounding online learning is phenomenal, but few actually address how a fundamental paradigm shift in Higher Education is implemented methodologically (Luctkar-Flude and Tyerman, 2021). What is usually described is a narrative description of the processual use of technological intervention, rather than any degree of alignment in terms of underpinning theoretical justification for implementation, or indeed the constructive alignment demonstrating best how processes of assessment can effectively be driven by complementary processes of teaching and learning (Moreira, 2020). The physicality of learning has also been altered beyond recognition, seeing people as upper torsos and faces has changed everyday interaction in the situated nature and context of learning, yet minimal evidence exists as to the long term impact of this on motivating, engaging and sustaining active processes of learning, teaching and assessment on an individual level (Park and Kim, 2020). By over reliance on the physicalism of the articulated voice and postural positions of the upper torso, executed in an atmosphere of scrutiny, learners have had to change their interaction so that their degree of interaction is heavily influenced and constrained (Obrad, 2020). Whilst predicting how global disease and inequality will influence the future of education, it is impossible to ignore potential challenges that lie ahead for Higher Education (Bevins et al, 2020). It is possible to inferentially predict that COVID-19 may be one of the first of a new generation of global pandemics that will need to be death with, alongside dramatic changes in overall global warming, which will also ensure that populations which are densely populated suffer most severely (Negev et al, 2021). Alongside the issue of pandemic disease is the prospect of global catastrophes and natural disasters occurring far more frequently and necessitating support and address now. The progressive redevelopment of existing technology to accommodate this is more than apparent, so that learners can engage physically in medical and healthcare settings with less extensively sized equipment and a greater capacity to seamlessly integrated extended reality into all practice (Yigitcanlar et al, 2020). Geographically there are other issues at play, in terms of the accessibility of technology across global outcomes, with the result that some countries cannot be guaranteed adequate internet access, bandwidth or the cost of the technology products may simply be prohibitively expensive (Horton, 2021). Being cognisant of this necessitates ensuring both affordability and accessibility across the globe if the differential inequity between countries is to be addressed on an ongoing basis. Being able to standardise and regulate experience for learners is also of fundamental importance if equity and parity of experience are to be assured across these programmes (Crouch et al, 2021).

CURRICULUM JUSTIFICATION, DESIGN AND DEVELOPMENT

Pedagogical design and its address within the context of Higher Educational institutional curricula often places processes of curriculum justification and design under scrutiny (Annala et al, 2021). This is largely attributable to the complex ambiguity that curriculum designers have to contend with, in terms of the technical capacity of XR equipment and the accompanying resources they necessitate (Aebersold and Dunbar, 2021). A key example of this is the multi-disciplinary perspectives that designed scenarios have to authentically represent within the context of health and medical education, where XR is implemented in practice (Antoniou et al, 2020). As a consequence of this, the concept of experiential learning has become a focus for the opportunity of ensuring that XR is relevant to real world application in practice, with the introduction of its continuum's integral parts (AR, VR and MR). The published evidence to date demonstrates that XR training has been shown to improve learner performance skills across an array of learning domains (cognitive, affective and psychomotor) within the context of instructional simulation (Tabatabei, 2020). Having moved firmly from proof of concept pilot studies, XR as an embedded part of health and medical curricula is being used across a wide variety of simulated contexts (Tang et al, 2020). In comparison to traditional didactic teaching methodologies the benefits are seen within the areas of student motivation, confidence and the capacity of learners to take measured risk within the context of a consequence free facilitative environment where constructive feedback on performance can inform reflexive praxis around complex ambiguity and clinical decision making. Acclimatisation to new contexts and settings, for military learners, for example is invaluable, where introduction to new unfamiliar climates and contexts is undertaken via constructivist experiential learning opportunity in interactive immersive scenarios, where the pace and timing of exposure can largely be controlled in line with learner need (Cobos, 2020). The addition of iteratively increasing levels of complex ambiguity as skill increases is another opportunity for the formal scaffolding of learning within customised immersive experiences (Orr et al, 2020). Depending on whether learning is about the magnification of micro- theoretical concepts such as, for example atomic level particles, blood corpuscles or synaptic junctions or whether learning is centred around macro social constructs such as social justice and equity in different contexts of culture or climate, immersive technology with XR has the potential to extend the reach within and between academic pedagogies and disciplines and as a direct consequence impact on the capacity and capability of multi-disciplinary and interdisciplinary professional working at the front line of patient care (Mitchell and Boyle, 2021). Confidence underpins learner motivation and in turn elevates levels of competence, which ensure this iterative cycle continues (Owens, 2021).

Roussin and Weinstock (2017) detailed the pedagogical challenges faced by educators and trainers leading simulation-based training in the context of healthcare and medical services. In relation to the theoretical underpinning of their work, they presented the complexities of managing programmes in relation to single and double- loop experiential learning and the impact of organising organisational hierarchies in relation to the need to gain experiential learning in practice. Whilst their work omits specific reference to the implicit value of tacit knowledge in crisis situations, the functional insight they provide in relation to situated learning is invaluable in relation to the overall administration of optimal multidisciplinary and interprofessional teamworking scenarios. Most significantly their research demonstrated the application of scaffolded learning to the point of autonomy, consistent with Vygotsky's Zone of Proximal Development (1978) but also Argyris' acknowledgement of the relevance of single and double loop learning and the need to challenge and reconcile assumptions relating to the acquisition of knowledge through experience. Both raise important issues in terms of the longitudinal provision in education with XR, in relation to the phasing and iterative presentation of learning outcomes, each serving to consolidate consequent stages of learning within and between cognitive, affective and psychomotor learning domains.

DRIVING AUTHENTIC LEARNING WITH PEDAGOGICAL DESIGN

Pedagogical design of the blurring of where reality and actuality co-exist within the context of digital immersion underpins the concept of validity in XR. While pedagogical research and applied praxis are still at the mercy of technology to a certain extent, as the virtual world becomes progressively more advanced, then so too will the capacity and capability for authenticity and validity within medical and healthcare education and training (Ligtart et al, 2021).

It is useful here, to consider the degree to which VR, AR and XR have been integrated across the health professions within differing signature pedagogies and the cognitive, psychomotor and affective learning domain skills necessitating address. It is here that some healthcare professions can be delineated in terms of their functional involvement in patient centred care. For example, dentistry and physiotherapy have relatively functional interventions, whilst the work of a podiatrist, due to the ergonomic positioning of a practitioner, entails more of an opportunity to engage psychosocially with patients during their appointments (King et al, 2018). Indeed academic debates have historically been posited about the functional basis of such healthcare professional roles as dentistry, since they are so functional in nature that people queried whether they could actually be regarded as a profession at all (Welie, 2004). The other implication is the stage of learning that medical and allied healthcare practitioners have reached in their career trajectories, where VR, AR and XR may be implemented most appropriately. The majority of published literature to date focuses on learning 'in situ' whereas the assessment of learning longitudinally in the context of real life praxis, is often evaluated with a degree of tokenism by those whose initiatives have introduced simulation in the first place.

The operationally definitive terms of VR, AR and XR are significant when considering the nature of the artificial environments that are created in the exploration of potentially risk filled scenarios, which emulate the real world (Alnagrat, Ismail and Idrus, 2021). This is primarily in relation to how artificial intelligence can be embedded within the context of virtual and simulated learning experiences, which also have to be optimally facilitated by staff skilled in the field of clinical simulation (Abbas, Kenth and Bruce, 2020). Central to progression in these aspects of a pedagogical paradigm shift, is the need for active dissemination and sharing of knowledge creation and acquisition that happens at the front line of medical and healthcare education where simulation in the context of XR are the expected and anticipated norms of undergraduate and postgraduate academic curricula across HEIs (Luo et al, 2021).

IMMERSION IN LEARNING EXPERIENCE

AR and VR enhance health professions education via immersion in learning experiences, positively influencing levels of engagement and motivation and by creating an atmosphere of interactive dialogue, which in terms of social inclusion can have a direct impact on the reduction of learner stress and anxiety (Brandon, Freiwirth and Hjersman, 2021). Encompassed by the umbrella term of XR, AR, MR and VR all bring a signature technological approach to applied praxis in the context of healthcare professions. In instances where different levels of sensorial intrusion are now widely used to extend the reach of pedagogic practice in medical and healthcare education and training, this has broad ramifications, not only on the practical delivery of emergent technology in practice but on their pedagogical theoretical justifications as well (Robert, 2021). In instances where the affordability and hence the extent of digital technology available determines accessibility in practice-based settings. In terms of a hierarchy of availability, AR is perhaps the most widely available and least invasive of all XR and can be easily accommodated by readily available display systems (Suryanti et al, 2020).

In instances where the need for the relevance of space and situatedness and context is of fundamental importance, then MR is the best platform for integration into available physical environments. In this sense MR fills the gap that VR leaves, in permitting users to physically interact with pre-identified physical spaces (Silén et al, 2008). Dimensionality is also of key importance in terms of whether the ability to facilitate visualisation in 3-D is something which can actively contribute to the acquisition of tacit knowledge and actively contribute to a more finely tuned intuitive response to any given scenario in medical and healthcare practice (Gerup, Soerensen and Dieckmann, 2020). MR effectively bridges the gap between AR and VR as a consequence of the development of the hardware capability of display screens and visualisation resources (Juraschek, 2018).

Research into XR pedagogical initiatives and methodological designs is usually characterised by relatively small-scale case studies, focused on the collection of qualitative data rather than tangible quantitative evidence about the impact of XR in practice (Hamilton, 2021).Those which have succeeded in this, tend to focus specifically on psychomotor skill or level of cognitive improvement rather than affective domain learning. The concept of tacit knowledge is also one which remains relatively underexplored and which remains almost a hidden bonus in developing the confidence of collective team hierarchies in clinical and medical practice. making generalisability of findings to other contexts and settings. Whilst this is a disadvantage, the potential for transferability of findings within and between similar situational contexts and settings across the global can be quite high in terms of overall content validity (Levitt, 2021).

The majority of XR technologies now extends the bridge between simulated environments and their polar opposites in physical reality. The rate of progressive developmental platforms has been amplified and magnified by the global COVID-19 pandemic, which has contributed to a paradigmatic shift in learners centred hybrid and hyflex learning and teaching opportunities across the medical and healthcare professions pedagogies (Acharya, 2021). As signature disciplines in their own right, these professions have maintained a certain degree of reticence to engage fully immersive technology within the context of clinical healthcare practice, since this completely detaches the clinician from their normal parameters of visual capacity. Whilst lenses are acceptable, they also permit and maintain human characteristics and gestures such as established eye contact and that degree of connection, which patients deserve and need (Jongerius et al, 2020). This has been particularly evidenced within the context of brain and cardiac surgery, both of which have optimally utilised these technological advances for the patients they serve.

TRADITIONS IN MEDICAL AND HEALTHCARE EDUCATION

Across the continuum of signature pedagogies that contribute directly to medical and allied health education, it is anatomy and mathematics which arguably transcend most disciplinary boundaries (Hayes and Capper, 2020). The visualisation techniques, which both permit and facilitate enhanced pedagogical teaching methodologies respectively appeared first in the context of simulation within the aviation industry at the beginning of the 20th Century. Their developmental progression over the last century and the early part of the 21st Century has ensured that levels of complex sensory and visual experience have now become a mainstay of medical and healthcare education and training programmes (Jentsch and Curtis, 2017). In the sense of providing students with the opportunity to undertake complex and risk inclined procedures, simulation is an invaluable resource. Within the context of safety, processes of experiential learning from practice can be fully exploited without there being any tangible, negative consequences in reality, so that unwanted outcomes can be illustrated and acknowledged without them actually ever having to come to fruition to do so.

Resources and student access to them have been a key issue during the pandemic, particularly for health and medical students for whom access to real- life anatomical models and cadavers may have been completely negated (Hilburg et al, 2020). For these students XR has ensured an opportunity for continued engagement with the discipline of anatomy and physiology across a range of contexts and settings. Since learning is extensive in relation to the need to develop a 3-D knowledge of bodily organs and systems, then the spatiality that XR offers also permits dynamic interaction, which otherwise would not be possible. In relation to the functional role of bodily organs and systems, XR has the added advantage that simulation of the dynamic motion of the body can be visualised as a learning resource, in contrast to cadavers, which are obviously non-functional (Ziker, Truman and Dodds, 2021). Within this simulation, it is also possible to identify, isolate and examine the individual functionality that specified aspects of these systems perform via repeated familiarisation. Ensuring learners iteratively progress from novice to expert within the use of XR of this nature, also ensures that learners can work in a risk free environment, which nevertheless serves to introduce them to the experiential learning which can form a solid foundation for their future professional careers in healthcare and medicine. In terms of pedagogic design and academic rigour the use of XR also provides an ideal opportunity to benchmark functional skills acquisition, alongside the real-time assessment of clinical practice and the opportunity for them to be exposed to sensory feedback from the situated learning they undertake (Kang et al, 2021).

BUILDING CAPABILITY FOR CLINICAL EDUCATORS WITH XR

The education and training of future medical and healthcare staff is not only dependent on disciplinary expertise but also the capacity to provide optimal learning experiences which in turn drive processes of assessment which are authentic and have real world validity and credibility (Voštinár et al, 2021). Future practitioners of all disciplines across the health and wellbeing continuum not only have to use evidence-based practice to discern clinical decision making, they also have to continually use scientific published evidence to iteratively update their continuing professional development in practice (Agha, 2021). As methodologies of pedagogic practice have become progressively more student there has been increasing emphasis on a move away from traditional rote learning to mechanisms of interactive, engaging processes of learning, which ensure deep rather than superficial learning across all aspects of education and training. Alongside this, is the recognition that learning driven purely by pressure to 'perform' within the context of examinations is futile in the truest sense of meaningful learning opportunity. In order to achieve this, XR can be regarded as a significant tool in the armoury of medical and healthcare educators who use this form of specialist resource to reinforce, motivate and enhance learning opportunities through authentically, strategically and constructively aligned academic curricula in Higher Education (Howell and Mikeska, 2021). Future practitioners also need the capacity to be educated in authentic situated learning contexts which are:

- Based on principles of diversity, equity and inclusion in terms of both optimal provision and optimal service to global, national, regional and local practice areas.
- Built on an ethos of compassion for all recipients and a respect for human life and wellbeing.
- Co-constructed with medical and healthcare service users and their families and carers.
- Designed on the basis of evidence-based healthcare practice and evidence-based processes of educational provision.
- Drivers of high quality multi-disciplinary and interprofessional patient centred teamworking.
- Effective in their capacity to drive education in relation to health and medical outcomes for patients at the front line of clinical care.
- Globally responsive and globally focussed
- Pedagogically designed and responsively designed on the basis of need and healthcare priorities in applied practice.
- Responsive in their capacity to dynamic and iterative change in healthcare landscapes.
- Specifically designed to value and promote autonomous learning, capacity for teamwork and proactive higher order critical thinking in relation to problem solving in health and medical care practice.

Within the context of XR integration, each pose individual challenges in relation to ensuring that digital technology is only ever seen as an adjunct to medical and healthcare education for the human race, not merely a functionalist or solely objective driver of it (Gandolfi, Kosko and Ferdig, 2021).

EXPERIENTIAL LEARNING THEORIES

The grander philosophical debates of perceived versus actual reality on an individual and collective basis are central to the processes of teaching and learning with XR. As a tool for the enhancement of understanding, meaning making and then critical reflection on practice, digital technology in invaluable as an adjunct to the human facilitation of knowledge, skills, attitudes and behaviours (Logeswaran et al 2021). The philosophical underpinning of experiential learning has its origins in constructivism, which is central to the acknowledgement of truth, either perceived or actual, and the capacity of all individuals to construct a perspective on truth based on their immersion in experience and the meaning they make of it (Koufidis et al, 2021). In this sense education is an entirely different experience for everyone who experiences the same phenomena and it is this individual experience and perspective meaning making, which lies at the heart of both collective and personal processes of transformation. The construction of a version of reality ensures that different perspective lenses can be applied to the same phenomena, so that scrutiny from a number of sources of triangulation can take place. Whether the experience differs collectively between adults and children in terms of capacity for meaning making through experiential learning was the source of seminal debate in the late 20th Century, with Knowles assertion that there was a distinction between andragogy, in terms of 'adult' ways of knowing and that of 'pedagogic' or child based learning. What is arguable more relevant is the concept of lifelong learning, across which learning takes place from the cradle to the grave, as a temporal mechanism of integrating the prospective with the retrospective and making inference from it as part of the integral processes of reflection and reflexivity (Loeng, 2021).

THEORETICAL UNDERPINNINGS OF XR PEDAGOGY

Experiential learning has become a byword for the placement experiences that medical and healthcare students undertake as an integral part of their undergraduate studies with patients, whose consent, briskly acquired provides novice learners with an opportunity to build confidence and be guided by an ever vigilant and highly respected disciplinary expert observer. In instances of postgraduate study, it may conjure the image of a professional moving from competence to proficiency and consequent mastery of their specific field of disciplinary context (Mortimore et al 2021). Medical training to the uninitiated is instilled with the imagery of cadaveric dissection as a means of visualising what lies beneath the skin that is to be negotiated across a respected lifelong career. In contrast to practice based experience at the front line of patient care in the context of care provision, though, the two are very different. It is here that whilst disciplinary knowledge and skill are invaluable to the expert educator, that skills of pedagogical praxis are equally important if the acquisition of knowledge which will underpin this lifelong career is to be assured and validated in practice. The theoretical underpinnings of learning and teaching have resonance in relation to the eventual capacity of medical and healthcare students not only to make meaning of experience but also to question that which cannot be taught, the tacit and reflexive response to intuition, which can only be derived from inner conscience and derived from processes of experiential learning in the psychomotor, cognitive and affective domains of learning, which can be tangible assessed and used to benchmark fundamental knowledge and skills acquisition (Birt et al, 2018). Similarly the capacity to transfer knowledge from the context of learning to the real world with patients who have an immediate need for assessment, diagnosis and consequent management is highly relevant to the potential to scaffold knowledge as clinical learners each move from the state of disciplinary novice to expert (Durning & Artino 2011)

MEANING MAKING IN HEALTHCARE PRACTICE

At the heart of capacity to learn and build on pre-existing experience is the theory of constructionist philosophy which when integrated alongside sociocultural perspectives from processes of active participation lies at the heart of all learning. The delineation between and linkage across theory and practice has become a fundamental goal of all involved in workplace education and training (Dennick, 2016). Since learning is both an individual and collective experience in the same sense as learning. What the Covid-19 pandemic detracted from was the fact that education is a social science, wholly reliant on interactivity and the derivation of meaning from multi-faceted and complex situational specificities, which when grouped as a collective constitute human experience. Being able to understand and frame the margin between knowledge and research entails a consideration of both the origin and consequent history of learning (Ten Cate and Billet, 2014). Alongside this, it is also necessary to consider how knowledge acquisition is gradually scaffolded through experience from novice to expert and to value those contributors to pedagogic practice who have acknowledged and formally recognised this (Graf et al, 2020). Whilst Kolb is often regarded as the seminal theorist of experiential learning, however there are several others of direct relevance to the pedagogical implementation of XR (Heong et al, 2020). Rooted in constructivist perspectives, Kolb's is of relevance since its focus lies in the translation of experience from external sources into epistemic cognition and meaning making on an individual basis. Kolb's theoretical perspectives are of importance when considering the processes of experiential learning, which in turn contribute to elements of subconscious bias that inevitably contribute to the professional identity of educators from specific signature pedagogies and disciplines. Social learning theory also plays a significant role in the development of experiential learning. It is a perspective upon which health and medicine have drawn heavily upon in the shaping and framing of new pedagogical perspectives. It frames learning outcomes in the context of their impact in applied praxis rather than in terms of their individual impact and acknowledges that these are often a natural by-product of distinctive social cultures and contexts. This also aligns with the concept of lifelong learning within which there is the acknowledgement that learning is dependent on levels of increasing experience (Hartman et al, 2020).

SCAFFOLDING LEARNING

XR provides an environment where the context of safety ensures that learners can iteratively be scaffolded through processes of knowledge acquisition and the basis of psychomotor skill competency and eventual mastery can be gained and evidenced in practice (Adefila et al, 2020).

One important aspect of the integration of XR though, is the degree to which it increases non-patient-based learning and the potential impact of this in relation to a lack of authentic human interaction across health and medical curricula. What this debate highlights are the significance of strategic curriculum design and justification across all programmes, where pedagogical constructive alignment is pivotal to outcomes-based assessment techniques and the credibility of their implementation. Similarly, where variations and combinations of XR are integrated across academic and clinical curricula then the technology selected ought to be aligned with the need for the acquisition of specific skills and techniques. The integration of XR and its components does ensure, however, that during the process of learning and the acquisition of new knowledge, skills and behaviours that ensure:

- Aims and objectives can be aligned with the opportunity for ongoing feedback and the opportunity to rehearse and develop new skill sets from novice to expert.
- Benchmarking of learner performance can be isolated into specific learning domains and assessed accordingly, with the potential of identifying individual learning need.
- Interruption and hence unnecessary and unwanted distraction, during the process of learning, can be avoided
- Patients can avoid any risk in terms of discomfort or the need to move regularly, as learners iteratively develop and refine new skills, where they can focus on domain specificity until a level of competency and eventual mastery is reached.
- That individual learning styles can be accommodated and encouraged by constructively aligning individual learning outcomes within each teaching session, where time permits.
- That psychomotor tasks can be repeated so that exposure, practical viability and accuracy can be iteratively increased.
- The opportunity for focused learner reflection on specific aspects of knowledge and skill acquisition and a reflexive approach for the address of individually recognised shortfalls.
- The theory-praxis gap can be gradually reduced by scaffolding learning and gradually increasing exposure to real life contexts where patients and their families are an integral part of authentic learning.

Non-technical skills such as interprofessional working and multi-disciplinary team working and the clinical attributes they necessitate in terms of optimal interpersonal communication and the management of the clinical environment characterise the skill sets necessary to ensure the achievement of holistic learning in proficient practice (Dehghani et al, 2021). Examples where this is now integrated in practice are in the skills and drills training, where it is also possible to integrate aspects of complex ambiguity and stress into situations, where a clear integration of psychomotor skill, affective and cognitive domain knowledge and application are necessary within any given scenario (DeMaria and Levine, 2013). It is these learning needs that high-fidelity clinical simulators address, so that once basic competence in a skill has been achieved then additional emotional stress and the need for instantaneous clinical decision making can be assessed. Whilst simulation is not an active replacement for the adrenaline rush faced in reality, it does offer an insight within learner centred experiential learning of the potentially uncertain scenarios that health and medical professionals often face in the real world. The portability of simulators such as 'SimMan' and 'SimMom' also provides the opportunity for context specific training opportunities where situated learning ca become an integral part of strategic curriculum justification, design and delivery (Viglialoro, 2021).

SUPPORTING CHANGE IN GLOBAL HEALTHCARE WORKFORCE PROVISION

Despite being one of the most needed and often underacknowledged parts of the global workforce, healthcare workers have virtually all been exposed to traditionalist mechanisms of education, which in terms of educational delivery have remained pedagogically unaltered for the best part of half a century (Karunathilake and Samarasekera, 2021). XR, as an integral part of a new technological age has been embedded within existing educational infrastructures, where traditional instruction mechanisms have shaped its implementation in relation to the pre-existing array of subject areas and academic disciplines represented by HEIs across the world. Stemming from the traditionalist apprenticeship models of learning, these learning approaches have been shaken to the core by a global pandemic that despite being predicted, came as a complete shock to global academic communities where health and medical education had to continue, despite education as a social science being altered beyond recognition in a space of six months, when national lockdowns shaped altered approaches to educational affordance and opportunity to learn (Chan, 2021). Whilst medical publications have an average currency of five years, clinicians of health and medical practice work for an average of forty years on the foundational knowledge attained almost half a century before. It is perhaps no surprise to learn then, that medical errors have become a progressively iterative problem across global health and medical practice, in situations where technology has developed to such an extent that new interventions are often almost obsolete before their initial implementation at the front line of patient care (Melnyk et al, 2021). Whilst these issues are concerning, they also pose the greatest opportunity for processes of progressive change for health and medical students whose curricula will inform the complex and ambiguous territories of professionalism that they will need to negotiate over the forthcoming years. This is an opportunity not only to focus and stabilise the quality and optimal provision of education for the next generations of healthcare practice, but also to ensure that medical education becomes more accessible, cost effective and most importantly places patients at the heart of compassionate human care. Exponentially in response to these challenges there has been a progressive switch to Problem Based Learning pedagogical approaches to medical and healthcare curricula across the globe. The immediacy of feedback and impact of professional facilitation of learning is central to the success of this approach in practice and ensures that the mindset of a critical enquirer is entrenched in learners who one day will become the next generation of medical and healthcare providers.

PATIENT CARER PUBLIC INVOLVEMENT IN CURRICULUM DELIVERY

The integration of patients and their families and carers, within the context of patient and carer public involvement (PCPI) initiatives is now an integral part of the majority of health and medical school curricula (Ocloo et al, 2021). Whilst they are invaluable in relation to the development of affective domain learning and in particular interpersonal and effective communication skills, the fact that these skills are inseparable from highly attuned cognitive and psychomotor skills in practice still exists. Where they are therefore of particular value is in the integration of these skills in conjunction with high fidelity simulation equipment, so that psychological fidelity can also be integrated into the acquisition of psychomotor technical skills training (Johnson et al, 2020; Hayes and Graham, 2020). This is of particular value in the transitioning between specifically designed learning environments, within which simulated learning takes place, and the eventual 'real life' praxis that students face. In terms of recreating learning environments which also reflect the multi-disciplinary and interprofessional working contexts within which health and medical staff find themselves on a daily basis, XR provides a useful mechanism of ensuring the psychological fidelity of scenarios used in learning. The origins of human factor analysis and historical emergence of XR training are well documented within the aviation industry, where contexts of flight simulation and the selective integration and conditions of flying can be reconstructed in terms of variability (Hawkins, 2017). One distinct variation in terms of the potential transferability of learning to 'real life' though, is the complex ambiguity and unpredictability of working with humans, whose predictability far outweighs anything an aeroplane, however complex can reflect. Unlike flying, therefore, those assessments regarded as 'high stake' in terms of potential outcome and risk, cannot be conducted with medical simulation equipment because of their relative potential variability in pathological and physiological status (Spurgeon et al, 2019).

Using teaching and learning to drive assessment is an acknowledged feature of student centred learning but we must never lose sight of the fact that XR, whilst being an adjunct and embedded part of health and medical curricula must never become the driver of learning in itself, lest the most important learning opportunities and factors may be lost to the prioritisation of technology over human need. Similarly, some higher education institutions aspire to owning the latest equipment, which is often declared obsolete before it can be pedagogically integrated with any degree of credibility across those academic curricula for which it was originally purchased. The focus of curriculum design and how teaching and learning ought to drive assessment rather than vice-versa must be advocated if the overall resultant levels of quality in patient care are to remain optimal (Burgess et al, 2020).

EXTENDED REALITY AND ASSESSMENT MECHANISMS IN HEALTH EDUCATION

Within the context of the assessment of healthcare and medical students, formative assessment that is subject to the regulations of Professional and Statutory Regulatory Boards such as allied health and medicine programmes, there is also the opportunity to effectively moderate assessment within and between educational institutions in terms of the parity and equity of assessment mechanisms. Where clinical educators and academics have to evidence the objectivity of processes of assessment, then XR is invaluable in terms of being able to standardise approaches to both formative and summative assessment techniques and their respective outcomes in educational practice (Wilson and Shankar, 2021). The COVID-19 pandemic has seen an exponential rise in the delivery of blended synchronous online and face to face teaching, which has been termed a hybrid learning approach. However, a newer term is the Hyflex curricula which have permeated the educational marketplace, with tailored offers of individual flexibility in learning patterns, which can accommodate more diverse student cohorts. Instructional resources delivered by XR are often an integral part of these flexible offers and it can be an optimal way of managing learning time for those adult learners who have additional family or working commitments to fulfil (Gagnon et al, 2020). Operationally defined, Hyflex models also adopt a hybrid approach but offer the opportunity to study flexibly rather than at a pre-set time. Delineating between models of actual attendance on campus is often indicated by the term hybrid, whereas the actual curriculum model is termed blended.

CONCLUSION

Progressive innovation across medical and healthcare professions is something which challenges traditional, conservative approaches to pedagogy, which ultimately contributes to the life and death decision making of clinicians at the front line of care. In this regard, it is important that technology is seen as a driver of pedagogic practice, rather than a methodology in itself. In this sense uptake of these new adjuncts is wholly dependent on medical and healthcare educators being open to change in approaches to education of subsequent generations of students and an acceptance that iterative and ongoing professional skills development is an integral part of adopting technology in practice. In practice this also necessitates the recruitment of staff with specialist technical skills who are responsible for the operationalisation of equipment, but who may not necessarily have specialist pedagogical skills in terms of curriculum design and implementation. So collaborative teamwork in the context of operational delivery of teaching sessions is pivotal. This investment, in terms of financial cost, collaborative working and mandatory iterative skills development for both academic and clinical educators, ensures that learning in a context safe from real-life risk with the potential for benchmarking the acquisition of knowledge and skills, is made possible in practice. The ongoing global COVID-19 pandemic has caused huge global disruption to traditional medical and healthcare education. Innovative responses in digital and technological tools have been quickly implemented with the aim of ensuring that learning can be maintained and sustained in order to ensure sufficient medical and healthcare graduates continue to qualify each year. Whilst change continues to ensure transformative approaches in those countries who can afford the fiscal implications of these developments, the gap between training providers globally also has the potential to widen in relation to optimal quality of medical and healthcare education. This is an obvious area for address if there is not to become a skills deficit in those countries where the affordance of digital technology as standard for learners and their academic and clinical teachers, is not yet possible. It is the acknowledgement and address of these key challenges which has the potential for a truly authentic paradigm shift in the application of XR in pedagogic design, scholarship and implementation to be achieved.

REFERENCES

Abbas, J. R., Kenth, J. J., & Bruce, I. A. (2020). The role of virtual reality in the changing landscape of surgical training. *The Journal of Laryngology and Otology*, *134*(10), 863–866. doi:10.1017/S0022215120002078 PMID:33032666

Acharya, S., Bhatt, A. N., Chakrabarti, A., Delhi, V. S., Diehl, J. C., van Andel, E., & Subra, R. (2021). Problem-Based Learning (PBL) in Undergraduate Education: Design Thinking to Redesign Courses. In *Design for Tomorrow—Volume 2* (pp. 349–360). Springer. doi:10.1007/978-981-16-0119-4_28

Adefila, A., Opie, J., Ball, S., & Bluteau, P. (2020). Students' engagement and learning experiences using virtual patient simulation in a computer supported collaborative learning environment. *Innovations in Education and Teaching International*, *57*(1), 50–61.

Aebersold, M., & Dunbar, D. M. (2021). Virtual and Augmented Realities in Nursing Education: State of the Science. *Annual Review of Nursing Research*, *39*(1), 225–242. doi:10.1891/0739-6686.39.225 PMID:33431644

Agha, S. (2021). Aligning continuing professional development (CPD) with quality assurance (QA): A perspective of healthcare leadership. *Quality & Quantity*, 1–15.

Alnagrat, A. J. A., Ismail, R. C., & Idrus, S. Z. S. (2021, May). Extended Reality (XR) in Virtual Laboratories: A Review of Challenges and Future Training Directions. *Journal of Physics: Conference Series, 1874*(1), 012031. doi:10.1088/1742-6596/1874/1/012031

Annala, J., Lindén, J., Mäkinen, M., & Henriksson, J. (2021). Understanding academic agency in curriculum change in higher education. *Teaching in Higher Education*, 1–18. doi:10.1080/13562517.2021.1881772

Antoniou, P., Arfaras, G., Pandria, N., Ntakakis, G., Bambatsikos, E., & Athanasiou, A. (2020). Real-time affective measurements in medical education, using virtual and mixed reality. In *International Conference on Brain Function Assessment in Learning* (pp. 87-95). Springer. 10.1007/978-3-030-60735-7_9

Argyris, C. (1991). Teaching smart people how to learn. *Harvard Business Review, 69*(3).

Bevins, F., Bryant, J., Krishnan, C., & Law, J. (2020). *Coronavirus: How should US higher education plan for an uncertain future.* McKinsey.

Birt, J., Stromberga, Z., Cowling, M., & Moro, C. (2018). Mobile mixed reality for experiential learning and simulation in medical and health sciences education. *Information (Basel), 9*(2), 31. doi:10.3390/info9020031

Brandon, E., Freiwirth, R., & Hjersman, J. (2021, May). Special Session—Student Engagement with Reduced Bias in a Virtual Classroom Environment. In *2021 7th International Conference of the Immersive Learning Research Network (iLRN)* (pp. 1-3). IEEE.

Burgess, A., van Diggele, C., Roberts, C., & Mellis, C. (2020). Key tips for teaching in the clinical setting. *BMC Medical Education, 20*(2), 1–7. PMID:33272257

Chan, S. (2021). *Digitally Enabling 'Learning by Doing' in Vocational Education: Enhancing 'Learning as Becoming' Processes.* Springer Nature. doi:10.1007/978-981-16-3405-5

Crouch, L., Rolleston, C., & Gustafsson, M. (2021). Eliminating global learning poverty: The importance of equalities and equity. *International Journal of Educational Development, 82*, 102250. doi:10.1016/j.ijedudev.2020.102250

Dehghani, M., Acikgoz, F., Mashatan, A., & Lee, S. H. (2021). A holistic analysis towards understanding consumer perceptions of virtual reality devices in the post-adoption phase. *Behaviour & Information Technology*, 1–19. doi:10.1080/0144929X.2021.1876767

DeMaria, S., & Levine, A. I. (2013). The use of stress to enrich the simulated environment. In *The comprehensive textbook of healthcare simulation* (pp. 65–72). Springer. doi:10.1007/978-1-4614-5993-4_5

Dennick, R. (2016). Constructivism: Reflections on twenty-five years teaching the constructivist approach in medical education. *International Journal of Medical Education, 7*, 200–205. doi:10.5116/ijme.5763.de11 PMID:27344115

Durning, S. J., & Artino, A. R. (2011). Situativity theory: a perspective on how participants and the environment can interact: AMEE Guide no. 52. *Medical Teacher, 33*(3), 188–199. doi:10.3109/0142159X.2011.550965 PMID:21345059

Gagnon, K., Young, B., Bachman, T., Longbottom, T., Severin, R., & Walker, M. J. (2020). Doctor of physical therapy education in a hybrid learning environment: Reimagining the possibilities and navigating a "new normal". *Physical Therapy, 100*(8), 1268–1277. doi:10.1093/ptj/pzaa096 PMID:32424417

Gandolfi, E., Kosko, K. W., & Ferdig, R. E. (2021). Situating presence within extended reality for teacher training: Validation of the extended Reality Presence Scale (XRPS) in preservice teacher use of immersive 360 video. *British Journal of Educational Technology, 52*(2), 824–841. doi:10.1111/bjet.13058

Gerup, J., Soerensen, C. B., & Dieckmann, P. (2020). Augmented reality and mixed reality for healthcare education beyond surgery: An integrative review. *International Journal of Medical Education, 11*, 1–18. doi:10.5116/ijme.5e01.eb1a PMID:31955150

Goh, P. S., & Sandars, J. (2020). A vision of the use of technology in medical education after the COVID-19 pandemic. *MedEdPublish, 9*(1), 9. doi:10.15694/mep.2020.000049.1

Graf, A. C., Jacob, E., Twigg, D., & Nattabi, B. (2020). Contemporary nursing graduates' transition to practice: A critical review of transition models. *Journal of Clinical Nursing, 29*(15-16), 3097–3107. doi:10.1111/jocn.15234 PMID:32129522

Hamilton, D., McKechnie, J., Edgerton, E., & Wilson, C. (2021). Immersive virtual reality as a pedagogical tool in education: A systematic literature review of quantitative learning outcomes and experimental design. *Journal of Computers in Education, 8*(1), 1–32. doi:10.100740692-020-00169-2

Hartman, E., Reynolds, N. P., Ferrarini, C., Messmore, N., Evans, S., Al-Ebrahim, B., & Brown, J. M. (2020). Coloniality-decoloniality and critical global citizenship: Identity, belonging, and education abroad. *Frontiers: The Interdisciplinary Journal of Study Abroad, 32*(1), 33–59. doi:10.36366/frontiers.v32i1.433

Hawkins, F. H. (2017). *Human factors in flight*. Routledge. doi:10.4324/9781351218580

Hayes, C., & Capper, S. (2020). Illustrating the transcendence of disciplinarity. In *Beyond Disciplinarity* (pp. 40–49). Routledge. doi:10.4324/9781315108377-4

Hayes, C., & Graham, Y. (2020). *Designing a Benchmarking Tool for Testing Posttest Confidence Levels in Emergency Obstetrics Training*. SAGE Publications. doi:10.4135/9781529709285

Hayes, C., Hinshaw, K., & Petrie, K. (2019). Reconceptualizing medical curriculum design in strategic clinical leadership training for the 21st century physician. In *Preparing Physicians to Lead in the 21st Century* (pp. 147–163). IGI Global. doi:10.4018/978-1-5225-7576-4.ch009

Heong, Y. M., Ping, K. H., Hamdan, N., Ching, K. B., Yunos, J. M., Mohamad, M. M., ... Azid, N. (2020). Integration of Learning Styles and Higher Order Thinking Skills among Technical Students. *Journal of Technical Education and Training, 12*(3), 171–179.

Hilburg, R., Patel, N., Ambruso, S., Biewald, M. A., & Farouk, S. S. (2020). Medical education during the coronavirus disease-2019 pandemic: Learning from a distance. *Advances in Chronic Kidney Disease, 27*(5), 412–417. doi:10.1053/j.ackd.2020.05.017 PMID:33308507

Hilty, D. M., Parish, M. B., Chan, S., Torous, J., Xiong, G., & Yellowlees, P. M. (2020). A comparison of in-person, synchronous and asynchronous telepsychiatry: Skills/competencies, teamwork, and administrative workflow. *Journal of Technology in Behavioral Science*, *5*(3), 273–288. doi:10.100741347-020-00137-8

Horton, S. (2021). Empathy Cannot Sustain Action in Technology Accessibility. *Frontiers of Computer Science*, *3*, 31.

Howell, H., & Mikeska, J. N. (2021). Approximations of practice as a framework for understanding authenticity in simulations of teaching. *Journal of Research on Technology in Education*, *53*(1), 8–20. doi:10.1080/15391523.2020.1809033

Humpherys, S. L., Bakir, N., & Babb, J. (2021). Experiential learning to foster tacit knowledge through a role play, business simulation. *Journal of Education for Business*, 1–7. doi:10.1080/08832323.2021 .1896461

Jentsch, F., & Curtis, M. (2017). *Simulation in aviation training*. Routledge. doi:10.4324/9781315243092

Johnson, C. E., Kimble, L. P., Gunby, S. S., & Davis, A. H. (2020). Using deliberate practice and simulation for psychomotor skill competency acquisition and retention: A mixed-methods study. *Nurse Educator*, *45*(3), 150–154. doi:10.1097/NNE.0000000000000713 PMID:31246693

Jongerius, C., Hessels, R. S., Romijn, J. A., Smets, E. M., & Hillen, M. A. (2020). The measurement of eye contact in human interactions: A scoping review. *Journal of Nonverbal Behavior*, *44*(3), 1–27. doi:10.100710919-020-00333-3

Juraschek, M., Büth, L., Posselt, G., & Herrmann, C. (2018). Mixed reality in learning factories. *Procedia Manufacturing*, *23*, 153–158. doi:10.1016/j.promfg.2018.04.009

Kang, J., Diederich, M., Lindgren, R., & Junokas, M. (2021). Gesture patterns and learning in an embodied XR science simulation. *Journal of Educational Technology & Society*, *24*(2), 77–92.

Karunathilake, I. M., & Samarasekera, D. D. (2021). Learning In The 21st Century— 'What's All the Fuss about Change?'. In Educate, Train and Transform: Toolkit on Medical and Health Professions Education (pp. 1-14).Routledge.

Kierkegaard, S. (2013). Kierkegaard's Writings, II, Volume 2: The Concept of Irony, with Continual Reference to Socrates/Notes of Schelling's Berlin Lectures. Princeton University Press.

King, O., Borthwick, A., Nancarrow, S., & Grace, S. (2018). Sociology of the professions: What it means for podiatry. *Journal of Foot and Ankle Research*, *11*(1), 1–8. doi:10.118613047-018-0275-0 PMID:29942353

Koufidis, C., Manninen, K., Nieminen, J., Wohlin, M., & Silén, C. (2021). Unravelling the polyphony in clinical reasoning research in medical education. *Journal of Evaluation in Clinical Practice*, *27*(2), 438–450. doi:10.1111/jep.13432 PMID:32573080

Levitt, H. M. (2021). Qualitative generalization, not to the population but to the phenomenon: Reconceptualizing variation in qualitative research. *Qualitative Psychology*, *8*(1), 95–110. doi:10.1037/qup0000184

Loeng, S. (2018). Various ways of understanding the concept of andragogy. *Cogent Education*, *5*(1), 1496643. doi:10.1080/2331186X.2018.1496643

Logeswaran, A., Munsch, C., Chong, Y. J., Ralph, N., & McCrossnan, J. (2021). The role of extended reality technology in healthcare education: Towards a learner-centred approach. *Future Healthcare Journal*, *8*(1), e79–e84. doi:10.7861/fhj.2020-0112 PMID:33791482

Luctkar-Flude, M., & Tyerman, J. (2021). The Rise of Virtual Simulation: Pandemic Response or Enduring Pedagogy? *Clinical Simulation in Nursing*, *57*, 1–2. doi:10.1016/j.ecns.2021.06.008

Luo, C., Lan, Y., Luo, X. R., & Li, H. (2021). The effect of commitment on knowledge sharing: An empirical study of virtual communities. *Technological Forecasting and Social Change*, *163*, 120438. doi:10.1016/j.techfore.2020.120438

Mathew, P. S., & Pillai, A. S. (2020). Role of Immersive (XR) Technologies in Improving Healthcare Competencies: A Review. *Virtual and Augmented Reality in Education, Art, and Museums*, 23-46.

McGrath, J. L., Taekman, J. M., Dev, P., Danforth, D. R., Mohan, D., Kman, N., ... Won, K. (2018). Using virtual reality simulation environments to assess competence for emergency medicine learners. *Academic Emergency Medicine*, *25*(2), 186–195. doi:10.1111/acem.13308 PMID:28888070

Melnyk, B. M., Tan, A., Hsieh, A. P., Gawlik, K., Arslanian-Engoren, C., Braun, L. T., Dunbar, S., Dunbar-Jacob, J., Lewis, L. M., Millan, A., Orsolini, L., Robbins, L. B., Russell, C. L., Tucker, S., & Wilbur, J. (2021). Critical care nurses' physical and mental health, worksite wellness support, and medical errors. *American Journal of Critical Care*, *30*(3), 176–184. doi:10.4037/ajcc2021301 PMID:34161980

Mitchell, R., & Boyle, B. (2021). Understanding the role of profession in multidisciplinary team innovation: Professional identity, minority dissent and team innovation. *British Journal of Management*, *32*(2), 512–528. doi:10.1111/1467-8551.12419

Moreira, D. (2020). Virtual networks and asynchronous communities: methodological reflections on the digital. In *Ethnography in Higher Education* (pp. 177–196). Springer VS. doi:10.1007/978-3-658-30381-5_11

Mortimore, G., Reynolds, J., Forman, D., Brannigan, C., & Mitchell, K. (2021). From expert to advanced clinical practitioner and beyond. *British Journal of Nursing (Mark Allen Publishing)*, *30*(11), 656–659. doi:10.12968/bjon.2021.30.11.656 PMID:34109817

Negev, M., Dahdal, Y., Khreis, H., Hochman, A., Shaheen, M., Jaghbir, M. T., Alpert, P., Levine, H., & Davidovitch, N. (2021). Regional lessons from the COVID-19 outbreak in the Middle East: From infectious diseases to climate change adaptation. *The Science of the Total Environment*, *768*, 144434. doi:10.1016/j.scitotenv.2020.144434 PMID:33444865

Obrad, C. (2020). Constraints and consequences of online teaching. *Sustainability*, *12*(17), 6982. doi:10.3390u12176982

Ocloo, J., Garfield, S., Franklin, B. D., & Dawson, S. (2021). Exploring the theory, barriers and enablers for patient and public involvement across health, social care and patient safety: A systematic review of reviews. *Health Research Policy and Systems*, *19*(1), 1–21. doi:10.118612961-020-00644-3 PMID:33472647

Okoye, K., Rodriguez-Tort, J. A., Escamilla, J., & Hosseini, S. (2021). Technology-mediated teaching and learning process: A conceptual study of educators' response amidst the Covid-19 pandemic. *Education and Information Technologies*, 1–33. PMID:34025205

Orr, N., Matthews, B., See, Z. S., Burrell, A., Day, J., & Seengal, D. (2021). Transdisciplinarity in extended reality (XR) research design: Technological transformation and social good (co-creation session at XR+ Creativity Symposium, University of Newcastle, 2020). *Virtual Creativity, 11*(1), 163-179.

Owens, K. P. (2021, July). Competency-Based Experiential-Expertise and Future Adaptive Learning Systems. In *International Conference on Human-Computer Interaction* (pp. 93-109). Springer.

Park, C., & Kim, D. G. (2020). Exploring the roles of social presence and gender difference in online learning. *Decision Sciences Journal of Innovative Education*, *18*(2), 291–312. doi:10.1111/dsji.12207

Robert, I. V. (2021). Formation and development of digital transformation of domestic education on the basis of systemic convergence of pedagogical science and technology. In *SHS Web of Conferences* (Vol. 101, p. 03017). EDP Sciences.

Roussin, C. J., & Weinstock, P. (2017). SimZones: An organizational innovation for simulation programs and centers. *Academic Medicine*, *92*(8), 1114–1120. doi:10.1097/ACM.0000000000001746 PMID:28562455

Silén, C., Wirell, S., Kvist, J., Nylander, E., & Smedby, Ö. (2008). Advanced 3D visualization in student-centred medical education. *Medical Teacher*, *30*(5), e115–e124. doi:10.1080/01421590801932228 PMID:18576181

Suryanti, S., Sutaji, D., Arifani, Y., Muyasaroh, M., & Zamzamy, M. (2020). Improved learning accessibility and professionalism of teachers in remote areas through mentoring development of teaching materials based on Augmented Reality. *Kontribusia*, *3*(1), 224–232. doi:10.30587/kontribusia.v3i1.1032

Tabatabai, S. (2020). COVID-19 impact and virtual medical education. *Journal of Advances in Medical Education & Professionalism*, *8*(3), 140–143. PMID:32802908

Tang, K. S., Cheng, D. L., Mi, E., & Greenberg, P. B. (2020). Augmented reality in medical education: A systematic review. *Canadian Medical Education Journal*, *11*(1), e81. PMID:32215146

Ten Cate, O., & Billett, S. (2014). Competency-based medical education: Origins, perspectives and potentialities. *Medical Education*, *48*(3), 325–332. doi:10.1111/medu.12355 PMID:24528467

van der Niet, A. G., & Bleakley, A. (2021). Where medical education meets artificial intelligence: 'Does technology care?'. *Medical Education*, *55*(1), 30–36. doi:10.1111/medu.14131 PMID:32078175

Viglialoro, R. M., Condino, S., Turini, G., Carbone, M., Ferrari, V., & Gesi, M. (2021). Augmented Reality, Mixed Reality, and Hybrid Approach in Healthcare Simulation: A Systematic Review. *Applied Sciences (Basel, Switzerland)*, *11*(5), 2338. doi:10.3390/app11052338

Voštinár, P., Horváthová, D., Mitter, M., & Bako, M. (2021). The look at the various uses of VR. *Open Computer Science*, *11*(1), 241–250. doi:10.1515/comp-2020-0123

Vygotsky, L. S. (1978). Zone of proximal development: A new approach. *Mind in society: The development of higher psychological processes*, 84-91.

Welie, J. V. (2004). Is dentistry a profession? Part 3. Future challenges. *Journal - Canadian Dental Association*, *70*(10), 675–678. PMID:15530264

Wilson, I., & Shankar, P. R. (2021). The COVID-19 pandemic and undergraduate medical student teaching/learning and assessment. *MedEdPublish*, 10.

World Health Organisation. (2021). *International Data Online Updates*. https://www.who.int/data

Yigitcanlar, T., Butler, L., Windle, E., Desouza, K. C., Mehmood, R., & Corchado, J. M. (2020). Can building "artificially intelligent cities" safeguard humanity from natural disasters, pandemics, and other catastrophes? An urban scholar's perspective. *Sensors (Basel)*, *20*(10), 2988. doi:10.339020102988 PMID:32466175

Zulkifli, A. F. (2019). Student-centered approach and alternative assessments to improve students' learning domains during health education sessions. *Biomedical Human Kinetics*, *11*(1), 80–86. doi:10.2478/bhk-2019-0010

ADDITIONAL READING

Cranmer, K., Brehmer, J., & Louppe, G. (2020). The frontier of simulation-based inference. *Proceedings of the National Academy of Sciences of the United States of America*, *117*(48), 30055–30062. doi:10.1073/pnas.1912789117 PMID:32471948

Hong, T., Langevin, J., & Sun, K. (2018, October). Building simulation: Ten challenges. *Building Simulation*, *11*(5), 871–898. doi:10.100712273-018-0444-x

Jeffries, P. (2020). *Simulation in nursing education: From conceptualization to evaluation*. Lippincott Williams & Wilkins.

Kadian, A., Truong, J., Gokaslan, A., Clegg, A., Wijmans, E., Lee, S., Savva, M., Chernova, S., & Batra, D. (2020). Sim2Real predictivity: Does evaluation in simulation predict real-world performance? *IEEE Robotics and Automation Letters*, *5*(4), 6670–6677. doi:10.1109/LRA.2020.3013848

Satin, A. J. (2018). Simulation in obstetrics. *Obstetrics and Gynecology*, *132*(1), 199–209. doi:10.1097/AOG.0000000000002682 PMID:29889745

KEY TERMS AND DEFINITIONS

Augmented Reality (AR): Is a technology capable of superimposing or overlaying a computer-generated image across a visual projection of the real world, providing a composite view of the two.

Extended Reality (XR): Is the term given to all real-and-virtual combined environments and human-machine interactions, which are functionally digitally generated by technology and wearable accessories.

Health Professions: Is the term used for workers who have been formally trained in the application of medical and healthcare principles underpinned by the core principles of care, compassion and evidence-based approaches to the care of people whose health necessitates assessment, diagnosis or management.

Hybrid Curriculum: Is the term used to describe how online learning is integrated with traditional face to face learning and teaching.

Hyflex Curriculum: Is an adaptation of hybrid learning where each class session and learning activity is offered in-person, synchronously online, and asynchronously online. With this approach learners make the decision of how they will participate with the learning opportunities afforded to them.

Immersion Technology: Is the digital equipment which provides the perception of being present in a created and non-physical world.

Mixed Reality (MR): Is the merging of virtual and actual reality to provide new mechanisms of visualizing given scenarios. The physical objects and digital objects can interact with each other in real time.

Paradigm: A set of concepts or thought patterns, incorporating specific theories, designated research methods, hypotheses, and typical standards of what is a legitimate claim to contribution to a specific field of theory or practice.

Pedagogy: Is the methodological process and study of applied teaching and learning within specific subjects and academic disciplines.

Sensory: Relates to the experience of sensation via the physical senses in terms of either perception or transmission.

Simulation: Is the integrated use of a computer model, which imitates reality in the context of study, where risk can be eliminated as part of initial scaffolded learning.

Virtual Reality (VR): Is the digitally generated simulation of a 3-D image or situated context or learning environment, within which a learner can be placed and with which they can interact by wearing electronic accessories such as eye goggles or gloves with sensors.

Chapter 5
Virtual Simulation:
A Flipped Classroom Teaching Tool for Healthcare Education

Emily Tarver

University of Mississippi Medical Center, USA

ABSTRACT

Virtual simulation is a learning tool that employs specific hardware and software technology for simulation-based provider training within a digital domain. Extended reality or XR software includes virtual reality (VR), augmented reality (AR), and mixed reality (MR) programs that represent a rapidly growing area within the field of virtual simulation. This training may provide either provider- or patient-centered learning modules, with dedicated hardware and software centered on skill-based, 3D modeling or case-based learning. Demand for these learning programs in healthcare education was fueled by the remote learning needs of the COVID-19 pandemic. In addition to this growing demand, there is a significant role for many virtual simulation software programs within the traditional classroom and lecture hall. This is a previously untapped resource for simulation education. The flipped classroom model provides an opportune framework for the incorporation of immersive, virtual simulation learning programs within spaces previously limited to the more passive, podium-based lecture.

INTRODUCTION

This chapter is organized into four sections. Section 1 provides an overview of the historical evolution of simulation technology that set the stage for the multitude of current XR programs. Section 2 offers a general review of virtual simulation as a flipped classroom alternative to the traditional lecture for healthcare trainees. Section 3 provides an overview of the flipped classroom pedagogy and details empiric evidence from multiple research studies that provide validation for this teaching methodology within healthcare education. Section 4 provides an outline of the organizational framework for virtual simulation. This framework includes both patient-focused and provider-focused applications within the healthcare setting, with additional insight on their utility within the flipped classroom model. Overall,

DOI: 10.4018/978-1-7998-8371-5.ch005

this chapter seeks to offer readers a detailed account of the variety of virtual simulation programs within healthcare education as well as their critical role within the traditional classroom and lecture hall within the flipped classroom model.

1. BACKGROUND

Virtual simulation for healthcare education is defined as a learning tool that employs specific hardware and software technology for simulation-based provider training within a digital domain. With either a provider- or patient-centered focus, the earliest virtual simulation programs have evolved over several decades and pioneered a pathway for the vast array of both hardware and software technology that is available today (Chang, 2020; Muguerza & Canelas, 2021). Despite significant technological advancements, much of these tools still reside within a dedicated simulation center or other formal training space. More recently, many simulation programs have adopted training software for remote, asynchronous learning.

The COVID-19 pandemic magnified our need in medical training for remote learning alternatives. Some have described this pandemic as an "unintended digital accelerator" of virtual learning technology due to the rapid need for remote learning resources in all sectors of education, including healthcare (Hennick, 2021 & Towers-Clark, 2021). While historically cost-prohibitive for many resource-limited programs, virtual simulation software will likely become more accessible and affordable in future years (Breining, 2018). Regardless of cost, quality virtual simulation should employ all best-practice principles of traditional, manikin-based simulation. In addition, many digital programs offer the unique advantages of remote learning flexibility, a broad diversity of learning content and fewer staffing needs. The vast array high- and mid-fidelity manikins, low-fidelity task trainers and digital, on-site teaching tools in traditional simulation remain a critical component of current healthcare training. Accelerated by the remote-learning needs of the COVID-19 pandemic, virtual simulation, a previously lesser component of traditional simulation, will likely evolve to become a more mainstream complement to this widely utilized practice.

The field of aviation, from the military to NASA to commercial airlines, has embraced flight simulators in aeronautics education for nearly a century (McKnight et al., 2020 & Oman et al., 2020). The earliest simulators in healthcare education emerged in the early 1900s with Mrs. Chase, in the field of nursing simulation. Mrs. Chase was one of the first manikins for classroom-based, clinical skills training at the Hartford Hospital Training School (Cockrell, 2021; Hyland, 2008). In the1950s, mostly developed by pioneers in the field of anesthesiology, physician educators began to utilize full-body manikins for healthcare education. Since these early training programs in both nursing and physician education, the widespread adoption of simulation in healthcare education has soared in the last few decades. Fully remote, virtual simulation has historically involved a smaller proportion of overall users but will likely grow in popularity in the coming decades. This trend will likely mirror the success of simulation in dedicated, physical training spaces (Pottle, 2020 & Kyaw et al., 2019). The International Data Corporation (IDC) has projected a six-fold increase in spending on XR technology between 2020 and 2024 (Hennick, 2020). An estimated twelve billion dollars were spent on this technology in 2020 and there is projection that spending will increase to over 70 billion dollars by 2024 (Hennick, 2020). This trend indicates that virtual simulation software may grow tremendously in the upcoming years within the world of healthcare simulation.

2. OVERVIEW OF VIRTUAL SIMULATION AS A FLIPPED CLASSROOM TEACHING TOOL

Unlike a simulation center or in-situ learning space, the traditional classroom and lecture hall remain untapped resources for more immersive learning experiences in healthcare education. Though in-person learning restrictions continue to wane, due to recovery from the COVID-19 pandemic, virtual simulation software will likely remain a useful tool for remote-learning. The digital footprint of fully remote, virtual simulation eliminates many logistic barriers to the integration of traditional simulation within our classrooms and lecture halls. Instruction with remote simulation as an immersive alternative to the traditional lecture represents an innovative use of this newer technology. Within the classroom or lecture hall, remote simulation software offers healthcare instructors a teaching tool that is more immersive and interactive than the traditional lecture. Flipped classroom incorporation of virtual learning software in healthcare education is a lesser known but valuable adjunct to a growing trend of educational methodologies that enhance the traditional lecture with more active learning experiences (Hew, K & Low, C, 2018; Riddell et al., 2017; Kraut et al., 2019; King et al., 2019). Additional examples of this more interactive learning approach include problem-based or case-based learning, gamification, and audience response systems.

In clinical training, fully remote, virtual simulation software provides a valuable range of immersive, 3D modeling and virtual patient learning modules. Quality haptics or tactile-feedback hardware for skills-based training is in an earlier stage of technical development than 3D modeling and virtual patient, case-based learning (Chang, 2020). Nonetheless, this remote, skills-based software for healthcare training has similar potential for widespread utility in the traditional classroom environment. As the haptics technology becomes more refined and affordable, it may greatly complement case-based learning and 3D modeling and offer valuable skills-based training within the traditional classroom setting (Chang, 2020).

Virtual learning software with 3D modeling has been useful in disciplines such as gross anatomy, where 3D imagery may enhance the learner's grasp of visually complex subject matter (Zhao et al., 2020; Triepels et al., 2020). In case-based learning, virtual learning software utilizes the virtual patient for training in a variety of areas. Training in high-acuity, low-occurrence (HALO) cases in clinical education is a useful area for case-based learning, both remote and classroom-based (Bremner, 2019). These types of clinical encounters are rare but critical cases for expert management in fields such as emergency medicine and critical care, where simulation may fill a significant learning gap. For case-based learning, participants within a traditional classroom environment may complete a scenario involving a virtual patient. Depending on the software, they may work solo or within a group. The learning software may involve artificial intelligence (AI) as a primary interface between the learner and program. This AI-driven software provides for many virtual patient and scenario modifications throughout the case and offers data-driven feedback at the conclusion of a case. The paradigm of AI-driven, virtual learning software is frequently a "plug and play" experience, where a live instructor may or may not participate. When an instructor is present, they may observe the case and provide a live debriefing at the conclusion of the case. In less AI-driven software, as an alternative model, the instructor may serve as a simulation operator during the case and dynamically modify patient vitals and other exam or environmental details throughout a specific case. Working alone or with co-faculty, the instructor can facilitate a post-case debrief within this latter framework as well.

Whether AI- or instructor-driven, each type of case-based learning software has utility within the flipped classroom model. Depending on instructor preference and the overall learning objectives, both AI and non-AI software programs remain viable options for flipped classroom learning and are currently available from multiple commercial vendors. A few of these include SimX©, Acadicus©, Oxford Medical Simulation©, Health Scholars©, GigXR© and UbiSim©. This is a rapidly expanding field and there are likely additional software offerings since the publication of this chapter. Regardless of software choice, if utilized within a flipped-classroom framework, there would ideally be protected time at the end of each case for a live, in-person, debriefing for all participants. A few notable developers of skills-based virtual learning software are OSSO VR© and Precision OS©. Both companies are innovators of VR training software for a variety of surgical and other procedural skills.

Within the domain of nursing simulation, the COVID-19 pandemic prompted a collaboration between nursing faculty and simulation experts within the Organization for Associate Degree Nursing (OADN) and Unbound Medicine, a digital publisher of healthcare training programs. Through this collaboration, they created an online database of virtual simulation software programs for nursing education. This database has become a trusted resource as a detailed organization and review of the most current virtual simulation programs for nursing simulation (Hyland & Hawkins, 2009; Cockrell, 2020).

3. THE FLIPPED CLASSROOM MODEL

The flipped classroom model has been utilized in both undergraduate medical education (UME) and graduate medical education (GME) as a useful teaching alternative to the traditional classroom lecture (Hew, K & Low, C, 2018; Riddell et al., 2017; Kraut et al., 2019; King et al., 2019). Key differences with GME learners include a stronger tendency for this group to seek learning as a means of improved patient care over simple knowledge attainment and/or better test scores (King et al., 2019).

Along the flipped classroom model, remote-learning, virtual simulation software may find meaningful use within the traditional classroom. Within a flipped classroom, healthcare educators can pre-assign learning materials and utilize critical lecture time to engage learners in a virtual learning software program to reinforce key learning objectives. In this way, the instructor can transition from "sage on the stage" to "guide on the side" via immersive learning exercises (Durgahee, 1998 & Coyne et al., 2019). A few examples of pre-classroom assignments are short videos, pre-recorded slide presentations and traditional reading assignments. For optimal flexibility, this teaching modality would allow one or more learners to participate within a specific virtual environment. With respect to virtual patient, case-based programs, the software would ideally have the dual flexibility of utilizing a screen-based or fully virtual mode to accommodate both user preferences and general learning objectives.

Most traditional software for case-based learning in healthcare education lives in the single- or multi-user "plug-and-play" modality. Remote participation is often asynchronous, where users log-on and complete a medical case in a virtual environment. Within these programs, there is usually AI-driven feedback after each case. These programs are a valuable training tool for case-based learning in healthcare education. While often costly, they are largely scalable and require minimal instructor involvement. They can be completed remotely and asynchronously which has great appeal for many current providers in healthcare education. There is a similar grouping of 3D modeling software programs that offer supplemental training in anatomy, physiology, pharmacology, and a variety of both pre-clinical and clinical subjects. These programs have similar utility within a flipped classroom model.

There are multiple, recent meta-analyses that have reported effective learning within the flipped classroom model (Hew, K & Low, C, 2018; Kraut et al., 2019; King et al., 2019, Foronda et al., 2020). One meta-analysis of 28 studies reports that the flipped classroom model is particularly effective for procedural learning and facilitates overall greater knowledge and skills acquisition. This report found that, at a minimum, the flipped-classroom methodology is non-inferior to the traditional classroom approach (Hew, K & Low, C, 2018).

Another flipped classroom meta-analysis within GME cites that the flipped classroom model employs higher cognitive domains such as analysis and evaluation within Bloom's Revised Taxonomy (Kraut et al., 2019). This meta-analysis of flipped classroom research cites that learner engagement and satisfaction requires thorough and comprehensive preparation by the healthcare instructor and reports that 30-minute video lectures are the optimal materials for pre-classroom assignments within the articles reviewed for this study (Kraut et al., 2019).

Another recent meta-analysis within the Journal of Graduate Medical Education (GME) reviewed 22 flipped classroom research studies and reported that the flipped classroom model is broadly applicable across a variety of GME settings. This meta-analysis reviewed studies that employed multiple types of pre-lecture materials, including pre-reading from articles or book chapters and pre-recorded multimedia presentations or video lectures. The pre- and post-test results within most of these studies report significant improvements in knowledge and/or skills attainment over the traditional classroom model (King et al., 2019). This article organizes the findings of these studies according to Kirkpatrick's Framework to assess the overall outcome of the flipped classroom pedagogy. Seven of these studies report a Level I improvement in overall learner perception, where flipped classroom learning achieved higher learner ratings. One-third of these articles report educational outcomes at the 2a level of Kirkpatrick's Framework, defined as changes in learner opinion. One-third of these articles report outcomes at the 2b Level, with an improvement in knowledge or skills. Two studies report level 3 outcomes, classified as changes in learner behavior. These behavioral outcomes include an increase in self-directed learning outside of class as well as self-reported pre-class preparation activities (King et al., 2019). Authors of this meta-analysis of the flipped classroom model in healthcare education report an overall high level of learner enthusiasm for this teaching method and document improvements in both knowledge and skills, making the flipped classroom an attractive alternative to the traditional classroom model (King et al., 2019).

A study by Foronda et al. reviewed 80 research studies on virtual simulation specifically for nursing education. It found that 69 studies (86%) report an overall improvement in learning outcomes with virtual simulation in nursing education. Specific learning outcomes within this study included the areas of knowledge/learning, skills training, learner satisfaction, critical thinking, and self-confidence (Foronda et al., 2020). Overall, this study presents a sizeable body of research that supports the utilization of virtual simulation for nursing education.

For healthcare educators who are interested in incorporating virtual simulation within a flipped classroom teaching model, many software developers offer free trials for limited use. The high development costs for XR technology make this teaching tool cost prohibitive for many healthcare educators. In tandem with the significant decline in the cost of XR hardware in recent years, XR software will likely follow a similar trajectory over time and become more affordable and widely available in the future. There are some free and low-cost virtual simulation programs for remote and classroom-based learning. One example of this is Virtual Resus Room© (VRR), developed by Sara Foohey, CCFP-EM, a simulation educator at the University of Toronto (Foohey, 2020). VRR© is not a traditional XR technology, but it offers screen-based virtual simulation utilizing Google Slides© for case-based learning. It was originally pioneered during the COVID-19 pandemic as a remote-simulation teaching tool. This program is free for all users and allows instructors to incorporate case-based simulation within a traditional lecture setting. While designed for remote use, it may also find utility for in-person, case-based learning along a flipped classroom framework. Pending additional resources for more costly virtual patient software, free tools such as Virtual Resus Room© might provide a valuable resource for flipped classroom integration of case-based learning within the traditional lecture space.

4. OVERVIEW OF XR (VR, AR, MR) SOFTWARE APPLICATIONS

The invention of the x-ray by W.C. Rontgen in 1895 heralded the dawn of technology-driven medical imaging as means of improving both healthcare education as well as patient care (Vavra et al., 2017). Virtual learning technology represents a recent continuum of this trend.

Virtual simulation is a broad subset of digital education, or e-learning, that utilizes any learning software or other digital technologies (Kyaw et al., 2019). Digital learning includes online or offline, computer-based training, XR technology, massive, open, online courses, mobile learning applications, gamification software and psychomotor skills trainers (Car et al., 2019). In Figure 1 we can observe the multiple subtypes of digital or E-learning software available for healthcare educators.

Figure 1. Subcategories of Digital or E-Learning

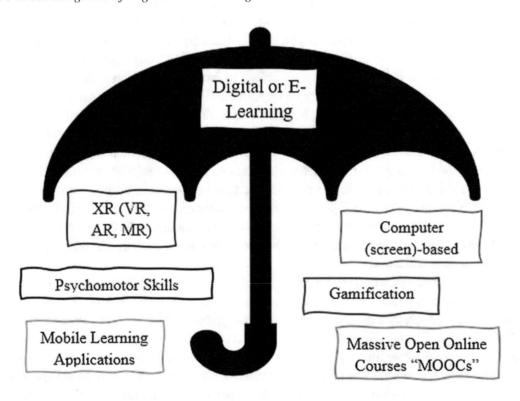

Specifically, virtual simulation encompasses any form of digital simulation software that may be accessed via a laptop or desktop computer, with or without adjuncts such as a head-mounted display (HMD), tablet, smartphone, or other hardware device. It may be single- or multi-user "plug and play", where the learner logs-on and participates in a case-based, skills-based or 3D imaging program, independent of a live instructor. Single- or multi-user software may also employ live, instructor involvement, with less automated feedback. Each of these applications have utility as flipped classroom teaching tools and their diversity of offerings will continue to grow in the coming years. Growth in this industry will likely drive down cost and make this technology accessible to more healthcare educators.

Virtual reality (VR) is one subcategory of digital learning. It includes any software that utilizes a head mounted display (HMD) to immerse the user in a fully alternative, digital environment. It may incorporate multiple sensory modalities such as visual, auditory and touch/vibration to achieve a maximal level of complete, digital immersion. VR software usually incorporates a virtual patient and one or more avatars or digital representations of a single or multiple users within the virtual environment. VR currently exists under three primary domains within healthcare training: 3D modeling, virtual patient/case-based training, and haptics/surgical simulation. Augmented reality (AR) is any software program that utilizes hardware such as an HMD, smartphone, tablet, or other programmed device to superimpose digital imagery upon the actual environment. With AR, both the live environment and superimposed digital imagery remain autonomous from each other within the same field of view. Mixed reality (MR) is any technology that blends both VR and AR to provide full immersion in a digital environment but preserves select elements from the non-digital space. In general, MR software facilitates more direct interaction between the digital and actual spaces than its AR counterpart. Extended reality (XR) is the overall term for any technology that employs either VR, AR or MR modalities. The organizational framework of the different types of XR software are detailed in Figure 2.

Figure 2. Virtual Reality (VR), Augmented Reality (AR) and Mixed Reality (MR) are examples of a broader category of extended reality (XR) technology within virtual simulation education.

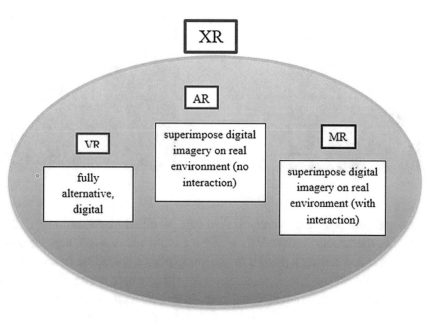

With increased affordability of XR hardware such as VR headsets, healthcare educators and clinicians have seen widespread growth in the utilization of these technologies for both patient-centered and provider-centered education and care. A systematic review and meta-analysis of VR for health professions education reviewed 31 research studies in this area between 1990 and 2017 (Kyaw et al., 2019). Researchers found that no studies in this area had been published before 2005, likely due to both software and hardware limitations at that time. They examined the impact of VR software training programs in areas such as knowledge, skills, and attitude. This report found an overall improvement in all three of these outcomes in learners who utilized VR software training programs in comparison to more traditional training approaches (Kyaw et al., 2019).

4.1 Patient-Focused Virtual Software

Currently, XR software is broadly categorized as either "provider-focused" or "patient-focused" (Chang, 2020). In Figure 3 we can observe examples of both provider- and patient-focused XR software.

Figure 3. Main uses of XR Technology

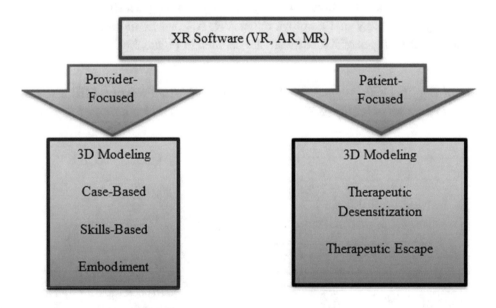

Patient-focused software is used in direct, clinical care, as either an educational or therapeutic tool. One example includes therapeutic escape VR, where a patient wears a VR headset and becomes immersed in an alternate reality during a painful or other unpleasant procedure or test. One of the earliest applications of therapeutic escape VR is called Snow World©, where burn patients are immersed in a virtual, fantasy world that is both whimsical and cold, to diminish the severe pain of therapeutic treatments such as frequent dressing changes (Hoffman, 2011). This was developed at the University of Washington Healthcare, Innovation and Technology Lab (HITLab) in collaboration with the Harborview Burn Center. In this software, when a burn patient wears a VR headset and enters Snow World©, they escape to a magical world of snow, flying through a music-filled, virtual canyon and throwing snowballs at penguins and snowmen (Hoffman, 2011).

The utilization of VR for therapeutic escape has also proven useful in the treatment of chronic pain. Practitioners in a Tennessee-based pain management clinic, in collaboration with VR developer Firsthand Technology, have designed a VR program for chronic pain treatment, like Snow World©. In one trial, forty patients in this clinic were treated with 60 VR sessions involving their therapeutic escape program and reported, on average, 60-75% less pain than before each treatment session (Clark 2017). For comparison, 1 dose of morphine offers, a 30% average pain reduction (Clark 2017). Multiple practitioners who utilize VR therapeutic escape report that this software has similar attention/distraction techniques as listening to music or watching a movie (Trost et al., 2021). For this reason, it has also been useful during procedures involving pediatric dentistry, pediatric venipuncture, and spinal cord injury (Trost et al., 2021).

In the area of pain-control, clinicians at St. George's Hospital in London piloted a study where VR software was utilized to alleviate pain and anxiety during wide-awake surgery ("VR Headsets," 2019). Patients in this study were undergoing upper extremity surgery with a regional nerve block and VR headsets were utilized to offer distracting sounds and imagery (beaches, forests, hilltops, and waterfalls) throughout the procedure. This pilot study examined the impact of VR therapeutic escape for pain and anxiety control in both a VR and control group. They tracked vital signs such as blood pressure and heart rate in all participants and examined subjective feedback via post-procedure surveys to assess the impact of VR therapeutic escape during an awake surgical procedure. This study showed that 100% of patients in the VR therapeutic escape arm reported an overall improvement in their hospital experience. Ninety-four percent reported that they felt more relaxed. Based on vital sign monitoring and patient feedback, there was an 80% reduction in pain and a 73% reduction in anxiety with the intraoperative use of VR therapeutic escape ("VR Headsets," 2019).

VR technology has also gained significant traction in the world of therapeutic desensitization. VR has been used for decades in the treatment of psychological ailments such as chronic anxiety, phobias, and post-traumatic stress disorder. As a further extension of this form of therapy, pioneers such as Hunter Hoffman, PhD, at the University of Washington HIT Lab, are linking therapeutic desensitization with VR headsets and fMRI to receive real-time neurofeedback and biofeedback. Hoffman and colleagues utilize fMRI data to monitor and adjust the effects of various immersive stimuli within the virtual environment (Hoffman et al., 2011; Maples-Keller et al., 2017; Hoffman et al., 20004; Gold et al., 2007).

There are also VR therapeutic desensitization programs for the treatment of autism spectrum disorder (ASD). Many of these programs provide therapy to autistic patients in areas such as social interaction, emotional recognition, empathy and problem-solving (Maples-Keller et al., 2017; Yang et al., 2018).

One of the earliest research studies on patient-focused VR, involving therapeutic desensitization, reviewed the use of this treatment for phobia therapy (Palmer, 2019). Since that study in the American Journal of Psychology, VR programs have been developed for the treatment of over two dozen different types of phobias. Skip Rizzo, PhD, director of the Medical Virtual Reality (MedVR) Lab at the University of Southern California and pioneer in the use of therapeutic-based applications of VR, has described VR software as "a controlled stimulus environment where you make things happen, monitor patient responses and activate emotions in ways far beyond what we could ever do in a clinical office" (Palmer, 2019). Dr. Rizzo lead the development of the VR therapeutic desensitization software, Bravemind©, utilizing VR Exposure (VRE) Treatment. This program is currently used at over 100 sites in the United States and produces the gradual repetition of a traumatic event for PTSD treatment. It has been used in military training, with Afghan and Iraqi city and desert environments, as well as scenarios relevant to combat medics. It has also created scenarios addressing PTSD from military sexual trauma (Palmer, 2019).

Since the development of Bravemind©, Dr. Rizzo has also collaborated with Barbara Rothbaum, PhD, a psychologist at Emory University, to create the VR Exposure treatment software known as STRIVE© or Stress Resilience in Virtual Environments. This program employs VR exposure therapy in military combat training by taking trainees through short virtual missions with stressful encounters that incorporates resilience debriefing with a virtual human mentor after the encounter. In this way, VR Exposure Treatment is utilized as a preventative measure for PTSD in combat training (Palmer, 2019).

Addiction therapy is an additional area of popularity for VR Exposure Treatment (Vavra et al., 2017; Yang et al., 2018; Palmer, 2019). VR treatment software has been useful for therapy in smoking cessation and a variety of other drug addictions. One study in the field of VR for addiction therapy found that VR smoking cues elicited cravings that were like those elicited by real-world cues (Bordnick et al., 2004; Maples-Keller et al., 2017).

In addition to a growing number of therapeutic applications, XR software has been utilized for patient education as well. During the COVID-19 pandemic, healthcare educators at George Washington University used VR software to show patients the more detailed pulmonary effects of COVID-19 (Hennick, 2020 & Iwanaga et al., 2021). Researchers and educators at this institution integrated the results of CT scans of 27 COVID-19 patients and found a strong correlation between certain lab results and the specific degree of damage inflicted by the viral infection. In this way, VR technology was utilized for research as well as patient and provider education within the same software domain.

The Stanford Virtual Heart© software, now piloted at multiple academic centers in the U.S., has also provided VR technology as a teaching tool for patients and trainees (Axelrod, 2017). This software utilizes 3D modeling to educate patients, family members and medical trainees on the complex structure of various congenital heart defects. With this software, patients and/or family members may don a VR headset and walk both around and through a virtual heart with various congenital defects as a better means of understanding these complex, 3D structures.

Patient-oriented XR programs for both therapeutic and educational aims have grown in popularity over the last three decades. They have made a significant impact in many areas of patient care. This growth was somewhat slow in the earlier years of XR development, mainly secondary to the high cost of XR software and hardware. In 2016, with the release of the Oculus Rift and Samsung Gear headsets, both less than four hundred U.S. dollars, a cost barrier for XR technology was removed (Chebanova, n.d.). When this occurred, therapeutic XR software also decreased in cost. In tandem with increased affordability of both hardware and software, XR-driven research has significantly increased and demonstrated greater empiric evidence for its utility (Chebanova, n.d.). As both hardware and software costs decline, the utilization of XR for patient-focused care will likely increase in the coming years. Healthcare trainees will likely gain most of their training on this software within the clinical environment. However, patient-oriented, therapeutic, and educational XR might also find utility in a flipped classroom model for healthcare education. Healthcare educators may utilize this software within the classroom setting to better educate learners on specific features and offer additional training before direct application in the clinical setting.

4.2 Provider-Focused Virtual Software

Across all disciplines of healthcare education, provider-focused virtual software is geared towards the learning needs of the healthcare provider and/or trainee. It has two broad domains, 3D visualization and virtual patient, procedural or case-based learning.

Some of our earliest virtual training programs were developed in the 1990s with the use of on-site surgical simulators such as the first VR arthroscopy simulator (McKnight, 2020). Hardware and software for these early virtual training programs was traditionally housed in a simulation center or other dedicated training space. Most of these programs were designed to provide auto-feedback to learners based on specific surgical skills and have not been utilized within the traditional classroom or lecture hall. Technology in this area has greatly advanced and provides training software that is accessible both remotely and within dedicated simulation space.

Current research in this field has established that VR improves surgical mastery outside of the OR (McKnight, 2020). The Stanford Surgical Simulator© in 2002 hallmarks the acceleration of haptics development in skills-based virtual training (Blumstein, 2019). This has evolved to an endoscopic sinus surgery simulation that uses CT scans from real patients to create 3D models for skills-based training (Blumstein, 2019). Similar technology has entered the clinical domain with the use of AR technology and HMDs that employ advanced imaging for intraoperative navigation (Blumstein, 2019). The development of remote-learning haptics for hands-on, skills-based training in virtual simulation will greatly augment the role of virtual simulation within a flipped classroom framework.

In skills-based learning with XR, educators at the David Geffen School of Medicine at the University of California Los Angeles (UCLA) have pioneered multiple training programs. One research study at this institution examined the educational impact of an orthopedic VR surgical simulation software program developed by Osso VR©. Within this study, learners who utilized the VR surgical training program demonstrated a 230% surgical performance improvement compared with traditional training methods (Blumstein, 2020). Researchers in this study examined 20 surgical trainees who were divided into traditional and Osso VR© training platforms for skills-based education in tibial intramedullary nailing. Researchers report that the VR learning group performed the procedure 20% faster than the traditionally trained group and completed 38% more correct steps throughout the procedure (Blumstein, 2020).

In addition to direct skills training, some VR applications allow for a 360-degree video recording of live surgical encounters. The VRinOR© application is one example of this offering. While less hands-on, it allows surgical trainees a more detailed view of specific surgical procedures in a more immersive, 3D environment (Kyaw et al., 2019).

In addition to skills-based training, the development of XR 3D modeling programs for healthcare education has grown exponentially before and during the COVID-19 pandemic. As one example, 3D modeling has been a useful remote learning tool within the field of gross anatomy. Before the advent of XR software as a supplement to gross anatomy training, the use of cadavers as the primary modality for medical training has been entrenched in medical education curricula since the 17th century (Iwanaga et al., 2021). Virtual learning technology in gross anatomy training was a critical remote learning tool during the COVID-19 pandemic, when in-person, cadaveric training was prohibited. Since a return to our more traditional form of teaching in this area, virtual learning technology will likely not replace but serve as a useful learning adjunct in this critical field of preclinical healthcare education. Like all remote-learning, virtual simulation software that utilizes 3D modeling has great utility within a flipped classroom model.

One meta-analysis of the use of virtual learning software with 3D anatomic models in gross anatomy training included a review of 21 research articles (Zhao et al., 2020). Twelve of these studies reported that the use of VR 3D software modeling was a significantly more effective learning method than the traditional use of 2D text and cadaveric training. Nine of these 21 articles reported an overall equivalence in the learning effectiveness of both offerings. In summary, this meta-analysis reported that medical students prefer to use 3D visualization XR software over the traditional use of cadaveric training in gross anatomy (Zhao et al., 2020).

As previously referenced, the Stanford Virtual Heart© program is a 3D modeling VR software program that provides useful patient and provider education on congenital heart defects (Chang, 2020; Axelrod, 2017). It has grown in popularity and has been piloted in over 20 learning institutions across the globe. Healthcare providers and educators in the field of pediatric cardiology use this VR software to teach students as well as patients and family members about the complex 3D structure of various congenital heart defects. It is one of the few VR educational programs that has found utility for both provider- and patient-centered education (Axelrod, 2017). With this program, users may wear a VR headset to explore a virtual heart from both an external and internal perspective to gain better understanding of the complexities of various types of congenital heart disease. Developers of this VR training program report that "VR is the most engaging way to learn anatomy, far surpassing textbooks, models, online videos and cadavers" (Axelrod, 2017).

In addition to a variety of XR programs that center on 3D modeling for healthcare education, case-based, virtual learning software represents the digital counterpart to our traditional, manikin-based simulation training. Dr. Todd Chang is a pioneering researcher in the field of VR software for case-based learning in pediatric emergency medicine. He has conducted research to quantify the level of physiologic stress induced by VR, case-based learning in high-acuity pediatric emergency medicine cases. He has quantified the learner's physiologic stress by measuring variables such as heart rate and salivary cortisol levels during a virtual learning case (Chang, 2019). He has reported a statistically significant increase in the level of physiologic stress that learners experience when immersed in a variety of emergent pediatric cases. Dr. Chang and his colleagues have reported that markers of physiologic stress increased among less experienced learners during these high-stakes, pediatric emergency cases. They also report that similar markers are present to a lesser degree with more seasoned providers (Chang, 2019). Dr. Chang has worked to develop a variety of pediatric critical care cases that utilize VR technology. These cases have adjustable levels of difficulty as well as AI-driven feedback for the learners at the end of every case.

Within this realm of provider-focused virtual learning software, Dr. Mel Slater has pioneered multiple "embodiment" training programs (Gillies, 2020; Banakau et at., 2016). These VR software programs frequently allow learners to don a headset and assume the physical identity of a different person based on factors such as age, sex, race and/or specific disabilities. VR embodiment software has allowed participants the ability to inhabit another person's body within a virtual world. This type of software has been ground-breaking in education on personal bias and identity perception within healthcare education (Slater, 2020). With respect to VR embodiment for empathy training, Dr. Slater writes that "Most people think of VR as being about being somewhere different, but it can also be about being someone different" (Slater, 2020). Dr. Slater has currently reported VR embodiment research in three different experiences. The first has involved allowing white people an embodiment experience as black people as a means of reducing implicit racism. He has developed additional VR software that allows male participants to embody a female victim of sexual harassment. He has also developed a VR program where participants embody themselves as Sigmund Freud and address their own mental health issues. The utilization of VR for embodiment experiences will continue to grow and provide critical training in healthcare education in areas such as empathy and implicit bias.

The use of VR technology for role playing may also become a valuable resource in healthcare education. There are several VR software programs that utilize virtual patient encounters as a means of role playing in healthcare education. This may be particularly useful in difficult patient encounters where patients or family members may demand unnecessary treatments such as antibiotics or narcotic pain medications. Role playing can also help in circumstances where providers need additional training in the delivery of difficult news such as death notification. Virtual patient case-based learning can also facilitate role playing to impart better communication skills with patients and/or family members with mental health or other physical impairments (King et al., 2019). Patients and family members at extremes of age may also have communication barriers that healthcare trainees can better overcome with role play in VR. In a similar way, the use of role play with VR may assist in training healthcare providers to develop more empathy for their patients and family members. Effective communication skills are critical for healthcare providers within all specialties and role playing with VR software may further assist in greater education in this area.

Within the realm of provider-centered education, both 3D modeling and virtual patient learning programs have tremendous utility in a flipped classroom model. An optimal learning program depends fully on the learning objectives of the specific course and serves to complement the more passive, lecture-based learning that occurs in the traditional classroom setting. Fully remote, virtual simulation software has great utility within the in-person, flipped classroom space. Its remote, digital footprint has great potential as a meaningful teaching tool for in-person learning because it allows healthcare instructors a means of incorporating our best practices of simulation education directly within the traditional classroom and lecture hall.

CONCLUSION

Virtual learning software provides a useful teaching tool for both provider- and patient-focused learning objectives. For provider-centered training, the utility of virtual simulation software far exceeds its remote-learning capabilities. It is also a valuable tool for live, classroom-based simulation in healthcare education, particularly within the flipped classroom model. The utilization of this software as an immersive learning alternative to the traditional medical lecture is currently in its infancy but closely follows current trends to transform our healthcare classroom into a more active and engaging learning space. The classroom environment is not a typical space for medical simulation, but virtual simulation challenges this paradigm and delivers our best practice principles of traditional simulation in this critical learning space.

Fundamentally, as virtual simulation technology continues to evolve within healthcare education, we must remain steadfast that all learning exercises must be tailored to best meet the specific learning objectives of any educational pursuit. A pioneer of simulation in healthcare education, David Gaba, states this best when he writes that "Simulation is a technique, not a technology, to replace or amplify real experiences with guided experiences that evoke or replicate substantial aspects of the real world in a fully interactive manner" (Gaba, 2007). Virtual simulation exemplifies this teaching approach and will bolster future efforts to replace the more passive, podium-based lectures of yesteryear with the best-practice, immersive and innovative learning of simulation education.

REFERENCES

Axelrod, D. (2017). *The Stanford Virtual Heart: Revolutionizing Education on Congenital Heart Defects.* Stanford Children's Health. https://www.stanfordchildrens.org/en/innovation/virtual-reality/stanford-virtual-heart

Banakou, D., Hanumanthu, P. D., & Slater, M. (2016). Virtual Embodiment of White People in a Black Virtual Body Leads to a Sustained Reduction in Their Implicit Racial Bias. *Frontiers in Human Neuroscience, 10*, 601. doi:10.3389/fnhum.2016.00601 PMID:27965555

Blumstein, G. (2019). Research: How Virtual Reality Can Help Train Surgeons. *Harvard Business Review.* https://hbr.org/2019/10/research-how-virtual-reality-can-help-train-surgeons

Blumstein, G., Zukotynski, B., Cevallos, N., Ishmael, C., Zoller, S., Burke, Z., Clarkson, S., Park, H., Bernthal, N., & SooHoo, N. F. (2020). Randomized Trial of a Virtual Reality Tool to Teach Surgical Technique for Tibial Shaft Fracture Intramedullary Nailing. *Journal of Surgical Education, 77*(4), 969–977. https://doi-org.ezproxy2.umc.edu/10.1016/j.jsurg.2020.01.002

Bordnick, P. S., Graap, K. M., Copp, H., Brooks, J., Ferrer, M., & Logue, B. (2004). Utilizing virtual reality to standardize nicotine craving research: A pilot study. *Addictive Behaviors, 29*(9), 1889–1894. doi:10.1016/j.addbeh.2004.06.008 PMID:15530734

Breining, G. (2018). Future or Fad? Virtual Reality in Medical Education. *AAMCNews.* https://www.aamc.org/news-insights/future-or-fad-virtual-reality-medical-education

Bremner, J. (2019). Simulation-Based Education: Bringing Theory and Practice Together. *Dal News.* https://www.dal.ca/news/2019/11/28/simulation_based_education--bringing-theory-and-practice-togethe.html

Car, J., Carlstedt-Duke, J., Tudor Car, L., Posadzki, P., Whiting, P., Zary, N., Atun, R., Majeed, A., & Campbell, J.Digital Health Education Collaboration. (2019). Digital Education in Health Professions: The Need for Overarching Evidence Synthesis. *Journal of Medical Internet Research, 21*(2), e12913. doi:10.2196/12913 PMID:30762583

Chang, T. P. (2020, April 30). *Practical & Academic Considerations for Integrating VR and AR into the Simulation Center Repertoire.* Children's Hospital Los Angeles. https://chla.webex.com/recordingservice/sites/chla/recording/playback/d410d5beaeae46bd9e8756024d091905

Chang, T. P., Beshay, Y., Hollinger, T., & Sherman, J. M. (2019). Comparisons of Stress Physiology of Providers in Real-Life Resuscitations and Virtual Reality-Simulated Resuscitations. *Simulation in Healthcare: Journal of the Society for Simulation in Healthcare, 14*(2), 104–112. doi:10.1097/SIH.0000000000000356

Chebanova, A. (n.d.). Making Use of Virtual Reality in Healthcare. *Steel Kiwi.* https://steelkiwi.com/blog/making-use-of-virtual-reality-in-healthcare/

Clark, B. (2017). Study: VR Twice as Effective as Morphine at Treating Pain. *TNW News.* https://thenextweb.com/news/study-vr-twice-as-effective-as-morphine-at-treating-pain

Cockrell, R. K., Fischer, K., Stevens, L., Robison, E. S., Cooney, T. A., Lagunas, M., & Rahman, S. (2021). OADN Virtual Simulation Reviews: Team Collaboration to Develop an Online Resource to Assist Nurse Educators. *Teaching and Learning in Nursing*, *16*(4), 352–356. Advance online publication. doi:10.1016/j.teln.2021.06.004

Coyne, L., Merritt, T. A., Parmentier, B. L., Sharpton, R. A., & Takemoto, J. K. (2019). The Past, Present, and Future of Virtual Reality in Pharmacy Education. *American Journal of Pharmaceutical Education*, *83*(3), 7456. doi:10.5688/ajpe7456 PMID:31065173

Durgahee, T. (1998). Facilitating reflection: From a sage on stage to a guide on the side. *Nurse Education Today*, *18*(2), 158–164. doi:10.1016/S0260-6917(98)80021-X PMID:9592516

Foohey, S. (2020). *Virtual Resus Room.* https://virtualresusroom.com/

Foronda, C. L., Fernandez-Burgos, M., Nadeau, C., Kelley, C. N., & Henry, M. N. (2020). Virtual Simulation in Nursing Education: A Systematic Review Spanning 1996 to 2018. Simulation in Healthcare. *Journal of the Society for Simulation in Healthcare*, *15*(1), 46–54. doi:10.1097/SIH.0000000000000411 PMID:32028447

Gaba, D. M. (2007). The future vision of simulation in healthcare. *Simulation in Healthcare, 2*(2), 126–135. https://doi-org.ezproxy2.umc.edu/10.1097/01.SIH.0000258411.38212.32

Gillies, M. (2020). Mel Slater: Becoming a Better Person Through VR Embodiment. *Medium.com* https://medium.com/virtual-reality-virtual-people/mel-slater-becoming-a-better-person-through-vr-embodiment-2c055058d8a4

Gold, J. I., Belmont, K. A., & Thomas, D. A. (2007). The neurobiology of virtual reality pain attenuation. *Cyberpsychology & Behavior*, *10*(4), 536–544. doi:10.1089/cpb.2007.9993 PMID:17711362

Headsets Relaxing Patients During VR Surgery at St. George's. (2019, December 26). Retrieved from https://www.stgeorges.nhs.uk/newsitem/vr-headsets-relaxing-patients-during-surgery-at-st-georges/

Hennick, C. (2020). How VR in Healthcare Delivers Pandemic Education and Outreach. *Healthtech Magazine.* https://healthtechmagazine.net/article/2020/10/how-vr-healthcare-delivers-pandemic-education-and-outreach

Hew, K. F., & Lo, C. K. (2018). Flipped classroom improves student learning in health professions education: A meta-analysis. *BMC Medical Education*, *18*(1), 38. doi:10.118612909-018-1144-z PMID:29544495

Hoffman, H. G., Chambers, G. T., Meyer, W. J., III, Arceneaux, L. L., Russell, W. J., Seibel, E. J., Richards, T. L., Sharar, S. R., & Patterson, D. R. (2011). Virtual reality as an adjunctive non-pharmacologic analgesic for acute burn pain during medical procedures. *Annals of Behavioral Medicine, 41*(2), 183–191. https://doi-org.ezproxy2.umc.edu/10.1007/s12160-010-9248-7

Hoffman, H. G., Sharar, S. R., Coda, B., Everett, J. J., Ciol, M., Richards, T., & Patterson, D. R. (2004). Manipulating presence influences the magnitude of virtual reality analgesia. *Pain*, *111*(1), 162–168. doi:10.1016/j.pain.2004.06.013 PMID:15327820

Hyland, J. R., & Hawkins, M. C. (2008). High-fidelity human simulation in nursing education: A review of literature and guide for implementation. *Teaching and Learning in Nursing, 4*(1), 14–21. doi:10.1016/j.teln.2008.07.004

Iwanaga, J., Loukas, M., Dumont, A. S., & Tubbs, R. S. (2021). A review of anatomy education during and after the COVID-19 pandemic: Revisiting traditional and modern methods to achieve future innovation. *Clinical Anatomy (New York, N.Y.), 34*(1), 108–114. doi:10.1002/ca.23655 PMID:32681805

King, A. M., Gottlieb, M., Mitzman, J., Dulani, T., Schulte, S. J., & Way, D. P. (2019). Flipping the Classroom in Graduate Medical Education: A Systematic Review. *Journal of Graduate Medical Education, 11*(1), 18–29. doi:10.4300/JGME-D-18-00350.2 PMID:30805092

Kraut, A. S., Omron, R., Caretta-Weyer, H., Jordan, J., Manthey, D., Wolf, S. J., Yarris, L. M., Johnson, S., & Kornegay, J. (2019). The Flipped Classroom: A Critical Appraisal. *The Western Journal of Emergency Medicine, 20*(3), 527–536. doi:10.5811/westjem.2019.2.40979 PMID:31123556

Kyaw, B. M., Saxena, N., Posadzki, P., Vseteckova, J., Nikolaou, C. K., George, P. P., Divakar, U., Masiello, I., Kononowicz, A. A., Zary, N., & Tudor Car, L. (2019). Virtual Reality for Health Professions Education: Systematic Review and Meta-Analysis by the Digital Health Education Collaboration. *Journal of Medical Internet Research, 21*(1), e12959. doi:10.2196/12959 PMID:30668519

Maples-Keller, J. L., Bunnell, B. E., Kim, S. J., & Rothbaum, B. O. (2017). The Use of Virtual Reality Technology in the Treatment of Anxiety and Other Psychiatric Disorders. *Harvard Review of Psychiatry, 25*(3), 103–113. doi:10.1097/HRP.0000000000000138 PMID:28475502

McKnight, R. R., Pean, C. A., Buck, J. S., Hwang, J. S., Hsu, J. R., & Pierrie, S. N. (2020). Virtual Reality and Augmented Reality-Translating Surgical Training into Surgical Technique. *Current Reviews in Musculoskeletal Medicine, 13*(6), 663–674. doi:10.100712178-020-09667-3 PMID:32779019

Muguerza, P., & Canelas, A. (2021). Breaking Boundaries. *PharmaTimes Magazine, 8*(6). http://www.pharmatimes.com/magazine/2021/june_2021/breaking_boundaries

Oman, S. P., Magdi, Y., & Simon, L. V. (2020). *Past Present and Future of Simulation in Internal Medicine.* StatPearls Publishing.

Palmer, C. (2019). *Real treatments in virtual worlds: Treating patients in virtual environments is now easier and less expensive, and the number of conditions that the technology can treat has grown.* American Psychological Association. https://www.apa.org/monitor/2019/09/cover-virtual-worlds

Pottle, J. (2019). Virtual reality and the transformation of medical education. *Future Healthcare Journal, 6*(3), 181–185. doi:10.7861/fhj.2019-0036 PMID:31660522

Riddell, J., Jhun, P., Fung, C. C., Comes, J., Sawtelle, S., Tabatabai, R., Joseph, D., Shoenberger, J., Chen, E., Fee, C., & Swadron, S. P. (2017). Does the Flipped Classroom Improve Learning in Graduate Medical Education? *Journal of Graduate Medical Education, 9*(4), 491–496. doi:10.4300/JGME-D-16-00817.1 PMID:28824764

Slater, M. (2020, May 11). Transforming the Self Through Virtual Reality. *Frontiers Science News.* https://blog.frontiersin.org/2020/05/05/frontiers-in-virtual-reality-online-seminar-series/

Towers-Clark, C. (2021). Medicine and Mindfulness: How VR is Helping Healthcare Through the Pandemic. *Forbes.* https://www.forbes.com/sites/charlestowersclark/2021/02/19/medicine--mindfulness-how-vr-training-is-helping-healthcare-through-the-pandemic/?sh=36ce916558b9

Triepels, C., Smeets, C., Notten, K., Kruitwagen, R., Futterer, J. J., Vergeldt, T., & Van Kuijk, S. (2020). Does three-dimensional anatomy improve student understanding? *Clinical Anatomy (New York, N.Y.)*, *33*(1), 25–33. doi:10.1002/ca.23405 PMID:31087400

Trost, Z., France, C., Anam, M., & Shum, C. (2021). Virtual reality approaches to pain: Toward a state of the science. *Pain, 162*(2), 325–331. doi:10.1097/j.pain.0000000000002060 PMID:32868750

Vávra, P., Roman, J., Zonča, P., Ihnát, P., Němec, M., Kumar, J., Habib, N., & El-Gendi, A. (2017). Recent Development of Augmented Reality in Surgery: A Review. *Journal of Healthcare Engineering, 4574172*, 1–9. Advance online publication. doi:10.1155/2017/4574172 PMID:29065604

Yang, Y., Allen, T., Abdullahi, S. M., Pelphrey, K. A., Volkmar, F. R., & Chapman, S. B. (2018). Neural mechanisms of behavioral change in young adults with high-functioning autism receiving virtual reality social cognition training: A pilot study. *Autism Research, 11*(5), 713–725. https://doi-org.ezproxy2.umc.edu/10.1002/aur.1941

Zhao, J., Xu, X., Jiang, H., & Ding, Y. (2020). The effectiveness of virtual reality-based technology on anatomy teaching: A meta-analysis of randomized controlled studies. *BMC Medical Education, 20*(1), 127. doi:10.118612909-020-1994-z PMID:32334594

KEY TERMS AND DEFINITIONS

AR: Any software program that utilizes hardware such as a head-mounted display, smart phone, tablet, or other programmed device to superimpose digital imagery upon the actual environment. Both the live environment and digital imagery remain autonomous from each other within the same field of view.

Embodiment: The use of VR technology to place the user in the physical body of a virtual human or other being, often used as a means of training to engender greater empathy for someone with different fundamental characteristics such as race, sex, age, and/or disability than the user

Flipped Classroom: A teaching methodology whereby instructors pre-assign material and utilize classroom time for active and immersive learning experiences as an alternative to the traditional, podium-based lecture.

HALO Case: This stands for High-Acuity, Low-Occurrence cases; these are rare, emergent cases, often used in simulation to narrow a knowledge gap for healthcare providers who would otherwise have little or no exposure for routine management.

Haptics: The use of technology that stimulates the senses of touch and motion, often for skills-based training in virtual simulation.

MR: Any technology that blends both VR and XR such that there is full immersion in a digital environment but with preservation of select elements from non-digital space.

VR: Any software that utilizes a headset or similar device to immerse the user in a fully alternative, digital environment. It may simulate multiple sensory modalities such as visual, auditory, sensory, or haptic and even olfactory elements to achieve a maximal level of complete, digital immersion.

XR: Overall term for any technology that employs either VR, AR, or MR modalities.

Chapter 6

Building an Extended Reality Pedagogical Continuum Through 180° First-Person Point-of-View Video:
From VR to Computer and Mobile Displays to AR

Maxime Ros
Montpellier University, France

Lorenz S. Neuwirth
iD https://orcid.org/0000-0002-8194-522X
SUNY Old Westbury, USA

ABSTRACT

The advancement of virtual reality (VR) technology for educational instruction and curricular (re)design have become highly attractive and newly demanding areas of both the technology and healthcare industries. However, the quickly evolving field is still learning about each of the associated VR technologies, whether they are evidence-based, and how they are validated to decrease cognitive load and in turn increase student/learner comprehension. Likewise, the instructional (re)design of the content that the student/learner is exposed to in VR, and whether it is immersive, and promotes memorable content and experiences can influence their learning outcomes. Here the Revinax® Handbook content library that is displayed in an immersive virtual reality application in first-person point-of-view (IVRA-FPV) is contrasted with third-person point-of-view (IVRA-TPV) through VR headsets to an individual, and computer displays to many individuals along with augmented reality (AR) are evaluated as emerging advancements in the field of VR and AR.

DOI: 10.4018/978-1-7998-8371-5.ch006

INTRODUCTION

Different VR Environments Examined Through Cognitive Load Theory: Advantages & Issues

Learning through Virtual Reality (VR) formats has shown to decrease the cognitive load of the student/learner by placing them within an environment that simulates real-world scenarios (Andersen et al., 2016). The intention to design instructional materials based upon the cognitive load theory (Leppink et al., 2015; Brachten et al., 2020; Sweller et al., 2011; Sweller, 2011; Paas et al., 2010a; 2010b; 2010c; Kirscher, 2002; Sweller, 1994) and the transient information effect (Wong et al., 2012; Leahy & Sweller, 2011) in an effort to reduce cognitive load has been an important topic for science, technology, engineering, and mathematics (STEM) disciplines (Nyachwaya & Gillaspie, 2016; Josephsen, 2015; Reedy, 2015; Schlairet et al., 2015; Yung & Paas, 2015; Sweller et al., 1990) and is even more critical for interdisciplinary studies (e.g., in medical education; Leppink, 2015; Hessler & Henderson, 2013). Moreover, there is a need to balance the student/learners cognitive load with the pedagogical learning outcomes in an educational effort to increase science text comprehension of the student/learner through visual imagery (Wouters et al., 2017; Leutner et al., 2009; Ayres & Paas, 2007a; 2007b; Hasler et al., 2007; Moreno, 2007).

The use of an intentional instructional design method to teach STEM and medical educational tools through VR has been an advantageous tool that serves to leverage technology (Yung & Paas, 2015; Van Merriënboer & Sweller, 2010) with training of complex cognitive tasks (Van Merriënboer & Sweller, 2005; Paas & Van Merriënboer, 1994), while simulating multiple pedagogical learning methods rich content with embedded images within the VR environment (Brachten et al., 2020; Cheng et al., 2015; Nelson & Erlandson, 2008) helps to overcome the limitations of working memory (Meguerdichian et al., 2016). Research in the areas of digital educational game development has shown that when such a balance is achieved it can increase student's learning and motivation, while decreasing their cognitive load (Hawlitschek & Joeckel, 2017; Leahy & Sweller, 2011). Thus, this type of cognitive load instructional method for learning offers the student/learner with the possibility to be fully focused and enhance their concentration when presented with information in a simulated form of the real-world through VR, unlike when learning from a textbook in which the student/learner must conceptualize the situation in their mind in order to project themselves into the learning context. Notably, VR environments were initially created using computer-generated images (CGI) or 360° videos (Kaminska et al., 2019). The main feature which engaged the student/learner to use CGI was their ability to interact with every aspect or component of the VR environment. Thus, such rich interactive experiences serve both to emphasize and facilitate the reification (i.e., the perceptual and spatial sense of the object within the environment) as defined by Fowler (2015).

Furthermore, Fowler's (2015) initial work in this area served as a one of the principled arguments and supporting evidence regarding how to conceptualize building relevant pedagogical VR environments that would benefit the student/learner. However, one critical limitation of Fowler's (2015) work was that it failed to provide access to the optimal point-of-view (POV) for enhancing translational learning. Additionally, a cost-benefit ratio has become a critical and practical limitation for designing, developing, and implementing these VR environments in a conservative yet intentional way to obtain a high-fidelity rendering (i.e., a realistic experience; Concannon et al., 2019). This situation has led VR instructional designers to carefully consider the pedagogical value of the VR environment and how they can maximize the student/learner interactivity within the VR environment while creating it at as low a cost as possible (Parham et al., 2019). This approach has directed the VR instructional designers to also consider how to cost-effectively deploy these VR pedagogical tools efficiently on various devices (e.g., smartphones, desktop, etc.), even out of extended reality. Alternatively, 360° videos can be used to approach levels of realism, but unfortunately fall short of achieving an optimal VR experience as 360° videos are based on footage from a real environment with the student/learner having limited interactions within that very environment.

The main limitation here is that it fails to provide access to the optimal point-of-view (POV) for enhancing translational learning: 1) the student/learner views the situation from a third-person point-of-view (TPV) that follows an action but does not actually take part in that very action; 2) regarding technical skills, TPV is not optimal as it fails to encompass the first-person point-of-view (FPV) of the expert (Fiorella et al., 2017). It is important to note here, that the FPV is a critical factor in promoting maximal student/learner comprehension as it serves to activate the neural circuitry of the mirror neuron system (Bohil et al., 2011; Van Gog et al. 2008; Wiedermann, 2003) that permits, in real-time and through the VR environment, both a rich and interactive sense of imitation learning (Anderson et al., 2001), but also the potential for vicarious reinforcement (Blascovich & McCall, 2010). Therefore, it is argued that the way(s) in which a VR environment is designed, developed, and displayed (i.e., the 3-Ds for effective VR pedagogical design) can facilitate blended learning applications by providing direct access to a multitude of resources. This is particularly important as it can give a student/learner such educational accessibility within any place and at any time (i.e., as a form of mental time and experience travel), through the use of different pedagogical techniques (e.g., videos, text, 3D reconstruction, etc.). As there is no limit to the extent by which integration for all of these pedagogical features could be presented to the student/learner, the current trend in the VR field is to add a range of complementary data (e.g., video, animated 3D objects, etc.) to make the experience more meaningful. However, this approach requires validation and evidence-based practices for which pedagogical methods are most effective based upon their instructional design through VR educational curricular delivery.

From the instructional designer perspective, the greatest risk is to add too many complementary datasets within a single VR environment in an inconsistent and/or illogical way(s) that may inadvertently overwhelm the student/learner, thereby counterintuitively increasing their cognitive load, and consequently reducing/impeding their intended learning of the materials being presented in VR (Ros et al., 2020). Thus, negatively augmenting the student's/learner's cognitive load in such a way will result in reduced technical skills training outcomes through procedural learning and conceptual flaws in the comprehension of the skills being taught. Without a proper instructional design in these VR environments, the field may be inadvertently left creating more less than practical environments that can constrain learning outcomes, produce inefficient pedagogical approaches, and result in a failure to upskill, reskill, and teach students/learners effectively through VR environments. This situation, may in turn, create additional learning gaps beyond what already exists for the next generation of diverse students/learners (for review, see Neuwirth et al., 2020; 2019; 2018a; 2018b; Mukherji et al., 2017). Furthermore, the situation may also create obscurities regarding the pedagogical effectiveness amongst the available VR pedagogical techniques, technologies, and platforms without carefully assessing and considering the limitations of the student's/learner's preparedness as an extraneous cognitive load limiting factor that will carry over into the VR environments.

THE INSTRUCTIONAL DESIGN OF THE REVINAX® HANDBOOK METHOD: CREATING AN IMMERSIVE TUTORIAL ENVIRONMENT

From the literature on VR environments, Fiorella (2017) showed that learning in FPV can serve to reduce learning errors by up to 50%. The Revinax® Handbook method uniquely takes advantage of the FPV pedagogical approach to facilitate motor programming (i.e., through the mirror neuron systems activation) and decreasing cognitive load on one hand, while alternatively using the immersive VR environment to increase a deeper level of understanding and comprehension that is gained by increasing the visual perspective and content of the material being learned (Andersen et al., 2016). Thus, it can be argued that the Revinax® Handbook method provides a uniquely integrated pedagogical approach to teaching students/learners through VR. Moreover, the Revinax® Handbook method creates an Immersive Virtual Reality Application (IVRA) based on FPV video (i.e., IVRA-FPV). Initially, the Revinax® Handbook method was designed as a hardware composed of two stabilized cameras, that was worn by an expert while they performed a specific skill and the procedural components it involved (Neuwirth & Ros, 2021; Ros & Trives, 2020; Ros et al., 2017). Through such a unique filming approach, the orientation of the cameras could be optimized to record what the expert actually saw from their FPV during the actual procedure so that the student/learner could encounter the same visual experience as the expert as they learned the material (**Fig. 1 A**) as well as from a slightly different angle simulating a shadowing-like experience in the third-person POV (IVRA-TPV) vantage point (**Fig. 1 B**).

Figure 1. Comparison of two different recording point-of-views (POVs). The surgeon is wearing a camera device to capture his First-Person-POV (IVRA-FPV; A), whereas an external participant is recording the same procedure from another angle (Third Person-POV (IVRA-TPV; B)
Source: © 2021, Ros & Neuwirth. Used with permission.

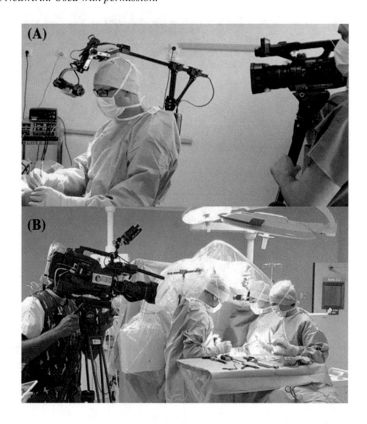

This IVRA-FPV approach offers the advantage and/or creative solution to replace and/or overcome the need to directly shadow an expert during a procedure, and compete with other students/learners to look over the shoulder of the expert, or be limited to the student's/learner's vantage point that is often too far away from the actual expert conducting the procedure within a larger class demonstration. The IVRA-FPV provides a pedagogical solution to address this problem by offering educators the ability to present the same educational content through both IVRA-TPV **(Fig. 2 A)** and IVRA-FPV **(Fig. 2 B)**. In doing so, a deeper level of understanding and comprehension is gained by increasing the visual perspective and content of the material being learned.

Figure 2. Representative illustration of one group learning in an IVRA-TPV displayed through a TV screen (A), when compared to another group learning in IVRA-FPV (B). The same scene displayed on the TV in (A) is being watched in (B)
Source: © 2021, Ros & Neuwirth. Used with permission.

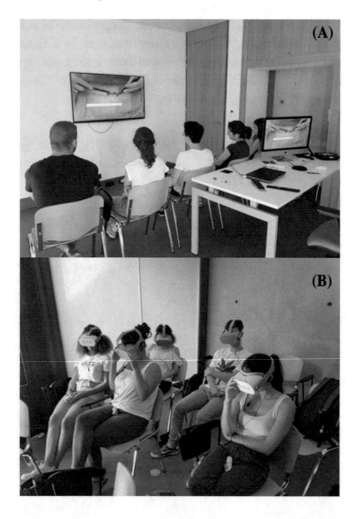

After recording this expert's FPV (i.e., using the 180° stereoscopic visual perspective of the expert), movie clips were then edited as concise and targeted chapters/learning modules and placed into the central part of the IVRA-FPV environment (**Fig. 3**). Typically, these chapters/learning modules would not exceed 20 minutes while within the IVRA-FPV experience. At the top of this central screen (**Fig. 3A**), the student/learner can select from the different chapters/learning modules at their leisure, within any sequence they choose, and can revisit a given chapter/learning module as many times as they deem necessary to meet their individualized learning needs. This pedagogical approach and instructional design has the advantage for the learner to go back and relearn content that wasn't clear to them without being left behind in a given class lecture that may move too quickly for some students/learners. This offers students/learners an ability to relearn and relive an IVRA-FPV experience to recapture the moment in time that they might have missed to prevent further widening of the academic achievement gap. Specific to the chapter/learning module being viewed on each side of the central screen (**Fig. 3 B & C**), additional complementary datasets are strategically placed (i.e., a lecture in the form of a slideshow, other video content/imagery, 3D models with free form rotation and movement through the object, etc.; **Fig. 3 C**) to complete the pedagogical instructional design and student/learner experience through IVRA-FPV. Finally, the student/learner can look downward to watch the actual procedure recorded from the experts FPV comprising the IVRA-FPA experience, which eliminates the limitations brought on by traditional shadowing procedures (**Fig. 3 D**).

Figure 3. A representative student/learner IVRA-FPV experience where they can choose chapters/learning modules by looking upwards (A), access additional learning content to refer to at their leisure and as frequently as needed (B), to access specific medical imagery/content and rotate images/content for unique concept formation and intervention approaches (C) and to watch the actual procedures from the FPV of an expert (D)
Source: © 2021, Ros & Neuwirth. Used with permission.

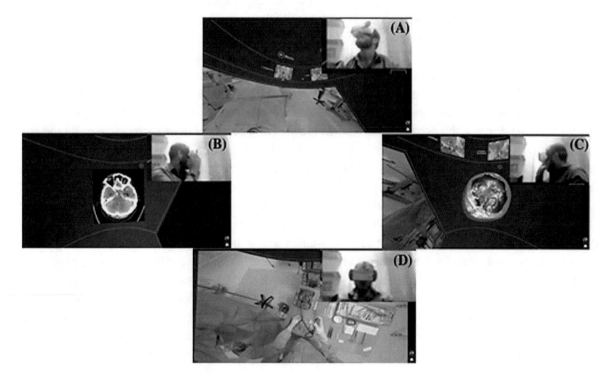

This instructional design of the IVRA-FPV gives the student/learner the simulated feeling of an as real as possible "lived" experience "through the eyes" of the expert. Thus, having direct and limitless access to the complementary datasets serve to further enhance the student's/learner's comprehension of the material while reducing learning errors in a more efficient manner. Following these developments, the Revinax® Handbook method was adapted to be displayed through mobile devices as well as desktop/laptop applications based on the same IVRA-FPV environment. However, these new display formats took into account the student/learner experience on these different devices - to make the content available at any time yet through more readily accessible technological means.

Immersive Tutorials: Uses and Outcomes Studies

Ros et al. (2021; 2020; 2017) performed different studies in a step-by-step approach to understand the interest, the impact, and to validate the use of the immersive tutorial. The main challenges to consider while performing these studies are to develop a comprehensive curriculum that directly links the pedagogical approach with the material, and measurable behavioral learning outcomes. First, it is important to acknowledge that the IVRA-FPV is a new tool that is being used for teaching, without knowing and/or appreciating its efficiency in promoting VR-dependent enhanced learning. However, despite the aforementioned, there is a real risk of negative pedagogy whereby the tool itself can be either counterproductive or lead to/influence incorrect memorization. This is why the IVRA-FPV learning approach was first tested using topics that were specialized and not generally apart of nor essential to a typical student's curriculum. The second aspect to consider is the actual material that would be used as a comparator to teach within the study (i.e., intra-study/internal validity) and to compare the results with other studies from the literature (i.e., extra-study/external validity). While reviewing the different studies around VR and education (Kaminska et al., 2019), it appears that the approaches being tested are quite different between their types and definitions of the VR that they employ (e.g., 360, CGI, etc.) along with the comparison between different pedagogical material (e.g., real life, videos, texts, etc.). Carefully considering these first two points, there was a unique opportunity to further determine the pedagogical application of the immersive tutorial through the Revinax® Handbook method as a complementary tool to traditional lecture methods. This was first done comparing the IVRA-FPV with the traditional lecture methods and showing that IVRA-FPV increased more learning and comprehension over traditional lectures (Ros et al. 2017; 2020). Finally, the behavioral challenge (i.e., reaction of the users/learners regarding the VR experience) comes from the participants of the study. Notably, not everyone experiences VR in the same way and certain head mounted displays (HMD) have extraneous variability in creating motion sickness (Concannon et al., 2019; Kamińska et al., 2019) which is not experienced by everyone. Second, even if the student/learner has already tried a range of VR pedagogical tools, and also considering that this may have been the first time the student/learner might have had access to the IVRA-FPV. This leads to two possible considerations, while ensuring that the studies were randomized: 1) on one hand, the participants from the group that did not have access to the IVRA-FPV felt less immersed and as a byproduct felt less willing to participate. Alternatively, students/learners that had access to the learning material needed more time to not learn per se, but rather explore, the immersive content and go over the "novelty effect" in order to focus on the lesson at hand. In order to resolve this inherent challenge as a function of novelty and acclimation to the technology itself (i.e., an extraneous variable), the best option was to consider some time before the learning outcomes assessment to make every student's/learner's ability to try another alternative immersive tutorial with the VR headset to assess their own personnel evaluation of the IVRA-FPV amongst other learning solutions.

INCREASED COMPREHENSION ABSENT OF AGE-RELATED EFFECTS

In a novel study that included 30 surgeons from a residency to advanced practitioners, Ros et al. (2017) collected survey feedback regarding their pedagogical interest and their willingness to have, access, and use the IVRA-FPV content. The results showed that 93% of participants answered in support that they would use the IVRA-FPV content to learn the material, whereas 97% indicated that they would use it to teach the material accordingly (Ros et al., 2017). Moreover, 97% of participants indicated that they would have understood the material faster, thereby influencing their ability to efficiently master the procedural skills that they were being taught through the IVRA-FPV pedagogical instruction. Interestingly, Ros et al. (2017) did not find any statistical differences related to age nor the IVRA-FPV experience, thereby suggesting the effect was due to the presentation of the pedagogy rather than the potential age effects of the participants. These findings suggest that the Revinax® Handbook method through the IVRA-FPV experience could serve as a invaluable tool, that may address or perhaps circumvent, any age-related academic learning and/or achievement gaps in students/learners for both initial and also continuing education aspirational goals. Moreover, these findings also suggest that even the most skilled professionals could engage others by creating FPV content on a particular skillset and demonstrate the specific training to educate the student/learner through an IVRA-FPV curriculum. It was postulated that this pedagogical intervention could provide support of utilizing the presentation of video-based content in curricular development of the IVRA-FPV since it utilizes a familiar environment that caters to the student's/learner's ability to adopt this pedagogical tool.

IMPROVED PRACTICAL QUESTIONS LEARNING OUTCOMES

In a second study, Ros et al. (2020) randomly assigned 175 early career medical students into two groups. The first group read an operative technique about a novel neurosurgical procedure, and the second group read the same technical note and then had access to the IVRA-FPV corresponding to aforementioned procedures. The participants were then asked to answer a survey with multiple-choice questions based upon the practical questions asked immediately after the intervention and during follow up 6-months thereafter. The findings revealed that the IVRA-FPV Group answered the practical questions significantly more accurately immediately following the intervention and at the 6-months follow up suggesting improved and more stable learning retention of the demonstrable skill overtime (Ros et al., 2020). These findings suggest that using IVRA-FPV pedagogical instruction may provide ample visual imagery, complementary content and scientific text through the side-viewed images with the ability to rotate images to access unique perspectives that ordinary textbooks and traditional lectures cannot provide to the student/learner. Further, this IVRA-FPV instructional design embeds the actual procedure with an unobstructed FPV for optimal learning which cannot be achieved through shadowing and/or engaging in group work to perform or mimic the procedures on a model, mannequin, cadaver, etc. Lastly, the ability to review and repeatedly review content that may not be captured easily by the student/learner in real-time increases a more efficient learning process, reduces the student's/learner's cognitive load, and ultimately increases there capacity for learning. Taken together, the IVRA-FPV instructional design and pedagogical approach is consistent reports on the predictive validity of cognitive load and perceived learning satisfaction (Kozan, 2016).

REDUCED PROCEDURAL TIME WITH 65% LESS ERRORS

In another study, Ros et al. (2021) randomly assigned 89 medical students in two groups: the first group benefited from a traditional lecture with a teacher explaining how to perform a lumbar puncture procedure, whereas the second group had only access to the IVRA-FPV. Then, each participant went into a separate room where they had an oral assessment on the theoretical questions, as well as the practical assessment by performing a lumbar puncture on a mannequin. Subsequently, their latency to complete the procedure as well as their number of errors was also measured. The Lecture Group answered the theoretical questions significantly more accurately, whereas VR group made more conceptual errors (34%), but interestingly there were no differences between the two groups regarding the generalization of the procedure on the mannequin, and yet their latency to perform the procedure was significantly reduced (60%) in the IVRA-FPV Group (Ros et al., 2021). By analyzing the errors made by both groups, Ros et al. (2021) showed that the IVRA-FPV method helped to decrease the number of procedural mistakes during the practical assessment by 65%. Taken together, this study revealed that having a teacher/instructor explain the conceptual theory and introduce the practical training to the students/learners through the IVRA-FPV can improve their training and practical skills competency through a brief pedagogical intervention in this instructional format.

LARGE SCALE MOBILE APPLICATIONS RAPID DEVELOPMENT AND DEPLOYMENT

In employing the IVRA-FPV at regular scale, Ros & Neuwirth (2020) conducted a longitudinal study over a period of two years using content that was developed by Revinax®, and through the Revinax® Handbook an additional complementary dataset library of tutorials was developed to be displayed through the IVRA-FPV format, which was then dedicated to healthcare professionals and nurses at much larger scale (i.e., thousands). During the first wave of the coronavirus (COVID-19) pandemic, the study by Ros & Neuwirth (2020) demonstrated how Revinax® expanded upon its previous library and created another eight new tutorials within a one-week time-period that was specifically dedicated to public health education in an effort to create a timely solution in educating healthcare workers and front-line responders to be upskilled and reskilled quickly in the evolving fight against COVID-19. The study by Ros & Neuwirth (2020) reported clearly that Revinax® worked uncompensated in a genuine humanitarian effort, to release the COVID-19 dataset library at no cost to the healthcare worker/front-line responder/student/learner, and this content was instructionally designed to be displayed on a dedicated mobile application to further increase its accessibility given the social/physical distancing challenges imposed by COVID-19. Interestingly, from these creative problem solving efforts, there were 12,500 healthcare professionals/front-line responders and students/learners in training that voluntarily downloaded and used the IVRA-FPV COVID-19 library content and application in 45 days (i.e., approximately a rate of 278 users per day). Ros & Neuwirth (2020) sent out a survey during 72 hrs of the COVID-19 content library deployment directly to these healthcare professionals/front-line responders and students/learners in training, and the results they obtained showed a 71.48% response rate. Overall, the COVID-19 content library users provided very positive feedback, whereby 94% indicated it increased their understanding of COVID-19 related health and safety issues, and 88% felt more confident in implementing the medical healthcare procedures taught through the content library, whereas 91% identified being upskilled or reskilled on COVID-19 medical healthcare procedures, respectively.

REMOTE TRAINING THROUGH DESKTOP/LAPTOP DISPLAYS

In a more recent study, Neuwirth & Ros (2021) evaluated two groups of undergraduate college students to learn a laboratory procedure (i.e., stereotactic surgery) in autonomy with a VR headset displaying the IVRA-FPV ($n = 26$) or with a teacher presenting the IVRA-FPV remotely through Zoom® using a desktop/laptop ($n = 32$). The participants then answered a survey and both groups stated that the pedagogical approach was innovative and engaging, with an immersive feeling perceived even through the remote desktop/computer displays (Neuwirth & Ros, 2021). The additional data that were displayed from a specific chapter helped them to understand the procedure and made this instructional design radically different than the usual training video that can be found. Here, the IVRA-FPV remotely through Zoom® using a desktop/laptop answered better to theoretical question (i.e., similar to the prior study's Lecture Group), whereas IVRA-FPV group answered better to practical question (i.e., similar to the prior study's procedural group).

AR DISPLAYS TO ASSIST DURING PROCEDURES

In 2017, the author did a trial (unpublished data) by giving access to a surgeon to the immersive tutorial on Augmented Reality (AR) glasses. The environment identical to the FPV video and was divided in chapters/modules supplemented with additional data (i.e., specific to the patient being operated: CT-scan and 3D model of the organ). The study found that expert/advanced practitioners (i.e., that did not necessarily need the immersive tutorial to complete familiar procedure), anecdotally self-reported that the additional data helped the expert/advanced practitioner to remain focused on the surgery. Moreover, the expert/advanced practitioner indicated that a clear benefit of the technology was that he could increase his attention to the surgical areas on the patient without ever having to lift his head or redirect his head away from the surgical field of vision. This was an important finding given that when and how frequent an expert/advanced practitioner looks away from the surgical field they must reorient themselves back to the procedure to reposition themselves where they last left off. It is argued that this/these specific point(s) in time during surgeries are where most unintentional errors may occur and the AR immersive experience could serve to reduce such inherent surgical errors in real-time. This particular issue becomes even more important when an expert/advanced practitioner may have to conduct many surgeries back-to-back and errors may increase linearly with time, number of surgeries to complete in a given shift, and the subsequent attentional and performance fatigue. Although AR may not overcome all of these concerns, they can at best leverage some, but long hours and number of surgeries in a given shift cannot be addressed by any technology at this time. Thus, AR instructional design for immersive tutorials to complement the experts/advanced practitioners years of experience may be most useful to refamiliarize themselves with surgical procedures they have not conducted in sometime, help to familiarize them with new surgical procedures they have yet to become skilled at, and perhaps help to refresh, support, or spot them during very familiar surgical procedures where they may be at increased risk for attentional and performance fatigue when conducting repeated surgeries over long hours.

BUILDING A PEDAGOGICAL CONTINUUM

In review of the aforementioned studies, a common theme has emerged that consistently shows the value and the efficiency of the Immersive Tutorial Instructional Design (ITID) as a relevant and effective learning solution. These ITIDs are developed from video-based recordings that begin from an individualized FPV small scale, and quickly, can be re-packaged into a content library through IVRA-FPV and AR to be developed rather swiftly and deployed at a large scale with broad ranging access for many types of students/learners. In keeping the ITID to be displayed through IVRA-FPV and AR, it creates a convenient real-world environment that makes the instructional method "believable" thereby increasing student/learner motivation, increasing familiarity to further promote later generalization into the real-world practical translation of the educational content, and promotes optimal engagement of the student/learner. This pedagogical approach and instructional design improves the student/learner to have an increased understanding of the different steps of each type of medical procedure, since they have already "lived through" the situation and its context, and this translates into the student/learner feeling that they are more confident to perform that very procedure in the future. Thus, this allows the student/learner to achieve these critical learning outcomes faster and with a fewer mistakes. Further, the pedagogical options can be visualized through **Fig. 4** to best conceptualize how the Revinax® Handbook has evolved rather quickly with evidence-based studies to validate it as an effective tool to teaching procedural medical content individually through: IVRA-FPV (**A**), in a group through IVRA-FPV (**B**), individually through computer displayed IVRA-FPV (**C**), in a group through computer displayed IVRA-FPV (**D**), individually through a mobile device through the computer displayed IVRA-FPV (**E**), individually through a mobile device through the computer displayed IVRA-FPV or the IVRA-FPV using a 2D to 3D conversion cardboard glasses over the mobile device (**F**), and through AR (**G**).

Figure 4. Illustrates the different options for students/learners to use the IVRA-FPV across different types of learning possibilities
Source: © 2021, Ros & Neuwirth. Used with permission.

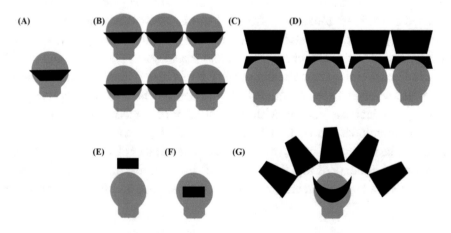

(A) shows the standard IVRA-FPV for an individual instruction with a HMD, (B) shows a group instruction using the IVRA-FPV with a HMD, (C) shows an individual instruction using a computer displayed IVRA-FPV, (D) shows a group instruction using a computer displayed IVRA-FPV, (E) shows an individual instruction using a mobile device as a form of computer displayed IVRA-FPV, (F) shows an individual instruction using a mobile device with a 2D to 3D conversion glasses attached to the mobile device to provide a mobile IVRA-FPV, and (G) shows an individual instruction for using AR with imagery that is accessible over the working area.

SUMMARY/CONCLUSION

The IVRA-FPV and the ITIDs methodologies for describing and developing a pedagogical curriculum have unique value for educators to consider. Although there are other VR applications out there, many fall short of providing evidence-based outcomes, clear learning outcomes, and ensuring adequate levels of immersion, or often ill define what they mean by immersion. Considering that other technologies offer some advantages to instructional design and pedagogy, few have provided a better complete product that continually meets the changing demands of the users as the Revinax® Handbook. As such, the immersive tutorial can be displayed in a number of ways to adapt to real-time challenges, cost and environmental constraints, can amplify the number of students/learners to be trained, can reduce training time and procedural errors, and can transmit information quickly on a global scale. Thus, the ability to develop, deploy, and display the IVRA-FPV on different platforms (i.e., mobile devices, AR glasses, etc.; **Fig. 4**) to support the experiential learning of current and next generation medical healthcare professionals is of significant value. Additionally, the content that is displayed through the AR glasses to support the student/learner while performing the procedure for the very first time, serves to reinsured them that they have the possibility and/or ability to (re)check the different steps of the procedure in real-time. Thus, further fostering a higher degree of attention, motivation, and decreasing cognitive load to retain more information from the procedure. The lectures that are supplementing the ITIDs can also be displayed on the student's/learner's desktop in a computer displayed IVRA-FPV format to help them to understand the theoretical parts of a lesson/procedure. The advantage for the student's/learner's to have access to a VR Headset can help them to memorize the content better for the practical aspects of the lesson/ procedure when in the IVRA-FPV. However, if cost is an issue, then the content can also be displayed on their smartphone to refresh them to learn the skills just before performing the procedure as another approach. Taken together, the portability, adaptability, and accessibility of the IVRA-FPV through the Revinax® Handbook provides an ideal set of solutions to learning in a modern world through VR for future generations of medical healthcare professionals.

REFERENCES

Andersen, S. A. W., Mikkelsen, P. T., Konge, L., Cayé-Thomasen, P., & Sørensen, M. S. (2016). Cognitive Load in Mastoidectomy Skills Training: Virtual Reality Simulation and Traditional Dissection Compared. *Journal of Surgical Education*, *73*(1), 45–50. doi:10.1016/j.jsurg.2015.09.010 PMID:26481267

Anderson, P. L., Rothbaum, B. O., & Hidges, L. (2005). Virtual reality: Using the virtual world to improve quality of life in the real world. *Bulletin of the Menninger Clinic*, *65*(1), 78–91. Advance online publication. doi:10.1521/bumc.65.1.78.18713 PMID:11280960

Ayres, P., & Paas, F. (2007a). Can the cognitive load approach make instructional animations more effective? *Applied Cognitive Psychology*, *21*(6), 811–820. doi:10.1002/acp.1351

Ayres, P., & Paas, F. (2007b). Making instructional animations more effective: A cognitive load approach. *Applied Cognitive Psychology*, *21*(6), 695–700. doi:10.1002/acp.1343

Blascovich, J., & McCall, C. (2010). Attitudes in virtual reality. In J. Forgas, W. Crano & J. Cooper (Eds.), The Psychology of Attitudes and Attitude Change. Google Books.

Bohil, C. J., Alicea, B., & Biocca, F. A. (2011). Virtual reality in neuroscience research and therapy. *Nature Reviews. Neuroscience*, *12*(12), 752–762. doi:10.1038/nrn3122 PMID:22048061

Brachten, F., Brünker, F., Frick, N. R. J., Ross, B., & Stieglitz, S. (2020). On the ability of virtual agents to decrease cognitive load: An experimental study. *Information Systems and e-Business Management*, *18*(2), 187–207. doi:10.100710257-020-00471-7

Cheng, T. S., Lu, Y. C., & Yang, C. S. (2015). Using the multi-display teaching system to lower cognitive load. *Journal of Educational Technology & Society*, *18*(4), 128–140.

Concannon, B. J., Esmail, S., & Roduta Roberts, M. (2019). Head-Mounted Display Virtual Reality in Post-secondary Education and Skill Training. *Frontiers in Education*, *4*(August), 1–23. doi:10.3389/feduc.2019.00080

Fiorella, L., Van Gog, T., Hoogerheide, V., & Mayer, R. E. (2017). It's all a matter of perspective: Viewing first-person video modeling examples promotes learning of an assembly task. *Journal of Educational Psychology*, *109*(5), 653–665. doi:10.1037/edu0000161

Fowler, C. (2015). Virtual reality and learning: Where is the pedagogy? *British Journal of Educational Technology*, *46*(2), 412–422. doi:10.1111/bjet.12135

Hasler, B. S., Kersten, B., & Sweller, J. (2007). Learner control, cognitive load and instructional animation. *Applied Cognitive Psychology*, *21*(6), 713–729. doi:10.1002/acp.1345

Hawlitschek, A., & Joeckel, S. (2017). Increasing the effectiveness of digital educational games: The effects of a learning instruction on student's learning, motivation and cognitive load. *Computers in Human Behavior*, *72*, 79–86. doi:10.1016/j.chb.2017.01.040

Hessler, K. L., & Henderson, A. M. (2013). Interactive learning research: Application of cognitive load theory to nursing education. *International Journal of Nursing Education Scholarship*, *10*(1), 133–141. doi:10.1515/ijnes-2012-0029 PMID:23813334

Josephsen, J. (2015). Cognitive load theory and nursing simulation: An integrative review. *Clinical Simulation in Nursing*, *11*(5), 259–267. doi:10.1016/j.ecns.2015.02.004

Kamińska, D., Sapiński, T., Wiak, S., Tikk, T., Haamer, R. E., Avots, E., Helmi, A., Ozcinar, C., & Anbarjafari, G. (2019). Virtual reality and its applications in education: Survey. *Information (Switzerland)*, *10*(10), 1–20. doi:10.3390/info10100318

Kirschner, P. A. (2002). Cognitive load theory: Implications of cognitive load theory on the design of learning. *Learning and Instruction*, *12*(1), 1–10. doi:10.1016/S0959-4752(01)00014-7

Kozan, K. (2016). The incremental predictive validity of teaching, cognitive and social presence on cognitive load. *The Internet and Higher Education*, *31*, 11–19. doi:10.1016/j.iheduc.2016.05.003

Leahy, W., & Sweller, J. (2011). Cognitive load theory, modality of presentation and the transient information effect. *Applied Cognitive Psychology*, *25*(6), 943–951. doi:10.1002/acp.1787

Leppink, J., & van den Heuvel, A. (2015a). The evolution of cognitive load theory and its application to medical education. *Perspectives on Medical Education*, *4*(3), 119–127. doi:10.100740037-015-0192-x PMID:26016429

Leppink, J., van Gog, T., Paas, F. G. W. C., & Sweller, J. (2015b). Cognitive load theory: Researching and planning teaching to maximise learning. Researching Medical Education. doi:10.1002/9781118838983.ch18

Leutner, D., Leopold, C., & Sumfleth, E. (2009). Cognitive load and science text comprehension: Effects of drawing and mentally imagining text content. *Computers in Human Behavior*, *25*(2), 284–289. doi:10.1016/j.chb.2008.12.010

Meguerdichian, M., Walker, K., & Bajaj, K. (2016). Working memory is limited: Improving knowledge transfer by optimizing simulation through cognitive load theory. *BMJ Simulation & Technology Enhanced Learning*, *2*(4), 131–138. doi:10.1136/bmjstel-2015-000098

Moreno, R. (2007). Optimising learning from animations by minimizing cognitive load: Cognitive and affective consequences of signaling and segmentation methods. *Applied Cognitive Psychology*, *21*(6), 765–781. doi:10.1002/acp.1348

Mukherji, B.R., Neuwirth, L.S. & Limonic. (2017). *Making the case for real diversity: Redefining underrepresented minority students in public universities*. Sage Open. doi:10.10.177/2158244017707796

Nelson, B. C., & Erlandson, B. E. (2008). Managing cognitive load in educational multi-user virtual environments: Reflection on design practice. *Educational Technology Research and Development*, *56*(5-6), 619–641. doi:10.100711423-007-9082-1

Neuwirth, L. S., Dacius, T. F. Jr, & Mukherji, B. R. (2018). Teaching neuroanatomy through a historical context. *Journal of Undergraduate Neuroscience Education*, *16*(2), E26–E31. PMID:30057504

Neuwirth, L. S., Ebrahimi, A., Mukherji, B. R., & Park, L. (2018). Addressing diverse college students and interdisciplinary learning experiences through online virtual laboratory instruction: A theoretical approach to error-based learning in biopsychology. In A. Ursyn (Ed.), *Visual Approaches to Cognitive Eductaion with Technology Integration.* https://www.igi-global.com/chapter/addressing-diverse-college-students-and-interdisciplinary-learning-experiences-through-online-virtual-laboratory-instructions/195070

Neuwirth, L. S., Ebrahimi, A., Mukherji, B. R., & Park, L. (2019). Addressing diverse college students and interdisciplinary learning experiences through online virtual laboratory instruction: A theoretical approach to error-based learning in biopsychology. *Virtual Reality in Education: Breakthroughs in Research and Practice*, 511-531. https://www.igi-global.com/chapter/addressing-diverse-college-students-and-interdisciplinary-learning-experiences-through-online-virtual-laboratory-instructions/195070

Neuwirth, L. S., & Ros, M. (2021). Comparisons between first person point-of-view 180° video virtual reality head-mounted display and 3D video computer display in teaching undergraduate neuroscience students stereotaxic surgeries. *Front. Virtual Reality, 2*, 706653. Advance online publication. doi:10.3389/frvir.2021.706653

Nyachwaya, J. M., & Gillaspie, M. (2016). Features of representations in general chemistry textbooks: A peek through the lens of the cognitive load theory. *Chemistry Education Research and Practice, 17*, 58–71. doi:10.1039/C5RP00140D

Paas, F. G. W. C., Renkl, A., & Sweller, J. (2010a). Cognitive load theory and instructional design: Recent developments. *Educational Psychologist, 38*(1), 1–4. doi:10.1207/S15326985EP3801_1

Paas, F. G. W. C., Tuovinen, J. E., Tabbers, H., & Van Gerven, P. W. M. (2010b). Cognitive load measurement as a means to advance cognitive load theory. *Educational Psychologist, 38*(1), 63–71. doi:10.1207/S15326985EP3801_8

Paas, F. G. W. C., van Gog, T., & Sweller, J. (2010). Cognitive load theory: New conceptualizations, specifications, and integrative research perspectives. *Educational Psychology Review, 22*(2), 115–121. doi:10.100710648-010-9133-8

Paas, F. G. W. C., & Van Merriënboer, J. J. G. (1994). Instructional control of cognitive load in the training of complex cognitive tasks. *Educational Psychology Review, 6*(4), 351–371. doi:10.1007/BF02213420

Parham, G., Bing, E.G., Cuevas, A., Fisher, B., Skinner, J., & Mwanahamuntu, M. (2019). Creating a low-cost virtual reality surgical simulation to increase surgical oncology capacity and capability. *Ecancer Medical Science*.

Reedy, G. B. (2015). Using cognitive load theory to inform simulation design and practice. *Clinical Simulation in Nursing, 11*(8), 355–360. doi:10.1016/j.ecns.2015.05.004

Ros, M., Debien, B., Cyteval, C., Molinari, N., Gatto, F., & Lonjon, N. (2020). Applying an immersive tutorial in virtual reality to learning a new technique. *Neuro-Chirurgie, 66*(4), 212–218. doi:10.1016/j.neuchi.2020.05.006 PMID:32623059

Ros, M., & Neuwirth, L. S. (2020). Increasing global awareness of timely COVID-19 healthcare guidelines through FPV training tutorials: Portable public health crises teaching method. *Nurse Education Today, 91*(104479), 1–6. doi:10.1016/j.nedt.2020.104479 PMID:32473497

Ros, M., Neuwirth, L. S., Ng, S., Debien, B., Molinari, N., Gatto, F., & Lonjon, N. (2021). The Effects of an Immersive Virtual Reality Application in First Person Point-of-View, Video-Based, on The Learning and Generalized Performance of a Lumbar Puncture Medical Procedure. *Educational Technology Research and Development, 69*(3), 1529–1556. Advance online publication. doi:10.100711423-021-10003-w

Ros, M., & Trives, J. V. (2020). *Point-of-view recording device*. US Patent App. 16/341,070.

Ros, M., Trives, J. V., & Lonjon, N. (2017). From stereoscopic recording to virtual reality headsets: Designing a new way to learn surgery. *Neuro-Chirurgie, 63*(1), 1–5. doi:10.1016/j.neuchi.2016.08.004 PMID:28233530

Ros, M., Weaver, L., & Neuwirth, L. S. (2020). Virtual reality stereoscopic 180-degree video-based immersive environments: Applications for training surgeons and other medical professionals. In J. E. Stefaniak (Ed.), *Cases on Instructional Design and Performance Outcomes in Medical Education*. IGI Global. doi:10.4018/978-1-7998-5092-2.ch005

Schlairet, M. C., Schlairet, T. J., Sauls, D. H., & Bellflowers, L. (2015). Cognitive load, emotion, and performance in high-fidelity simulation among beginning nursing students: A pilot study. *The Journal of Nursing Education, 54*(3). Advance online publication. doi:10.3928/01484834-20150218-10 PMID:25692940

Sweller, J. (1994). Cognitive load theory, learning difficulty, and instructional design. *Learning and Instruction, 4*(4), 295–312. doi:10.1016/0959-4752(94)90003-5

Sweller, J. (2011). Chapter two – cognitive load theory. *Psychology of Learning and Motivation, 55*, 37–76. doi:10.1016/B978-0-12-387691-1.00002-8

Sweller, J., Ayres, P., & Kalyuga, S. (2011). Measuring cognitive load. In *Cognitive Load Theory. Explorations in the Learning Sciences, Instructional Systems and Performance Technologies* (Vol. 1, pp. 71–85). Springer., doi:10.1007/978-1-4419-8126-4_6

Sweller, J., Chandler, P., Tierney, P., & Cooper, M. (1990). Cognitive load as a factor in the structuring of technical material. *Journal of Experimental Psychology, 119*(2), 176–192. doi:10.1037/0096-3445.119.2.176

Van Gog, T., Paas, F., Marcus, N., Ayres, P., & Sweller, J. (2008). The mirror neuron system and observational learning: Implications for the effectiveness of dynamic visualizations. *Educational Psychology Review, 21*(1), 21–30. doi:10.100710648-008-9094-3

Van Merriënboer, J. J. G., & Sweller, J. (2005). Cognitive load theory and complex learning: Recent developments and future directions. *Educational Psychology Review, 17*(2), 147–177. doi:10.100710648-005-3951-0

Van Merriënboer, J. J. G., & Sweller, J. (2010). Cognitive load theory in health professional education: Design principles and strategies. *Medical Education, 44*, 85–93. doi:10.1111/j.1365-2923.2009.03498.x PMID:20078759

Wiedermann, J. (2003). Mirror neurons, embodied cognitive agents and imitation learning. *Computer Information, 22*, 545–559.

Wong, A., Leahy, W., Marcus, N., & Sweller, J. (2012). Cognitive load theory, the transient information effect and e-learning. *Learning and Instruction, 22*(6), 449–457. doi:10.1016/j.learninstruc.2012.05.004

Wouters, P., Paas, F. G. W. C., & Van Merriënboer, J. J. G. (2017). How to optimize learning from animated models: A review of guidelines based on cognitive load. *Review of Educational Research, 78*(3), 645–675. doi:10.3102/0034654308320320

Yung, H. I., & Paas, F. (2015). Effects of computer-based visual representation on mathematics learning and cognitive load. *Journal of Educational Technology & Society, 18*(4), 70–77.

Section 3
Physical Intervention

Chapter 7
Application of Virtual/ Augmented Reality in Surgical Procedures:
Bibliographical Review in Recent Developments

Israel Barrutia Barreto
Innova Scientific, Peru

Dometila Mamani Jilaja
Altiplano National University, Peru

Fabrizio Del Carpio Delgado
National University of Moquegua, Peru

Gino Frank Laque Córdova
Altiplano National University, Peru

Renzo Antonio Seminario Córdova
https://orcid.org/0000-0001-6992-5990
Innova Scientific, Peru

ABSTRACT

This chapter seeks to explore from the reflexivity approach the current state of virtual and augmented technologies in various surgical procedures, analyzing the most relevant technological progress as well as the latest practical applications that have been developed. Bibliographic, documentary, and descriptive were the methodologies of research; the information was collected from various scientific articles from indexed journals and websites, using keywords such as "virtual reality," "augmented reality," and "surgical procedure" in search engines. Furthermore, technological progress in various branches that include surgery is explored in this chapter, which is focused on the research and technology application of virtual and augmented reality as well as the challenges.

DOI: 10.4018/978-1-7998-8371-5.ch007

INTRODUCTION

Although it is important, the access to surgical care has been highly uneven in the world's population for a long time. In 2015, the number of people without access to affordable and quality surgical care increased to 67% of the world's population (Alkire *et al.*, 2015), a situation that has not improved with the pandemic that currently afflicts the world (Nepogodiev, 2020). For that, many entities have searched to establish surgery as an integral part of global health, in other words, everyone can access surgical care in an equitable way (Dare *et al.*, 2014). Worldwide, surgical diseases cover one third of the total amount of diseases that are presented. To the present day, this has generated efforts to reduce the great number of people who do not have access to affordable and secure surgery (Mazingi *et al.*, 2020).

Given the complexity of carrying out a surgical procedure, a great responsibility falls on the performance level of the surgeon, due to risks that imply to carry out a surgical intervention in a patient, such as loss of physical integrity or life itself (Hernández-Sánchez, 2017). However, the only reliable form that students have to acquire experience in surgery is to accumulate hours of practice; which is why there exists a direct relationship between the surgical experience of the surgeon and the intervention's success in a patient (Norman *et al.*, 2018). In addition, it is important to consider that surgeons also get older, a natural process for everyone. However, the ageing in a surgeon negatively affects its surgical abilities, so it could have serious repercussions in the integrity of patients (Speare, 2018).

With the finality to improve these procedures, various studies have been carried out during the last 60 years, and as result considerable progress have been made in important fields such as cardiovascular surgery, organ transplantation, joint replacement, minimally invasive surgery, etc. (McCulloh *et al.*, 2018). Furthermore, and maintaining ethics in the research, researchers should focus on generating surgical innovation, in such a way that can optimize benefits and minimize damages that can appear (Birchley *et al.*, 2020). With the exponential progress of technology and the experienced computational power during the last years, new technologies were implemented in medicine. Among these are virtual and augmented reality, immersive technologies that will be common in the medical field during the next decade (Tarassoli, 2019).

In this context, the objective of the present book chapter is to explore, from the reflexivity approach, the progress of virtual and augmented reality technologies in last years, oriented to its research and application in different surgical procedures, as well as challenges that are currently presented to a massive use of this tools in the future.

BACKGROUND

Virtual and Augmented Reality

Virtual Reality can be defined as virtual objects within a simulation or artificial recreation of some situation or real-life setting created by a computer, causing in the user a sense of immersion through sense stimulations (Rebbani *et al.*, 2021). Although there are different definitions, virtual reality mainly focuses on concepts of presence, telepresence and immersion (Kardong-Edgren *et al.*, 2019). To interact with such a virtual environment, users need to use input elements that go from a keyboard or joystick, until a specialized glove. Output elements go from monitors until glasses or virtual reality headset, capable of allowing the user see, hear, smell or feel what happens within this realistic form simulation (*Cipresso et al.*, 2018).

On the other hand, augmented reality can be defined as the mix of virtual reality with real world using the integration of virtual elements in the user environment (Rebbant *et al.*, 2021). Systems of augmented reality commonly require a geospatial datum to locate the virtual element, a visual marker, a camera, a display screen and a good capacity of processing for charts, animations and images (Cipresso *et al.*, 2018). Doing so, the traditional concept of experience has been revolutionized, beyond the acquired commonly by our senses or through instruments. These so-called simulated experiences recently are acquiring great importance in diverse fields, especially in medicine (Gutiérrez, 2020).

Besides these two mentioned realities, there is usually talk about a third, known as mixed reality. Although usually confused with augmented reality, for a long time there was no clear definition of what was, even generating several contradictions among scientists (Speicher *et al.*, 2019). In recent research, a more up-to-date definition of mixed reality makes a difference in the fact that these systems integrate virtual reality in the physical world, instead of just layering it (Lungu *et al.*, 2021).

Surgical Procedures

Surgery is defined as a branch of medicine that modifies the human anatomy in a non-reversible way using invasive procedures. This includes various organs, apparatus and systems in the body, depending on the problem (Hernández-Sánchez, 2017). Among the main surgical procedures are vascular, heart and general surgeries, of which the first two have a great risk of post-operative mortality in comparison with the last (Kummer *et al.*, 2020). It should be noted that all surgical intervention carries a risk in the patient, even requiring post-operative care. Some factors of risk are old age, poor health, urgency, etc. (Myles & Mawine, 2020).

Post-operative care results in an important part of an intervention by the fact that even after this may occur a series of negative effects in patient's health, mainly within 24 hours after due to residual effect of regional or general anesthesia (Dávila *et al.*, 2021). This discomfort appearing product for a surgical procedure or its complications are known as post-operative pain. Although there is a progress in post-operative pain's control using drugs and techniques, this is not yet handled the right way, including in developed nations (Pérez-Guerrero *et al.*, 2017).

According to the Lancet Commission on Global Surgery, around 313 million surgical interventions are carried out per year at the global level, whose success rate is measured through the number of postoperative deaths (Nepogodiev *et al.*, 2019). Annually in the United States, 1.5 million of patients suffer some medical complication during a surgery, while 150 thousand die in 30 days of such intervention (Bihorac *et al.*, 2019). On the other hand, patients who die after an operation cover 7.7% of the total number of deaths globally, being the third cause of deaths most important in the world, after heart diseases and heart attacks (Nepogodiev *et al.*, 2019).

MAIN FOCUS OF THE CHAPTER

Current Situation of Surgery

In recent years, modern surgery has experienced quick progress in different ways. On the one hand, it extended the execution of minimally invasive surgeries, in which interventions were performed using long and flexible surgical instruments introduced by small incisions or natural orifices, instead of large incisions in open surgeries (Runciman *et al.*, 2019). Although this technique became popular due to the large number of clinical benefits it presented, it is accompanied by a loss of direct vision and tactile feedback in the responsible surgeon, being necessary methods of indirect vision to carry out the operation (Bernhardt *et al.*, 2017).

Technological advances, on the other hand, allowed the creation of advanced devices which perform more quick and clear diagnostics. Among the most recent innovations are vision 8k, 3D cameras, 3D printing, telesurgery using robotic systems, 5G mobile phone, etc. (Di Nardo *et al.*, 2020). This implementation of technological advances in the execution of surgical procedures, known as robotic surgery, has experienced a strong diffusion in recent years in a wide range of surgical procedures (Sheetz *et al.*, 2020). This tendency has been subject of attention lately due to its ability to reduce the amount of surgeon's unintentional inaccuracies during an operation and, consequently, get more accurate results (Gumbs *et al.*, 2020).

However, it should be noted the disastrous effect that had pandemic in surgical procedures. Seeking to support patients of COVID-19, a lot of non-urgent operations were postponed and others canceled directly, in search to have available beds to these new patients (Myles & Maswime, 2020). Eventually, this decision generated a crisis about the access to surgical care, because patients not only were seen affected by an economic crisis, but their diseases were still developing due to lack of a correct treatment. Was this context which allowed the generation of innovators strategies to fight challenges of this crisis (Billig & Sears, 2020).

VIRTUAL AND AUGMENTED REALITY POTENTIAL IN SURGERY

Both virtual and augmented reality have the potential to bring digital health care to the practice, having the potential to allow the integration, visualization, interaction and diffusion of health information in real time. Although it is already implemented in other fields, it is still necessary to implement in a wide way the use of these technologies in health care (Desselle *et al.*, 2020).

Medical Training

For decades, the only way that medicine's students have to acquire technical experience was working in the operating theatres under supervision of experienced surgeons (Li *et al.*, 2017). In addition, with the introduction of the robotic in surgical field, surgeons saw the necessity of training in handling of these new equipment. In this context, in recent years the interest between surgeons to search more efficient alternatives to receive these training has grown (Lee *et al.*, 2011). The current situation in surgical studies requires more effective and efficient methods to perform this training, due to a higher workload in medicine's students for the progressive decrease of total hours of residence (Lee & Lee, 2018).

Consequently, virtual reality has been strongly explored for several years by doctors and researchers. These have approached the study effects of a simulation using virtual reality in fields such as physical rehabilitation, pain management, surgical training, anatomic education, among others (Li *et al.*, 2017). Through the implementation of these technologies, it is possible to develop digital models of learning in areas such as basic science, learning based on scenarios, crisis management, etc. (Desselle *et al.*, 2020). It should also be noted that the augmented reality's ability to convey information in real time would allow one surgeon to advise another in the development of complex surgeries, even being a great distance from the place (Kerr, 2020).

Virtual and augmented reality application in surgeries remains a study object and its utility is still under investigation in depth. This due to previous results showed the application of virtual reality technology in medical training can be highly effective in some specialties, and have no important effect in others (Samadbeik *et al.*, 2018).

Surgical Procedures

Augmented reality systems have important applications in surgical procedures mainly for their ability to provide the surgeon a great amount of information in real time using processed images by computer (Vávra *et al.*, 2017). These virtual reality systems also allow this data visualization in real time, but also, a simulator with this technology can be used by surgeons to training tasks or one more effective prior planning of surgical procedures (Kim *et al.*, 2017).

For these reasons, there exists an interest growing in implementing these technologies in surgery, looking to improve the security and the effectiveness of surgical procedures. In the same way, the augmented reality has proven useful in the execution of surgical procedures, such as orthopedic surgery, of pancreas, neurosurgeries (Desselle *et al.*, 2020). In addition, the increase in robotic assistants to different types of surgery encouraged the need for more training methods, where the virtual reality is also useful implemented in novel simulators (Schreuder *et al.*, 2014).

VIRTUAL AND AUGMENTED REALITY APPLICATIONS

Technologies of virtual and augmented reality have been strongly studied during recent years to their application in several areas within the surgery. Below are some of the most relevant applications.

Robotic Surgery

Some technological advances oriented to surgical procedures can be manually controlled by surgeons. The correct use of these technological advances requires previous training, for which is useful a simulation through virtual reality (Diana & Marescaux, 2015).

Minimally Invasive Surgery

Also called laparoscopy, in this area can be used the augmented reality to create a virtual layer over what observe the surgeon. Doing so, is enabled to project the virtual planning and relevant information of the procedure directly on the patient, therefore the doctor can keep sight constantly in its work area, without necessity to search such information in near monitors (Meulstee et al., 2019).

Oral and Maxillofacial Surgery

The main application area of virtual and augmented reality within odontology. Within this area, surgeons can work with corrections of dental or facial deformities, post resection maxillofacial reconstruction of cancer to facial fractures (Ayoub & Pulijala, 2019).

Plastic Surgery

In all surgical procedures it is important to have detailed and precise knowledge of the patient's anatomical structure. In plastic surgery, this necessity is even more important because the surgery results are directly connected with the external appearance of the patient (Kim et al., 2017).

Orthopedic Surgery

Orthopedic surgery, just like trauma, mainly covers processes such as reduction of bone fractures or arthroscopies. To carry out such processes, it is required to implement plates or implants for proper repair of the infected area (Negrillo-Cárdenas et al., 2020).

Neurosurgery

Branch of surgery that is focused on neurosurgical diseases such as hydrocephalus, brain trauma, brain tumors, etc. Procedures in neurosurgery require a large number of personnel, dedicated spaces and specialized post-operative care (Servadei et al., 2018).

Spine Surgery

Branch of surgery that include procedures as kyphoplasty, foraminotomy and laminectomy in regions as cervical, thoracic and lumbar spine (Steinberger & Qureshi, 2020). These interventions are considered high-risk for causing damage to the spine, nerves or vascular (Yuk *et al.*, 2020).

Table 1 lists some possible benefits of the applications of virtual and augmented reality technologies in branches of surgery mentioned above.

Table 1. Possible virtual and augmented reality applications in branches of surgery

Area	Application	Reference
Robotic Surgery	Augmented reality technology to improve security and efficacy of surgical procedures assisted by images guided-robots.	Diana y Marescaux (2015).
	Training to develop surgical skills with robotic instruments.	Bric *et al.* (2016).
Minimally Invasive Surgery	Ergonomic solutions to keep the surgeon's attention in its work using portable augmented reality systems.	Cutolo (2018).
	Performance of surgical procedures in reduced time and workload.	Glas (2017).
Oral and Maxillofacial Surgery	Support in the intervention planning due to the importance of structures of this zone, included nerves and long veins.	Kwon *et al.* (2018).
	Support in procedures as jaw reconstruction, distraction osteogenesis, orthognathic surgery, salivary gland operations, facial graft transplant, etc.	Joda *et al.* (2019).
Plastic Surgery	Anatomy visualization and more natural appearance of the patient using 3D simulation.	Kim *et al.* (2017).
	Predicting outcomes of aesthetic procedures using virtual reality systems.	Sayadi *et al.* (2019).
Orthopedic Surgery	Prior planning to the intervention using a virtual realignment of fractured bone to be repaired.	Negrillo-Cárdenas *et al.* (2020).
	Direct visualization in the work area of appropriate trajectories for implant insertion.	Jud *et al.* (2020).
Neurosurgery	Neuronavigation using a 3D model with anatomic details projected in the field and updated in real time.	Meola *et al.* (2017).
	Identify deep intracranial structures with facilities using augmented reality.	Guha *et al.* (2017).
Spine Surgery	Virtual reality application to preoperative and postoperative visualization of complex conditions in spine.	Yuk *et al.* (2020).
	Augmented reality application to assistance is patient anatomy visualization and predefined drilling paths in real time.	Vadalà *et al.* (2020).

Virtual and Augmented Reality Deployment

Deployment of virtual and augmented reality technologies in surgical procedures has long been explored, deriving in the development of available commercial products to different tasks (Hertz *et al.*, 2018). Most of these new systems have been the object of various studies to verify its functionality and utility in surgical procedures. On the other hand, there are systems that, although not originally conceived for surgery application, have also been studied to explore the possibility of applying them in that field.

The main field of virtual reality application consists in the development of simulators with this technology. For a long time, the only way to improve the performance in these interventions was working in the operations area, learning at the cost of risking patients' lives (Cuschieri, 2006). A great number of prior studies already confirmed advantages to practice medicine procedures with virtual simulators, without mention that the integrity of any patient was not put at risk, product of obvious inexperience in medicine students (De Visser *et al.*, 2011).

This led to a strong deployment of these simulators in the last decade, mainly in several programs of minimally invasive surgery training. These simulators have a great number of training modules with realistic recreations of the human anatomy and relevant surgical tasks, as well as the necessary feedback (Lee & Lee, 2018).

The most popular robotic assistant in recent decades has been the surgical system da Vinci, a platform for minimally invasive surgeries assisted by robots. This system is already massively implemented in more than 60 countries around the world and has been used in millions of surgeries to the present day (Azizian *et al.,* 2019). The fourth version of this assistant was released in 2014 under the name of Da Vinci Xi Surgical System (Van der Schans *et al.*, 2020), and a more up-to-date version was released in 2017 under the name Da Vinci X, whose components are appreciated in Figure 1.

Being this important assistant to get a good performance in the work of surgeons, it has its own simulator of virtual reality to training tasks with more than 30 exercises to improve skills in the use of such robotic platform (Walliczek *et al.*, 2016).

Figure 1. Da Vinci X Surgical System.
Source: Azizian et al. (2019).

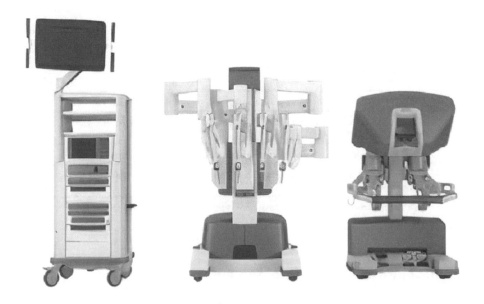

Regarding augmented reality, these systems have assisted surgeons for decades, being used for the first time in 1986 in neurosurgery. The efficacy of augmented reality systems in its beginnings was limited to the grade of interest structures deformation, a situation that was changing with the evolution of computers (Bernhardt *et al.*, 2017). Lately, the implementation of this technology has focused on the development of head-mounted displays (HMDs). Commercial models of this type have been developed, many of which have cameras, videos and accelerometers that follow the positions of the surgeon's head, and include some of them detect gestures of hands or the direction of his gaze (McKnight *et al.*, 2020).

One of the most famous devices of augmented reality in recent years is Google Glass, developed by Google Inc. This portable device had various characteristics that gave them great utility in several areas, both related and unrelated to surgery (Wei *et al.*, 2018). Its importance within surgery was that it incorporated a digital display in the vision of the user without limiting the natural vision of his environment, among other characteristics such as built-in camera, Bluetooth and Wi-Fi connection, web search, etc. (Chang *et al.*, 2016). Although this product is currently discontinued, during its lifetime it was the chosen device to research augmented reality in surgery thanks to its high quality, which was difficult to replicate by the portable devices that come after (McKnight *et al.*, 2020).

In table 2 studies carried out on some of the most important commercial products concerning to the application of virtual or augmented reality technologies in surgical procedures were explored.

Table 2. Studies on commercial products in virtual and augmented reality surgery

Product	Area	Results	Reference
Da Vinci Surgical Skills Simulator	Laparoscopy	Training in laparoscopy with the simulator can improve a surgeon's skills with a correct academic program.	Davila *et al.* (2018).
		Previous experience does not generate a significant difference in surgeons' performance in the simulator, being of intuitive use.	Moglia *et al.* (2018).
Google Glass	Shoulder surgery	Remote communication with expert surgeons for advice on decisions during full shoulder replacement surgery.	Chang *et al.* (2016).
	Prostatectomy	Improvement in monitoring of vital signs during this operation, but without effect in technical skills of surgeons.	Iqbal *et al.* (2016).
	Plastic surgery	Plastic surgeons rated the device as comfortable and useful to capture images of quality during operations.	Sinkin *et al.* (2016).
RobotiX Mentor	Robotic surgery	Positively rated by novice students of surgery as a useful tool to improve their skills in robotic surgery.	Whittaker *et al.* (2016).
		To allow a correct training in advance procedures of suture, independent of the previous experience.	Leijte *et al.* (2020).
	Thoracic lobectomy	It is a supporting tool useful to training in thoracic lobectomies thanks to specialized modules of the simulator.	Whittaker *et al.* (2019).
HoloLens	Orthopedic surgery	The utility of an augmented reality device was validated in the development of a hybrid simulator to hip arthroplasty.	Condino *et al.* (2018).
	Laparoscopy	Known as a visual support tool which can improve the performance of novice surgeons in laparoscopy operations.	Al Janabi *et al.* (2019).
ClarifEye	Spine surgery	Live intraoperative feedback with augmented reality during surgical interventions minimally invasive in the spine.	Hamilton-Basich (2021).

RECOMMENDATIONS

At the end of the development of a new technology system, this needs to go through a validation process to determine if its operation is expected according to what is needed. Although there exist various criteria to verify the functionality of a system, to systems of virtual and augmented reality, is common that first related studies be oriented to verify in the device three of the five types validation: of criteria, content and construct (Schijven & Jakimowicz, 2003; Hertz *et al.*, 2018; Whittaker *et al.*, 2019; McKnight *et al.*, 2020):

- The criterion validation focuses on measuring the correct index of realism and acceptance perceived for the user with regard to the new technology in question.
- The content validation focuses on analyzing the new device's efficacy as an instructive apparatus. This can be done using a bibliographic research or interviews to expert surgeons in the corresponding field.

- The construct validation focuses on analyzing the skill of such devices to differentiate novices from experts. This is achieved using experiments with a group of participants from different levels of experience.

In contrast, a product which has already been released at the market does not need to go through this validation again because its finality and its characteristics are public information revealed by the developer company. This information is sufficient for researchers to speculate about alternative uses of the product in question, based on existing deficiencies in these new areas. On this basis, the challenge consists in validate and refuse these speculations using the testing with a group of qualified participants (Wei *et al.*, 2018; Al Janabi *et al.*, 2019).

FUTURE RESEARCH DIRECTIONS

Technologies of virtual and augmented reality are on their way of having a greater presence on the surgical stage, next to the constant evolution of computational and miniaturization power (Tarassoli, 2019). Systems of virtual reality are in constant progress, which within the surgery field can mean an important improvement in the realism and precision of future simulators for the training of medical personnel (Rizzetto *et al.*, 2020). This idea is supported for the current tendency referent to these technologies, which indicate that its importance would see increased over the next few years regarding research and publication about its use in surgery (Muñon-Saavedra *et al.*, 2020).

On the other hand, augmented reality would be used mainly as a human-computer interface, working together with surgeons to further enhance its performance (Vávra *et al.*, 2017). Although its benefits have already been analyzed, portable devices of augmented reality still need to establish it as a useful technology in the field because there are still practical and ethical challenges related with the medical implementation of these devices (McKnight *et al.*, 2020). These systems of augmented reality become intertwined with surgical robotic systems as their use becomes more widespread, increasing chances of success of any surgical procedure (Azizian et al., 2019).

CONCLUSION

This book chapter shows how the execution of surgical procedures have been influenced in recent years thanks to technology advancements. In recent years, there has been great interest to improve methods of training in surgery, especially with the appearance of new procedures and the introduction of technological advances oriented to improve the efficiency of surgical interventions. With the global pandemic that is currently being experienced and its negative effects generally in medicine, technologies such as virtual and augmented reality have become more important as innovative elements to improve several surgical processes and be able to deal with new challenges.

With its potential, virtual reality will be capable of revolutionizing medicine studies using the development of all kinds of simulators, with the ability to train surgeons in the execution of different procedures and in the use of robotic equipment thanks to its high level of realism. Augmented reality, although already massified in certain grades thanks to big companies, is still a strong candidate to its massification in the surgery field due to its ability to give vital information to the surgeon in a comfortable and fast way. A great interest in the research related to these technologies can be appreciated, which has remained latent for many years and has generated a great number of discoveries and innovations.

This joint work of scientists, doctors, patients, software developers and device manufactures, promises to revolutionize health care in a future using virtual powerful technologies. For that, it can be inferred that they will be tools widely used within medicine in a few years, a product of the research currently carried out by various entities. As the potential of these tools is clear, it will be a matter of doctors and researchers trying to take advantage of it using the development of new technologies and the research of new applications, in such a way that the work of doctors will make it easier and the treatment of patients more effective.

REFERENCES

Al Janabi, H., Aydin, A., Palaneer, S., Macchione, N., Al-Jabir, A., Khan, M., Dasgupta, P., & Ahmed, K. (2019). Effectiveness of the HoloLens mixed-reality headset in minimally invasive surgery: A simulation-based feasibility study. *Surgical Endoscopy*, *34*(3), 1143–1149. doi:10.100700464-019-06862-3 PMID:31214807

Alkire, B., Raykar, N., Shrime, M., Weiser, T., Bickler, S., Rose, J., Nutt, C., Greenberg, S., Kotagal, M., Riesel, J., Esquivel, M., Uribe-Letiz, T., Molina, G., Roy, N., Mearat, J., & Farmer, P. (2015). Global access to surgical care: A modelling study. *The Lancet. Global Health*, *3*(6), e316–e323. doi:10.1016/S2214-109X(15)70115-4 PMID:25926087

Ayoub, A., & Pulijala, Y. (2019). The application of virtual reality and augmented reality in Oral & Maxillofacial Surgery. *BMC Oral Health*, *19*(1), 1–8. doi:10.118612903-019-0937-8 PMID:31703708

Azizian, M., Liu, M., Khalaji, I., & DiMaio, S. (2019). The da Vinci Surgical System. In The Encyclopedia of medical robotics: Volume 1 Minimally Invasive Surgical Robotics (pp. 3-28). World Scientific. doi:10.1142/9789813232266_0001

Bernhardt, S., Nicolau, S., Soler, L., & Doignon, C. (2017). The status of augmented reality in laparoscopic surgery as of 2016. *Medical Image Analysis*, *37*, 66–90. doi:10.1016/j.media.2017.01.007 PMID:28160692

Bihorac, A., Ozrazgat-Baslanti, T., Ebadi, A., Motaei, A., Madkour, M., Pardalos, P., Lipori, G., Hogan, W., Efron, P., Moore, F., Moldawer, L., Wang, D., Hobson, C., Rashidi, P., Li, X., & Momcilovic, P. (2019). MySurgeryRisk: Development and validation of a machine-learning risk algorithm for major complications and death after surgery. *Annals of Surgery*, *269*(4), 652–662. doi:10.1097/SLA.0000000000002706 PMID:29489489

Billig, J., & Sears, E. (2020). The compounding access problem for surgical care: Innovations in the post-COVID era. *Annals of Surgery*, *272*(2), e47–e48. doi:10.1097/SLA.0000000000004085 PMID:32675492

Birchley, G., Ives, J., Huxtable, R., & Blazeby, J. (2020). Conceptualising surgical innovation: An eliminativist proposal. *Health Care Analysis*, *28*(1), 73–97. doi:10.100710728-019-00380-y PMID:31327091

Bric, J., Lumbard, D., Frelich, M., & Gould, J. (2016). Current state of virtual reality simulation in robotic surgery training: A review. *Surgical Endoscopy, 30*(6), 2169–2178. doi:10.100700464-015-4517-y PMID:26304107

Chang, J., Tsui, L., Yeung, K., Yip, S., & Leung, G. (2016). Surgical vision: Google Glass and surgery. *Surgical Innovation, 23*(4), 422–426. doi:10.1177/1553350616646477 PMID:27146972

Cipresso, P., Giglioli, I., Raya, M., & Riva, G. (2018). The past, present, and future of virtual and augmented reality research: A network and cluster analysis of the literature. *Frontiers in Psychology, 9*, 2086. doi:10.3389/fpsyg.2018.02086 PMID:30459681

Condino, S., Turini, G., Parchi, P., Viglialoro, R., Piolanti, N., Gesi, M., Ferrari, M., & Ferrari, V. (2018). How to build a patient-specific hybrid simulator for orthopaedic open surgery: Benefits and limits of mixed-reality using the Microsoft HoloLens. *Journal of Healthcare Engineering, 2018*, 1–12. Advance online publication. doi:10.1155/2018/5435097 PMID:30515284

Cuschieri, A. (2006). Nature of human error. Implications for surgical practice. *Annals of Surgery, 244*(5), 642–648. doi:10.1097/01.sla.0000243601.36582.18 PMID:17060751

Cutolo, F. (2018). Augmented Reality in Image-Guided Surgery. Encyclopedia of Computer Graphics and Games, 1-11. doi:10.1007/978-3-319-08234-9_78-1

Dare, A., Grimes, E., Gillies, R., Greenberg, S., Hagander, L., Meara, J., & Leather, A. (2014). Global surgery: Defining an emerging global health field. *Lancet, 384*(9961), 2245–2247. doi:10.1016/S0140-6736(14)60237-3 PMID:24853601

Davila, D., Helm, M., Frelich, M., Gould, J., & Goldblatt, M. (2018). Robotic skills can be aided by laparoscopic training. *Surgical Endoscopy, 32*(6), 2683–2688. doi:10.100700464-017-5963-5 PMID:29214515

Dávila, M., Ceh, J., Balseca, S., & Rendón, M. (2021). Cuidado de enfermería durante el postoperatorio inmediato. *Revista Eugenio Espejo, 15*(2), 18-27. https://bit.ly/3iuDEoE

De Visser, H., Watson, M., Salvado, O., & Passenger, J. D. (2011). Progress in virtual reality simulators for surgical training and certification. *The Medical Journal of Australia, 194*(S4), S38–S40. doi:10.5694/j.1326-5377.2011.tb02942.x PMID:21401487

Desselle, M., Brown, R., James, A., Midwinter, M., Powell, S., & Woodruff, M. (2020). Augmented and virtual reality in surgery. *Computing in Science & Engineering, 22*(3), 18–26. doi:10.1109/MCSE.2020.2972822

Di Nardo, D., Eberspacher, C., & Palazzini, G. (2020). Technology spreading in healthcare: A novel era in medicine and surgery? *Journal of Gastric Surgery, 2*(2), 45–48. doi:10.36159/jgs.v2i2.26

Diana, M., & Marescaux, J. (2015). Robotic surgery. *Journal of British Surgery, 102*(2), e15–e28. doi:10.1002/bjs.9711 PMID:25627128

Glas, H. (2017). *Image guided surgery and the added value of augmented reality* (Master's thesis). University of Twente. https://bit.ly/3xXsgIh

Guha, D., Alotaibi, N., Nguyen, N., Gupta, S., McFaul, C., & Yang, V. (2017). Augmented reality in neurosurgery: A review of current concepts and emerging applications. *The Canadian Journal of Neurological Sciences, 44*(3), 235–245. doi:10.1017/cjn.2016.443 PMID:28434425

Gumbs, A., De Simone, B., & Chouillard, E. (2020). Searching for a better definition of robotic surgery: Is it really different from laparoscopy? *Mini-invasive Surgery, 4*. Advance online publication. doi:10.20517/2574-1225.2020.110

Gutiérrez, A. (2020). ¿Un mundo nuevo? Realidad virtual, realidad aumentada, inteligencia artificial, humanidad mejorada, Internet de las cosas. *Arbor, 196*(797), a572–a572. doi:10.3989/arbor.2020.797n3009

Hamilton-Basich, M. (2021). *Philips Launches ClarifEye Augmented Reality Surgical Navigation.* Axis Imaging News. https://bit.ly/36QGmj1

Hernández-Sánchez, R. (2017). El cirujano. *Revista de Sanidad Militar, 71*(2), 177–184. https://bit.ly/3xXV8QX

Hertz, A., George, E., Vaccaro, C. & Brand, T. (2018). Head-to-head comparison of three virtual-reality robotic surgery simulators. *Journal of the Society of Laparoendoscopic & Robotic Surgeons, 22*(1). doi:10.4293/JSLS.2017.00081

Iqbal, M., Aydin, A., Lowdon, A., Ahmed, H., Muir, G., Khan, M., Dasgupta, P., & Ahmed, K. (2016). The effectiveness of Google GLASS as a vital signs monitor in surgery: A simulation study. *International Journal of Surgery, 36*, 293–297. doi:10.1016/j.ijsu.2016.11.013 PMID:27833004

Joda, T., Gallucci, G., Wismeijer, D., & Zitzmann, N. (2019). Augmented and virtual reality in dental medicine: A systematic review. *Computers in Biology and Medicine, 108*, 93–100. doi:10.1016/j.compbiomed.2019.03.012 PMID:31003184

Jud, L., Fotouhi, J., Andronic, O., Aichmair, A., Osgood, G., Navab, N., & Farshad, M. (2020). Applicability of augmented reality in orthopedic surgery–A systematic review. *BMC Musculoskeletal Disorders, 21*(1), 1–13. doi:10.118612891-020-3110-2 PMID:32061248

Kardong-Edgren, S., Farra, S., Alinier, G., & Young, H. (2019). A call to unify definitions of virtual reality. *Clinical Simulation in Nursing, 31*, 28–34. doi:10.1016/j.ecns.2019.02.006

Kerr, R. (2020). Surgery in the 2020s: Implications of advancing technology for patients and the workforce. *Future Healthcare Journal, 7*(1), 46–49. doi:10.7861/fhj.2020-0001 PMID:32104765

Kim, Y., Kim, H., & Kim, Y. (2017). Virtual reality and augmented reality in plastic surgery: A review. *Archives of Plastic Surgery, 44*(3), 179–187. doi:10.5999/aps.2017.44.3.179 PMID:28573091

Kummer, B., Hazan, R., Merkler, A., Kamel, H., Willey, J., Middlesworth, W., Yaghi, S., Marshall, R., Elkind, M., Boehme, A., & Boehme, A. (2020). A multilevel analysis of surgical category and individual patient-level risk factors for postoperative stroke. *The Neurohospitalist, 10*(1), 22–28. doi:10.1177/1941874419848590 PMID:31839861

Kwon, H., Park, Y., & Han, J. (2018). Augmented reality in dentistry: A current perspective. *Acta Odontologica Scandinavica, 76*(7), 497–503. doi:10.1080/00016357.2018.1441437 PMID:29465283

Lee, G., & Lee, M. (2018). Can a virtual reality surgical simulation training provide a self-driven and mentor-free skills learning? Investigation of the practical influence of the performance metrics from the virtual reality robotic surgery simulator on the skill learning and associated cognitive workloads. *Surgical Endoscopy*, *32*(1), 62–72. doi:10.100700464-017-5634-6 PMID:28634632

Lee, J., Mucksavage, P., Sundaram, C., & McDougall, E. (2011). Best practices for robotic surgery training and credentialing. *The Journal of Urology*, *185*(4), 1191–1197. doi:10.1016/j.juro.2010.11.067 PMID:21334030

Leijte, E., de Blaauw, I., Rosman, C., & Botden, S. (2020). Assessment of validity evidence for the RobotiX robot assisted surgery simulator on advanced suturing tasks. *BMC Surgery*, *20*(1), 1–11. doi:10.118612893-020-00839-z PMID:32787831

Li, L., Yu, F., Shi, D., Shi, J., Tian, Z., Yang, J., Wang, X., & Jiang, Q. (2017). Application of virtual reality technology in clinical medicine. *American Journal of Translational Research*, *9*(9), 3867–3880. https://bit.ly/3rs5plE PMID:28979666

Lungu, A. J., Swinkels, W., Claesen, L., Tu, P., Egger, J., & Chen, X. (2021). A review on the applications of virtual reality, augmented reality and mixed reality in surgical simulation: An extension to different kinds of surgery. *Expert Review of Medical Devices*, *18*(1), 47–62. doi:10.1080/17434440.2021.1860750 PMID:33283563

Mazingi, D., Navarro, S., Bobel, M., Dube, A., Mbanje, C., & Lavy, C. (2020). Exploring the impact of COVID-19 on progress towards achieving global surgery goals. *World Journal of Surgery*, *44*(8), 2451–2457. doi:10.100700268-020-05627-7 PMID:32488665

McCulloch, P., Feinberg, J., Philippou, Y., Kolias, A., Kehoe, S., Lancaster, G., Donovan, J., Petrinic, T., Agha, R., & Pennell, C. (2018). Progress in clinical research in surgery and IDEAL. *Lancet*, *392*(10141), 88–94. doi:10.1016/S0140-6736(18)30102-8 PMID:29361334

McKnight, R., Pean, C., Buck, J., Hwang, J., Hsu, J., & Pierrie, S. (2020). Virtual reality and augmented reality—Translating surgical training into surgical technique. *Current Reviews in Musculoskeletal Medicine*, *13*(6), 663–674. doi:10.100712178-020-09667-3 PMID:32779019

Meola, A., Cutolo, F., Carbone, M., Cagnazzo, F., Ferrari, M., & Ferrari, V. (2017). Augmented reality in neurosurgery: A systematic review. *Neurosurgical Review*, *40*(4), 537–548. doi:10.100710143-016-0732-9 PMID:27154018

Meulstee, J., Nijsink, J., Schreurs, R., Verhamme, L., Xi, T., Delye, H., Borstlap, W., & Maal, T. (2019). Toward holographic-guided surgery. *Surgical Innovation*, *26*(1), 86–94. doi:10.1177/1553350618799552 PMID:30261829

Moglia, A., Ferrari, V., Melfi, F., Ferrari, M., Mosca, F., Cuschieri, A., & Morelli, L. (2018). Performances on simulator and da Vinci robot on subjects with and without surgical background. *Minimally Invasive Therapy & Allied Technologies*, *27*(6), 309–314. doi:10.1080/13645706.2017.1365729 PMID:28817346

Muñoz-Saavedra, L., Miró-Amarante, L., & Domínguez-Morales, M. (2020). Augmented and virtual reality evolution and future tendency. *Applied Sciences (Basel, Switzerland)*, *10*(1), 322. doi:10.3390/app10010322

Myles, P., & Maswime, S. (2020). Mitigating the risks of surgery during the COVID-19 pandemic. *Lancet, 396*(10243), 2–3. doi:10.1016/S0140-6736(20)31256-3 PMID:32479826

Negrillo-Cárdenas, J., Jiménez-Pérez, J., & Feito, F. (2020). The role of virtual and augmented reality in orthopedic trauma surgery: From diagnosis to rehabilitation. *Computer Methods and Programs in Biomedicine, 191,* 105407. doi:10.1016/j.cmpb.2020.105407 PMID:32120088

Nepogodiev, D. (2020). Global guidance for surgical care during the COVID-19 pandemic. *British Journal of Surgery, 107*(9), 1097–1103. doi:10.1002/bjs.11646 PMID:32293715

Nepogodiev, D., Martin, J., Biccard, B., Makupe, A., Bhangu, A., Ademuyiwa, A., ... Morton, D. (2019). Global burden of postoperative death. *Lancet, 393*(10170), 401. doi:10.1016/S0140-6736(18)33139-8 PMID:30722955

Norman, G., Grierson, L., Sherbino, J., Hamstra, S., Schmidt, H., & Mamede, S. (2018). Expertise in medicine and surgery. In K. Ericsson, R. Hoffman, A. Kozbelt, & A. Williams (Eds.), *The Cambridge handbook of expertise and expert performance* (pp. 331–355). Cambridge University Press. doi:10.1017/9781316480748.019

Pérez-Guerrero, A., Aragón, M., & Torres, L. (2017). Dolor postoperatorio: ¿hacia dónde vamos? *Revista de la Sociedad Española del Dolor, 24*(1), 1-3. https://bit.ly/3hTSxlc

Rebbani, Z., Azougagh, D., Bahatti, L., & Bouattane, O. (2021). Definitions and Applications of Augmented/Virtual Reality: A Survey. *International Journal (Toronto, Ont.), 9*(3), 279–285. doi:10.30534/ijeter/2021/21932021

Rizzetto, F., Bernareggi, A., Rantas, S., Vanzulli, A., & Vertemati, M. (2020). Immersive Virtual Reality in surgery and medical education: Diving into the future. *American Journal of Surgery, 220*(4), 856–857. doi:10.1016/j.amjsurg.2020.04.033 PMID:32386709

Runciman, M., Darzi, A., & Mylonas, G. (2019). Soft robotics in minimally invasive surgery. *Soft Robotics, 6*(4), 423–443. doi:10.1089oro.2018.0136 PMID:30920355

Samadbeik, M., Yaaghobi, D., Bastani, P., Abhari, S., Rezaee, R., & Garavand, A. (2018). The applications of virtual reality technology in medical groups teaching. *Journal of Advances in Medical Education & Professionalism, 6*(3), 123. https://bit.ly/3xXshMB PMID:30013996

Sayadi, L., Naides, A., Eng, M., Fijany, A., Chopan, M., Sayadi, J., Shaterian, A., Banyard, D., Evans, G., Vyas, R., & Widgerow, A. (2019). The new frontier: A review of augmented reality and virtual reality in plastic surgery. *Aesthetic Surgery Journal, 39*(9), 1007–1016. doi:10.1093/asjjz043 PMID:30753313

Schijven, M., & Jakimowicz, J. (2003). Construct validity. *Surgical Endoscopy, 17*(5), 803–810. doi:10.100700464-002-9151-9 PMID:12582752

Schreuder, H., Persson, J., Wolswijk, R., Ihse, I., Schijven, M., & Verheijen, R. (2014). Validation of a novel virtual reality simulator for robotic surgery. *TheScientificWorldJournal, 2014,* 1–10. Advance online publication. doi:10.1155/2014/507076 PMID:24600328

Servadei, F., Rossini, Z., Nicolosi, F., Morselli, C., & Park, K. (2018). The role of neurosurgery in countries with limited facilities: Facts and challenges. *World Neurosurgery*, *112*, 315–321. doi:10.1016/j.wneu.2018.01.047 PMID:29366998

Sheetz, K., Claflin, J., & Dimick, J. (2020). Trends in the adoption of robotic surgery for common surgical procedures. *JAMA Network Open*, *3*(1), e1918911–e1918911. doi:10.1001/jamanetworkopen.2019.18911 PMID:31922557

Sinkin, J., Rahman, O., & Nahabedian, M. (2016). Google Glass in the operating room: The plastic surgeon's perspective. *Plastic and Reconstructive Surgery*, *138*(1), 298–302. doi:10.1097/PRS.0000000000002307 PMID:27348661

Speare, J. (2018). El retiro del cirujano: ¿Por qué, cuándo y cómo debe retirarse un cirujano? *Anales Médicos de la Asociación Médica del Centro Médico ABC*, *63*(1), 73–79. https://bit.ly/3kI4RqH

Speicher, M., Hall, B., & Nebeling, M. (2019, May). What is mixed reality? In *Proceedings of the 2019 CHI Conference on Human Factors in Computing Systems* (pp. 1-15). 10.1145/3290605.3300767

Steinberger, J., & Qureshi, S. (2020). The Role of Augmented Reality and Virtual Reality in Contemporary Spine Surgery. *Contemporary Spine Surgery*, *21*(8), 1–5. doi:10.1097/01.CSS.0000689552.57650.21

Tarassoli, S. (2019). Artificial intelligence, regenerative surgery, robotics? What is realistic for the future of surgery? *Annals of Medicine and Surgery (London)*, *41*, 53–55. doi:10.1016/j.amsu.2019.04.001 PMID:31049197

Vadalà, G., De Salvatore, S., Ambrosio, L., Russo, F., Papalia, R., & Denaro, V. (2020). Robotic spine surgery and augmented reality systems: A state of the art. *Neurospine*, *17*(1), 88–100. doi:10.14245/ns.2040060.030 PMID:32252158

Van der Schans, E., Hiep, M., Consten, E., & Broeders, I. A. (2020). From Da Vinci Si to Da Vinci Xi: Realistic times in draping and docking the robot. *Journal of Robotic Surgery*, *14*(6), 835–839. doi:10.100711701-020-01057-8 PMID:32078114

Vávra, P., Roman, J., Zonča, P., Ihnát, P., Němec, M., Kumar, J., Habib, N., & El-Gendi, A. (2017). Recent development of augmented reality in surgery: A review. *Journal of Healthcare Engineering*, *2017*, 1–9. Advance online publication. doi:10.1155/2017/4574172 PMID:29065604

Walliczek, U., Förtsch, A., Dworschak, P., Teymoortash, A., Mandapathil, M., Werner, J., & Güldner, C. (2016). Effect of training frequency on the learning curve on the da Vinci Skills Simulator. *Head & Neck*, *38*(S1), E1762–E1769. doi:10.1002/hed.24312 PMID:26681572

Wei, N., Dougherty, B., Myers, A., & Badawy, S. (2018). Using Google Glass in surgical settings: Systematic review. *JMIR mHealth and uHealth*, *6*(3), e9409. doi:10.2196/mhealth.9409 PMID:29510969

Whittaker, G., Aydin, A., Raison, N., Kum, F., Challacombe, B., Khan, M. S., Dasgupta, P., & Ahmed, K. (2016). Validation of the RobotiX mentor robotic surgery simulator. *Journal of Endourology*, *30*(3), 338–346. doi:10.1089/end.2015.0620 PMID:26576836

Whittaker, G., Aydin, A., Raveendran, S., Dar, F., Dasgupta, P., & Ahmed, K. (2019). Validity assessment of a simulation module for robot-assisted thoracic lobectomy. *Asian Cardiovascular & Thoracic Annals*, 27(1), 23–29. doi:10.1177/0218492318813457 PMID:30417680

Yuk, F. J., Maragkos, G. A., Sato, K., & Steinberger, J. (2020). Current innovation in virtual and augmented reality in spine surgery. *Annals of Translational Medicine*, 9(1), 94. Advance online publication. doi:10.21037/atm-20-1132 PMID:33553387

ADDITIONAL READING

Barteit, S., Lanfermann, L., Bärnighausen, T., Neuhann, F., & Beiersmann, C. (2021). Augmented, Mixed, and Virtual Reality-Based Head-Mounted Devices for Medical Education: Systematic Review. *JMIR Serious Games*, 9(3), e29080. doi:10.2196/29080 PMID:34255668

Dennler, C., Bauer, D., Scheibler, A., Spirig, J., Götschi, T., Fürnstahl, P., & Farshad, M. (2021). Augmented reality in the operating room: A clinical feasibility study. *BMC Musculoskeletal Disorders*, 22(1), 1–9. doi:10.118612891-021-04339-w PMID:34006234

Elnikety, S., Badr, E., & Abdelaal, A. (2021). Surgical training fit for the future: The need for a change. *Postgraduate Medical Journal*. Advance online publication. doi:10.1136/postgradmedj-2021-139862 PMID:33941663

Godzik, J., Farber, S., Urakov, T., Steinberger, J., Knipscher, L., Ehredt, R., Tumialán, L., & Uribe, J. (2021). "Disruptive Technology" in Spine Surgery and Education: Virtual and Augmented Reality. *Operative Neurosurgery*, 21(Supplement_1), S85–S93. doi:10.1093/ons/opab114 PMID:34128065

Heinrich, F., Huettl, F., Schmidt, G., Paschold, M., Kneist, W., Huber, T., & Hansen, C. (2021). HoloPointer: A virtual augmented reality pointer for laparoscopic surgery training. *International Journal of Computer Assisted Radiology and Surgery*, 16(1), 161–168. doi:10.100711548-020-02272-2 PMID:33095424

Ivanov, V., Krivtsov, A., Strelkov, S., Gulyaev, D., Godanyuk, D., Kalakutsky, N.,... Yaremenko, A. (2021). Surgical navigation systems based on augmented reality technologies. https://arxiv.org/abs/2106.00727

Kovoor, J., Gupta, A., & Gladman, M. (2021). Validity and effectiveness of augmented reality in surgical education: A systematic review. *Surgery*, 170(1), 88–98. doi:10.1016/j.surg.2021.01.051 PMID:33744003

Lungu, A. J., Swinkels, W., Claesen, L., Tu, P., Egger, J. & Chen, X. (2021). A review on the applications of virtual reality, augmented reality and mixed reality in surgical simulation: an extension to different kinds of surgery. *Expert Review of Medical Devices, 18*(1), 47-62. .2021.1860750 doi:10.1080/17434440

Pears, M., & Konstantinidis, S. (2021). The Future of Immersive Technology in Global Surgery Education. *Indian Journal of Surgery*, 1-5. Advance online publication. doi:10.100712262-021-02998-6 PMID:34230785

Yeung, A., Tosevska, A., Klager, E., Eibensteiner, F., Laxar, D., Stoyanov, J., Glisic, M., Zeiner, S., Kulnik, S., Crutzen, R., Kimberger, O., Kletecka-Pulker, M., Atanasov, A., & Willschke, H. (2021). Virtual and augmented reality applications in medicine: Analysis of the scientific literature. *Journal of Medical Internet Research*, *23*(2), e25499. doi:10.2196/25499 PMID:33565986

KEY TERMS AND DEFINITIONS

Anatomy: Science that studies living beings, including human structure. It covers the study of the shape, topography, location, disposition, and relationship between the bodies of which it is composed.

Augmented Reality: Technology that offers interactive experiences by overlaying virtual elements over the user perception about the reality and allows an interaction in real time with them.

Medicine: Health science that focuses on the prevention, diagnostic, prognostic, and treatment of different health issues. Advanced studies are required for a person to practice medicine.

Simulation: The process of designing a model that resembles a real system and using it to describe its behavior, construct theories and hypotheses based on the observations, or foresee future behavior.

Surgery: Practice involving mechanical manipulation of anatomic structures for a medical purpose, is for removal or repair of any part of the body. The different kinds of surgery are classified according to urgency in three categories: emergency, urgent and elective.

Surgical Care: They occur in the post-surgical stage and consist of monitoring the patient's recovery after a surgical intervention and until he is fit to be discharged.

Technology: Consists in the creation of goods or services oriented to the resolution of problems using a body of scientific knowledge. These inventions can use it to transform the environment, solve problems, etc.

Virtual Reality: Realistic scenes and objects environments that are generated using computer technology and generate a sense of immersion in the user. Between their main uses are entertainment, medicine, and education.

Chapter 8
Improvements of Virtual and Augmented Reality for Advanced Treatments in Urology

Ranjit Barua
ⓘ https://orcid.org/0000-0003-2236-3876
CHST, Indian Institute of Engineering Science and Technology, Shibpur, India

Surajit Das
R. G. Kar Medical College and Hospital, India

ABSTRACT

Present signs of development in virtual and augmented reality have offered an important amount of inventive outfits into the customer market. Virtual reality (VR) technology has now affected the optimistic features of treatment. Surgeries in especially urology are constantly emerging, and the virtual reality model has become an important supplement in urologist teaching and training lists. This chapter provides a summary of the significance and varieties of virtual reality methods, their present applications in the area of urology (surgery), and upcoming implications.

1. INTRODUCTION

The idea of virtual reality (VR) includes the computational environs with which an operator can interact prominently (Hamacher et al., 2018). In medical uses, virtual reality is now being applied, particularly in the region of surgical simulation (Sutherland et al., 2019). As expertise improvements, virtual reality simulation will show a significant training role for together occupants and urologists previously in practice (Chinnock et al., 1994). This chapter inspects the history of virtual reality (VR), present advances, and its upcoming inferences for the area of urology. The idea of virtual reality (VR) includes the generation of computational environments with which an operator can involve directly (Linte et al., 2013). However,

DOI: 10.4018/978-1-7998-8371-5.ch008

several of the theoretical and applied basics of virtual reality (VR) were previously considered and trained in the 1980s, the enormously developed configurations of demonstrations, interactivity, instruments, and calculating power currently accessible in strategies recommend an innovative area of presentations to the medicinal-surgical region and also to urology in particular (Hamacher et al., 2018) (Moro et al., 2017). This development is also moving the medical science and health care specifically the surgical area (Tepper et al., 2017) (Ali et al., 2018). Fig.1. shows the involvement of VR/AR in modern medical science. Urology knowledge and surgical performs are continually developing and the simulation has become a significant match in urologist training programs (Hamacher et al., 2018). Virtual reality methods for the image-guided surgical procedure have been confirmed prospectively in the area of urology by ancillary direction for numerous complaints (Johnston et al., 2018). A growing number of preoperative imaging modalities have been applied to make complete surgical road maps (Del Pozo et al., 2019). The outlining of these surgical plans with the surgical idea of actual life has been created in dissimilar techniques like acoustic, electromagnetic, visual, etc. recommending the mixture of numerous methods to deliver a greater outcome (Sutherland et al., 2019). A real-time electromagnetic sensors was used percutaneous kidney access, which solves the inherent limitations of conventional approaches of kidney access, permitting exact, harmless, fast, and sucessful puncture of the renal collecting system (Lima et al., 2017). One of the difficulties of steering methods is soft-tissue deformations, needful positive images (Ali et al., 2018).

Figure 1. Involvement of VR and AR in modern medical science.

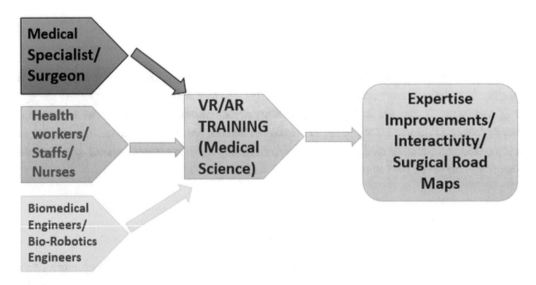

While the direction-finding surgeries deliver results equivalent to or better than traditional methods, most of the effort has been completed in comparatively minor groups of patients, therefore, the demanding studies with superior sample sizes (Smigelski et al., 2020). Virtual reality (VR) is a 3D, computational created environment that can be opened by a virtual reality headset, permitting individuals to engage themselves in this virtual world (Shah et al., 2001) (Sutherland et al., 2019). Augmented reality (AR) arrangements layer virtual evidence over a live camera feed into a receiver, or by a tablet device or smartphone (Sutherland et al., 2019). The improved step of revolution and successive decrease in the cost of types of machinery has revealed the opportunity to use virtual reality and augmented reality uses in conventional medical practice and education (Schenkman et al., 2008). This simulator could recover the knowledge curve for upcoming surgeons whereas decreasing patients' contact to possible risk or trauma (Hamacher et al., 2016). Fig. 2 shows how the virtual and augmented reality involves in modern urological surgery (Kidney stone remove). An increasing amount of imaging modalities of preoperative have been applied to create full surgical plans (Tepper et al., 2017). The conception of difficult anatomy and can simulate difficulties to advantage train the specialist for utmost possibilities. With supplementary medical events, they have the possibility to grow rapidly and accurateness (Nedas et al., 2004). This is additionally developed by the beginning of new technology, that emphases on trace/force feedback consciousness, for instance, a stylus which is capable of simulator a needle or scalpel and permits the beginner to improve an accepting of exactly how it senses to cut over dissimilar tissue (Breda et al., 2016). Right now, this technology is like a renaissance in medical science.

Figure 2. Contribution of the virtual and augmented reality in modern urological surgery for the removal of kidney stone.

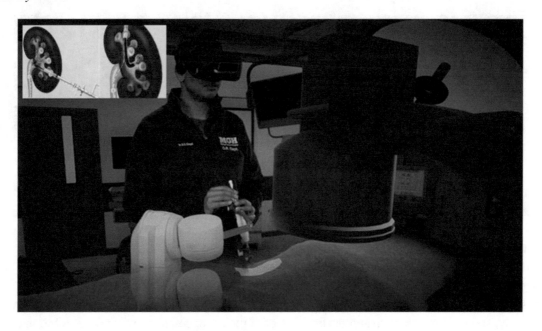

2. PRINCIPLES OF AUGMENTED REALITY

Augmented reality (AR) is an improved category of the real world that is achieved via the practice of digital visual features, sound, or other sensory stimuli delivered via technology (Hamacher et al., 2016). The projection of augmented reality is completed probably by using presentations, cameras, projectors, trackers, or additional particular apparatus (Childs et al., 2019). The key principle of a basic augmented reality system for urological study is shown in Fig. 3. The simplest technique is to cover a Computer-Generated image on an actual-world image taken by a camera and presenting the arrangement of these on a laptop/computer, video projector, or tablet (Moro et al., 2017) (Gutiérrez-Baños et al., 2015). If it is difficult to set up a video projector in the surgical operation room, a movable video projection device has been considered (Ferreira Reis et al., 2018). The main benefit of augmented reality is that the specialist is not enforced to look away from the operating spot as opposed to shared visualization performances (Mu et al., 2020). Presently, the applications of augmented reality are limited by the necessary basics of preoperative three-dimensional reconstructions of images (Nakamoto et al., 2012). It is potential to make these reestablishments by utilizing the commercial or customize software from the DICOM (digital imaging and communications in medicine) format (Smigelski et al., 2020) (Porpiglia et al., 2018). The feature of reconstruction is subject to the excellence of feedback data and the accurateness of the reconstruction method (Pokorny et al., 2019). Such reconstructions can be applied for virtual investigation of objective regions, scheduling an actual surgical methodology in improvement, and for improved coordination and navigation in the working area (Dickey et al., 2016) (Childs et al., 2019).

Figure 3. Augmented reality in modern urological study.

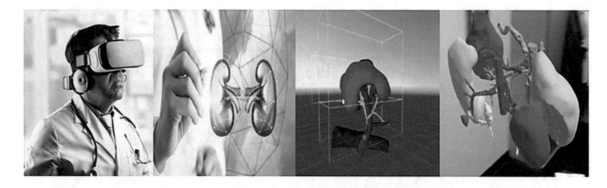

An additional opportunity is to usage a different HMD device (head-mounted display) or "smart glasses" that look like spectacles (Rahman et al., 2020). They use head tracking, distinctive projectors, and distance cameras to demonstrate Computer-Generated images on the glass, efficiently making the mirage of augmented reality (Hattab et al., 2020). Numerous augmented reality arrangements with a head-mounted display device have previously been established with success (Gautam et al., 2009) (Smigelski et al., 2020). Applying a head-mounted display device is advantageous as there is practically no obstacle in the surgeon's view related to a conventional presentation; it is not essential to transfer the display, and the essence of an appropriate line-of-sight arrangement between the exhibition and the surgeon is not as emphasized (Kong et al., 2017). The category and quantity of displayed information rely on the supplies of the process and individual preferences of the medical team (Aydin et al., 2016). Augmented reality is particularly valuable in imagining precarious structures for example nerves, major vessels, or additional vital organs (Hamacher et al., 2016). By planning these configurations straight onto the patient, augmented reality rises safety and decreases the time essential to complete the process. An additional advantageous feature of augmented reality is the capability to regulator the impenetrability of displayed substances (Pfefferle et al., 2020). Maximum head-mounted displays permit the wearer to exit all demonstrated images, becoming completely impervious, therefore eliminating any probable interruptions in an alternative (Rahman et al., 2020). Additionally, it is conceivable to operate speech recognition to make voice instructions, allowing a hands-free controller of the method (Smigelski et al., 2020). This is particularly significant in surgery as it permits surgeons to regulator the scheme without the essential help or breaks hygienic protocols. Additional stimulating preference is to practice signal recognition, permitting the team to cooperate with the hardware even on disinfected surfaces or in the airborne via physical activities (Hamacher et al., 2018).

3. USES IN CLINICAL PRACTICE

Virtual and augmented reality is the modern technique of superimposing CG (computer-generated) data content over a real vision of the world (Fig. 4). Augmented reality incorporates digital data with the user's background in actual time and is becoming more available and reasonable for surgical training, pediatric MRI evaluation, imaging, visualization of peripheral vasculature, dentistry, helping the visually impaired, and nurse training (Ma et al., 2021) (Peinado et al., 2018). The preoperative three-dimensional rebuilt images can be altered and arranged for display in augmented reality systems. Normally, augmented reality is applied for modifying exclusively desired incisions and surgical areas (Yu et al., 2018), optimum engagement of trocars, (Simpfendörfer et al., 2011) or to commonly develop the safety by presenting spots of main organ modules (Smigelski et al., 2020). An additional advantage of augmented reality is the capability to support surgeons in difficult topography subsequently radiotherapy or neoadjuvant chemotherapy or (Uppot et al., 2019). Augmented reality may be applied to imagine and enhance the surgical work of resection (Pfefferle et al., 2020). In various techniques, the augmented reality-supported surgery is similar to additional approaches of aid and the practice of such strategies be contingent on the specialist's preference (Kosieradzki et al., 2020). Virtual and augmented reality methods are the most beneficial throughout a surgery of internal organs i.e., brain, kidney, liver, and pancreas with slight movement and tissue deformation as the minimum amount of tracing and processing control are essential (Solbiati et al., 2020). Considering these specifics, the maximum frequently directed regions in augmented reality investigation are the brain and another major organ (Bettati et al., 2020), hepato-biliary system (Quero et al., 2019), orthopedic surgery (Verhey et al., 2020), and pancreas (Marzano et al., 2013). On the other hand, augmented reality may recompense the absence of tactile response typically practiced throughout laparoscopic surgery by offering the surgeon with visual evidence, therefore successful hand-eye direction and alignment, even in modern robotic surgery (Pratt et al., 2018). Numerous researchers projected to use this method in laparoscopic processes with success (Collins et al., 2021). Neurosurgical processes have engaged augmented reality methods effectively. It has been described that augmented reality had a main influence in 16.7% of neurovascular surgeries (Meola et al., 2017), permitting an advanced rate of accurate localization of cuts and shorter operational interval compared to a conventional 2D method (Yu et al., 2018). Neurosurgeons advantage mostly from accurate localization of separate blood vessels, gyros, major neuronal tracts, and the possibility to design the surgical corridor, for example, in neurovascular surgery (Guha et al., 2017), epilepsy surgery (House et al., 2020), or in the elimination of superficial tumors (Mascitelli et al., 2018).

Figure 4. Uses of virtual reality in urological training and observation.

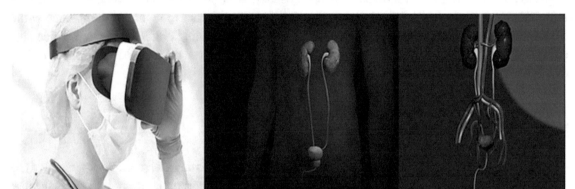

Augmented reality has also shown to be beneficial in the course of orthopedic surgeries and recon-structions, particularly as it permits to observation reconstructions directly on top of the patient's body that decreases the amount of interferences instigated by observing at an outer display (Keating et al., 2021). The list of processes effectively applying augmented reality varieties from MIS (minimally invasive surgeries) to bone resections, trauma reconstructions (Laverdière et al., 2019), osteotomies (Viehöfer et al., 2020), Kirschner wire placement (Fischer et al., 2016), arthroscopic surgery, tumour removal (Lan et al., 2018), or joint replacement. Percutaneous involvements only involve a surface needle of the insert point that can be presented by this technology (Drewniak et al., 2011). A fluoroscopic dual-laser-based method was applied by Liang et al., 2012, for insertion direction with acceptable accuracy. Though, the incapability to observe the complexity of insert forces the practice of further techniques. However, the usage of augmented reality confines the radiation experience throughout fluoroscopy and the quantity of time needed to complete the task (Alexander et al., 2020) whereas lessening the risk of excessive hemorrhage. It is also used to make a convenient imagining of scattered radiation for the period of a minimally invasive surgery (MIS) (Auloge et al., 2020), allowing to quantity and imagine the total of radiation established. Augmented reality can modification the workflow of forming orthopaedic implants, switching 3D printing of a customize model (Müller et al., 2020). It is also potential to engagement augmented reality in orthopaedic robot-assisted surgeries (McKnight et al., 2020).

It is more challenging to practice augmented reality in abdominal surgery because the amount of organ movement is important; yet, it is presently used through pancreatic and liver surgeries as it permits enhanced prognosis of large vessels (Sveinsson et al., 2021) or effective locates owing to the relatively stagnant nature of these organs. By matching the remodeled data with preoperative ultrasound, augmented reality can be applied for intraoperative management in the course of liver resections (Golse et al., 2021). It can also contribute to the surgeon with the setting up of laparoscopic ports (Teatini et al., 2020) or phrenotomy areas (Pessaux et al., 2015). Also, the kidneys seem to be appropriate for the treatment of augmented reality, for example, confirmed by Muller et al., 2020 through nephrolithotomy, where the augmented reality was applied to create the percutaneous renal access. An augmented reality system has been planned to precisely notice a sentinel node by a preoperative 'single-photon emission computed tomography (SPECT) scan of the neighboring lymph nodes, which permits to exactly steer to the sentinel node and achieve a resection even in complex topography (Valdés Olmos et al., 2014). Augmented reality has also been effectively engaged throughout urological dealings (Shirk et al., 2020), and Splenectomies in children (Tao et al., 2021). With the growing exactness of augmented reality methods, they can be securely applied even in otorhinolaryngologic surgery (Rose et al., 2019), endocrine surgeries (Hallet et al., 2015), vascular surgery (Fida et al., 2018), eye surgery (Ropelato et al., 2019), and dental implantology (Joda et al., 2019); though, their particular effectiveness in such surgical treatment is not accurately calculated remaining to the difficult structures (Zorzal et al., 2020). An augmented reality system for transcatheter aortic valve establishment was planned and effectively used by Currie et al., 2016, presenting similar accurateness to conventional fluoroscopic direction technique, therefore, evading impending difficulties of difference agent administration. The use of augmented reality in modern surgery is increasing rapidly, as a result of its capability to without difficulty integrate this system directly obsessed by the operators' comfort, which permits the surgeon to steer more rapidly and better recognize vital structures (Collins et al., 2021) (Gautam et al., 2009) (Smigelski et al., 2020). The computer-generated estimate can be shown independently or as an overlap of actual video as required by the surgeon.

4. VIRTUAL REALITY AND SIMULATION IN UROLOGY EDUCATION

A great variety of educational virtual and augmented reality needs in urology can be investigated in dissimilar categories of uses, software, and hardware. They are typically all advanced for a precise objective and improved to one devoted attention in urology education. Throughout their learning, the upcoming urologists have to obtain wide-ranging information and increasingly grow the services essential for the occupation. The instruction of specialists, healthcare team fellows is a vital part of urology training. This technology is applied in urology education in three main areas: theoretic information, practical and nontechnical skills. In urology knowledge and surgical performs (like removal of kidney stone) are continually developing and virtual reality-oriented computational simulation has become an important enhancement to current urology approaches in the exercise prospectuses of urologists (Fig. 5). Though, new improvements in urology also entail training and computational simulation for extensive use. To attain this virtual reality and computational model, the analysis could play a significant character. Training with computational simulators is recognized and lessons show that virtual reality models contribute to developed presentation in the operational room (Wake et al., 2020). A comprehensive overview of existing urological computational simulation techniques and also associated standards for different models was discussed (Borgmann et al., 2017). Several of these computational simulations are previously measure by urological training courses, moreover in agendas for urological exercise courses or committed practical workshops. The main cause for the requirement of nontechnical skills is a common fact that urologists generally do not work alone. They are often surrounded by a team of other doctors and experts, nurses, and medical staff. Functioning proficiently and well in a group is the main strategy to success. So these nontechnical skills are frequently significant for the effect of several involvements, and they are vital in emergency cases. Practical assistances rank among the most significant for surgeons and consultants. The main methods suggest exercise with computational simulators. While learning MIS (minimum invasive surgery) approaches, for example, Percutaneous Nephrolithotomy (PCNL), Laparoscopy operation, Ureteroscopy (URS), etc. surgeons essential to study to deal with the effect of fulcrum (Siff et al., 2018). This effect is an outcome of entering the body via minor incisions and forcing a rotation at the particular area where instruments (surgical) move in the body. These methods are used to control the instruments (surgical) for which it needs concentrated training. Particularly, in this case, the exactness of haptic response is important, meanwhile, forces and track of movement are counter-intuitive (Hamacher et al., 2016). The progress of these psychomotor abilities is important.

Figure 5. Application of modern virtual reality process in removal of kidney stone (LabOnLaptop).

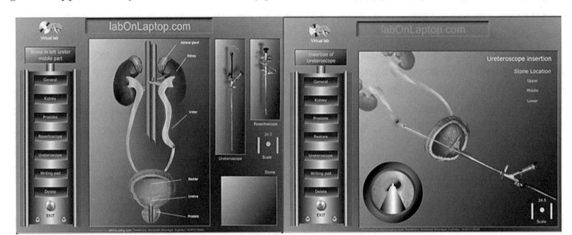

5. CONCLUSION

Present technical improvement is the main support behind a new development of virtual and augmented reality uses. Though comprehended and advanced over a time ago, numerous applications have increasingly found their technique to clinical practice. As minimally invasive surgery has advanced in a way which upgrades the urological surgical involvements, robots and working aids have become more corporate in the surgical room. Throughout the present time, these implements may have familiarized a modification in standard that also influences the work of surgeons. Even though observing at the best computational methods, it is significant to mention that the abilities and experience of urologists cannot just be taught through simulation only. A very vital portion is the response from a professional and the practice that can be increased over companionship. This is exact for even urology prospectuses over and above aforesaid workshops or training camps. Computational simulation cannot add this attachment or contribution, however, it can advantage to overcome problems for instance time and expanse, and make the interaction of a guide and a urologist informal and intensified. Virtual reality integrated communication abilities can make new potentials for telemedicine, teleguiding, and telesurgery. Scientifically improved solidarities can provision the learner by giving information, knowledge, and comment from an expert deprived of the expert in fact requiring to be on site. These tools could support and enable human interactions and advisor processes throughout the learning program. The complete benefits of virtual reality and computational simulation can be noticed as establishment capability and abilities for the urologist beginners. Therefore, an enhancement in the excellence of health care could be attained by the continued learning of healthcare specialists. The conclusion of these surgical plans with the precise knowledge of actual life has been produced in dissimilar approaches, mentioning the arrangement of several techniques to deliver an improved result.

CONFLICT OF INTEREST

The authors declare that there is no conflict of interest.

ACKNOWLEDGMENT

The authors would like to thank IIEST-Shibpur, Centre for Healthcare Science and Technology lab, and Dept. of Urology, R.G. Kar Medical College and Hospital, and thanks to Mrs. Nibedita Bardhan for language proof reading.

REFERENCES

Alexander, C., Loeb, A. E., Fotouhi, J., Navab, N., Armand, M., & Khanuja, H. S. (2020). Augmented Reality for Acetabular Component Placement in Direct Anterior Total Hip Arthroplasty. *The Journal of Arthroplasty*, *35*(6), 1636–1641.e3. doi:10.1016/j.arth.2020.01.025 PMID:32063415

Ali, S., Qandeel, M., Ramakrishna, R., & Yang, C. W. (2018). Virtual Simulation in Enhancing Procedural Training for Fluoroscopy-guided Lumbar Puncture: A Pilot Study. *Academic Radiology*, *25*(2), 235–239. doi:10.1016/j.acra.2017.08.002 PMID:29032887

. Auloge, P., Cazzato, R. L., Ramamurthy, N., de Marini, P., Rousseau, C., Garnon, J., Charles, Y. P., Steib, J. P., & Gangi, A. (2020). Augmented reality and artificial intelligence-based navigation during percutaneous vertebroplasty: a pilot randomised clinical trial. *European Spine Journal*, *29*(7), 1580–1589.

Aydin, A., Raison, N., Khan, M. S., Dasgupta, P., & Ahmed, K. (2016). Simulation-based training and assessment in urological surgery. *Nature Reviews. Urology*, *13*(9), 503–519. doi:10.1038/nrurol.2016.147 PMID:27549358

Bettati, P., Chalian, M., Huang, J., Dormer, J. D., Shahedi, M., & Fei, B. (2020). Augmented Reality-Assisted Biopsy of Soft Tissue Lesions. *Proceedings of SPIE—the International Society for Optical Engineering*, *11315*. 10.1117/12.2549381

Borgmann, H., Rodríguez Socarrás, M., Salem, J., Tsaur, I., Gomez Rivas, J., Barret, E., & Tortolero, L. (2017). Feasibility and safety of augmented reality-assisted urological surgery using smartglass. *World Journal of Urology*, *35*(6), 967–972. doi:10.100700345-016-1956-6 PMID:27761715

Breda, A., & Territo, A. (2016). Virtual Reality Simulators for Robot-assisted Surgery. *European Urology*, *69*(6), 1081–1082. doi:10.1016/j.eururo.2015.11.026 PMID:26688370

Childs, B. S., Manganiello, M. D., & Korets, R. (2019). Novel Education and Simulation Tools in Urologic Training. *Current Urology Reports*, *20*(12), 81. doi:10.100711934-019-0947-8 PMID:31782033

Chinnock, C. (1994). Virtual reality in surgery and medicine. *Hospital Technology Series*, *13*(18), 1–48. PMID:10172193

Collins, T., Pizarro, D., Gasparini, S., Bourdel, N., Chauvet, P., Canis, M., Calvet, L., & Bartoli, A. (2021). Augmented Reality Guided Laparoscopic Surgery of the Uterus. *IEEE Transactions on Medical Imaging*, *40*(1), 371–380. doi:10.1109/TMI.2020.3027442 PMID:32986548

Currie, M. E., McLeod, A. J., Moore, J. T., Chu, M. W. A., Patel, R., Kiaii, B., & Peters, T. M. (2016). Augmented reality system for ultrasound guidance of transcatheter aortic valve implantation. *Innovations*, *11*(1), 31–39. doi:10.1097/imi.0000000000000235 PMID:26938173

Del Pozo Jiménez, G., Rodríguez Monsalve, M., Carballido Rodríguez, J., & Castillón Vela, I. (2019). Virtual reality and intracorporeal navigation in urology. Realidad virtual y navegación intraquirúrgica en urología. *Archivos Espanoles de Urologia*, *72*(8), 867–881. PMID:31579046

Dickey, R. M., Srikishen, N., Lipshultz, L. I., Spiess, P. E., Carrion, R. E., & Hakky, T. S. (2016). Augmented reality assisted surgery: A urologic training tool. *Asian Journal of Andrology*, *18*(5), 732–734. doi:10.4103/1008-682X.166436 PMID:26620455

Drewniak, T., Rzepecki, M., Juszczak, K., Kwiatek, W., Bielecki, J., Zieliński, K., Ruta, A., Czekierda, Ł., & Moczulskis, Z. (2011). Obrazowanie guza nerki w trakcie zabiegow nerkooszczednych: Model zwierzecy i zastosowanie kliniczne [Augmented reality for image guided therapy (ARIGT) of kidney tumor during nephron sparing surgery (NSS): animal model and clinical approach]. *Folia Medica Cracoviensia*, *51*(1-4), 77–90. PMID:22891540

Ferreira Reis, A., Wirth, G. J., & Iselin, C. E. (2018). Réalité augmentée en urologie: Actualité et avenir [Augmented reality in urology: present and future]. *Revue Medicale Suisse*, *14*(629), 2154–2157. PMID:30484972

Fida, B., Cutolo, F., di Franco, G., Ferrari, M., & Ferrari, V. (2018). Augmented reality in open surgery. *Updates in Surgery*, *70*(3), 389–400. doi:10.100713304-018-0567-8 PMID:30006832

Fischer, M., Fuerst, B., Lee, S. C., Fotouhi, J., Habert, S., Weidert, S., Euler, E., Osgood, G., & Navab, N. (2016). Preclinical usability study of multiple augmented reality concepts for K-wire placement. *International Journal of Computer Assisted Radiology and Surgery*, *11*(6), 1007–1014. doi:10.100711548-016-1363-x PMID:26995603

Gautam, G., Benway, B. M., Bhayani, S. B., & Zorn, K. C. (2009). Robot-assisted partial nephrectomy: Current perspectives and future prospects. *Urology*, *74*(4), 735–740. doi:10.1016/j.urology.2009.03.041 PMID:19616827

Golse, N., Petit, A., Lewin, M., Vibert, E., & Cotin, S. (2021). Augmented Reality during Open Liver Surgery Using a Markerless Non-rigid Registration System. *Journal of Gastrointestinal Surgery*, *25*(3), 662–671. doi:10.100711605-020-04519-4 PMID:32040812

Guha, D., Alotaibi, N. M., Nguyen, N., Gupta, S., McFaul, C., & Yang, V. (2017). Augmented Reality in Neurosurgery: A Review of Current Concepts and Emerging Applications. *The Canadian journal of neurological sciences. Le journal canadien des sciences neurologiques, 44*(3), 235–245.

Gutiérrez-Baños, J. L., Ballestero-Diego, R., Truan-Cacho, D., Aguilera-Tubet, C., Villanueva-Peña, A., & Manuel-Palazuelos, J. C. (2015). Urology residents training in laparoscopic surgery. Development of a virtual reality model. *Actas Urologicas Espanolas*, *39*(9), 564–572. doi:10.1016/j.acuroe.2015.09.003 PMID:26068072

Hallet, J., Soler, L., Diana, M., Mutter, D., Baumert, T. F., Habersetzer, F., Marescaux, J., & Pessaux, P. (2015). Trans-thoracic minimally invasive liver resection guided by augmented reality. *Journal of the American College of Surgeons*, *220*(5), e55–e60. doi:10.1016/j.jamcollsurg.2014.12.053 PMID:25840539

Hamacher, A., Kim, S. J., Cho, S. T., Pardeshi, S., Lee, S. H., Eun, S. J., & Whangbo, T. K. (2016). Application of Virtual, Augmented, and Mixed Reality to Urology. *International Neurourology Journal*, *20*(3), 172–181. doi:10.5213/inj.1632714.357 PMID:27706017

Hamacher, A., Whangbo, T. K., Kim, S. J., & Chung, K. J. (2018). Virtual Reality and Simulation for Progressive Treatments in Urology. *International Neurourology Journal*, *22*(3), 151–160. doi:10.5213/inj.1836210.105 PMID:30286577

Hattab, G., Arnold, M., Strenger, L., Allan, M., Arsentjeva, D., Gold, O., Simpfendörfer, T., Maier-Hein, L., & Speidel, S. (2020). Kidney edge detection in laparoscopic image data for computer-assisted surgery: Kidney edge detection. *International Journal of Computer Assisted Radiology and Surgery*, *15*(3), 379–387. doi:10.100711548-019-02102-0 PMID:31828502

House, P. M., Pelzl, S., Furrer, S., Lanz, M., Simova, O., Voges, B., Stodieck, S., & Brückner, K. E. (2020). Use of the mixed reality tool "VSI Patient Education" for more comprehensible and imaginable patient educations before epilepsy surgery and stereotactic implantation of DBS or stereo-EEG electrodes. *Epilepsy Research*, *159*, 106247. doi:10.1016/j.eplepsyres.2019.106247 PMID:31794952

Joda, T., Gallucci, G. O., Wismeijer, D., & Zitzmann, N. U. (2019). Augmented and virtual reality in dental medicine: A systematic review. *Computers in Biology and Medicine*, *108*, 93–100. doi:10.1016/j.compbiomed.2019.03.012 PMID:31003184

Johnston, A., Rae, J., Ariotti, N., Bailey, B., Lilja, A., Webb, R., Ferguson, C., Maher, S., Davis, T. P., Webb, R. I., McGhee, J., & Parton, R. G. (2018). Journey to the centre of the cell: Virtual reality immersion into scientific data. *Traffic (Copenhagen, Denmark)*, *19*(2), 105–110. doi:10.1111/tra.12538 PMID:29159991

Keating, T. C., & Jacobs, J. J. (2021). Augmented Reality in Orthopedic Practice and Education. *The Orthopedic Clinics of North America*, *52*(1), 15–26. doi:10.1016/j.ocl.2020.08.002 PMID:33222981

Kong, S. H., Haouchine, N., Soares, R., Klymchenko, A., Andreiuk, B., Marques, B., Shabat, G., Piechaud, T., Diana, M., Cotin, S., & Marescaux, J. (2017). Robust augmented reality registration method for localization of solid organs' tumors using CT-derived virtual biomechanical model and fluorescent fiducials. *Surgical Endoscopy*, *31*(7), 2863–2871. doi:10.100700464-016-5297-8 PMID:27796600

Kosieradzki, M., Lisik, W., Gierwiało, R., & Sitnik, R. (2020). Applicability of Augmented Reality in an Organ Transplantation. *Annals of Transplantation*, *25*, e923597. doi:10.12659/AOT.923597 PMID:32732862

Lan, L., Xia, Y., Li, R., Liu, K., Mai, J., Medley, J. A., Obeng-Gyasi, S., Han, L. K., Wang, P., & Cheng, J. X. (2018). A fiber optoacoustic guide with augmented reality for precision breast-conserving surgery. *Light, Science & Applications*, *7*(1), 2. doi:10.103841377-018-0006-0 PMID:30839601

Laverdière, C., Corban, J., Khoury, J., Ge, S. M., Schupbach, J., Harvey, E. J., Reindl, R., & Martineau, P. A. (2019). Augmented reality in orthopaedics: A systematic review and a window on future possibilities. *The Bone & Joint Journal*, *101-B*(12), 1479–1488. doi:10.1302/0301-620X.101B12.BJJ-2019-0315.R1 PMID:31786992

Liang, J. T., Doke, T., Onogi, S., Ohashi, S., Ohnishi, I., Sakuma, I., & Nakajima, Y. (2012). A fluorolaser navigation system to guide linear surgical tool insertion. *International Journal of Computer Assisted Radiology and Surgery*, *7*(6), 931–939. doi:10.100711548-012-0743-0 PMID:22627882

Lima, E., Rodrigues, P. L., Mota, P., Carvalho, N., Dias, E., Correia-Pinto, J., Autorino, R., & Vilaça, J. L. (2017). Ureteroscopy-assisted Percutaneous Kidney Access Made Easy: First Clinical Experience with a Novel Navigation System Using Electromagnetic Guidance (IDEAL Stage 1). *European Urology*, *72*(4), 610–661. doi:10.1016/j.eururo.2017.03.011 PMID:28377202

. Linte, C. A., Davenport, K. P., Cleary, K., Peters, C., Vosburgh, K. G., Navab, N., Edwards, P. E., Jannin, P., Peters, T. M., Holmes, D. R., & Robb, R. A. (2013). On mixed reality environments for minimally invasive therapy guidance: systems architecture, successes and challenges in their implementation from laboratory to clinic. *Computerized medical imaging and graphics: the official journal of the Computerized Medical Imaging Society, 37*(2), 83–97.

Ma, R., Reddy, S., Vanstrum, E. B., & Hung, A. J. (2021). Innovations in Urologic Surgical Training. *Current Urology Reports*, *22*(4), 26. doi:10.100711934-021-01043-z PMID:33712963

Marzano, E., Piardi, T., Soler, L., Diana, M., Mutter, D., Marescaux, J., & Pessaux, P. (2013). Augmented reality-guided artery-first pancreatico-duodenectomy. *Journal of Gastrointestinal Surgery*, *17*(11), 1980–1983. doi:10.100711605-013-2307-1 PMID:23943389

Mascitelli, J. R., Schlachter, L., Chartrain, A. G., Oemke, H., Gilligan, J., Costa, A. B., Shrivastava, R. K., & Bederson, J. B. (2018). Navigation-Linked Heads-Up Display in Intracranial Surgery: Early Experience. *Operative Neurosurgery (Hagerstown, Md.)*, *15*(2), 184–193. doi:10.1093/ons/opx205 PMID:29040677

McKnight, R. R., Pean, C. A., Buck, J. S., Hwang, J. S., Hsu, J. R., & Pierrie, S. N. (2020). Virtual Reality and Augmented Reality-Translating Surgical Training into Surgical Technique. *Current Reviews in Musculoskeletal Medicine*, *13*(6), 663–674. doi:10.100712178-020-09667-3 PMID:32779019

Meola, A., Cutolo, F., Carbone, M., Cagnazzo, F., Ferrari, M., & Ferrari, V. (2017). Augmented reality in neurosurgery: A systematic review. *Neurosurgical Review*, *40*(4), 537–548. doi:10.100710143-016-0732-9 PMID:27154018

Moro, C., Štromberga, Z., Raikos, A., & Stirling, A. (2017). The effectiveness of virtual and augmented reality in health sciences and medical anatomy. *Anatomical Sciences Education*, *10*(6), 549–559. doi:10.1002/ase.1696 PMID:28419750

Mu, Y., Hocking, D., Wang, Z. T., Garvin, G. J., Eagleson, R., & Peters, T. M. (2020). Augmented reality simulator for ultrasound-guided percutaneous renal access. *International Journal of Computer Assisted Radiology and Surgery*, *15*(5), 749–757. doi:10.100711548-020-02142-x PMID:32314227

Müller, F., Roner, S., Liebmann, F., Spirig, J. M., Fürnstahl, P., & Farshad, M. (2020). Augmented reality navigation for spinal pedicle screw instrumentation using intraoperative 3D imaging. *The Spine Journal*, *20*(4), 621–628. doi:10.1016/j.spinee.2019.10.012 PMID:31669611

Nakamoto, M., Ukimura, O., Faber, K., & Gill, I. S. (2012). Current progress on augmented reality visualization in endoscopic surgery. *Current Opinion in Urology*, *22*(2), 121–126. doi:10.1097/MOU.0b013e3283501774 PMID:22249372

Nedas, T., Challacombe, B., & Dasgupta, P. (2004). Virtual reality in urology. *BJU International*, *94*(3), 255–257. doi:10.1111/j.1464-410X.2004.04975.x PMID:15291846

Peinado, F., Fernández, A., Teba, F., Celada, G., & Acosta, M. A. (2018). El urólogo del futuro y las nuevas tecnologías [The urologist of the future and new technologies]. *Archivos Espanoles de Urologia*, *71*(1), 142–149. PMID:29336344

Pessaux, P., Diana, M., Soler, L., Piardi, T., Mutter, D., & Marescaux, J. (2015). Towards cybernetic surgery: Robotic and augmented reality-assisted liver segmentectomy. *Langenbeck's Archives of Surgery*, *400*(3), 381–385. doi:10.100700423-014-1256-9 PMID:25392120

Pfefferle, M., Shahub, S., Shahedi, M., Gahan, J., Johnson, B., Le, P., Vargas, J., Judson, B. O., Alshara, Y., Li, Q., & Fei, B. (2020). Renal biopsy under augmented reality guidance. *Proceedings of SPIE—the International Society for Optical Engineering, 11315*.

Pokorny, M., & Yaxley, J. (2019). Three-dimensional Elastic Augmented Reality for Robot-assisted Laparoscopic Prostatectomy: Pushing the Boundaries, but Cutting it Fine. *European Urology*, *76*(4), 515–516. doi:10.1016/j.eururo.2019.04.025 PMID:31053374

Porpiglia, F., Fiori, C., Checcucci, E., Amparore, D., & Bertolo, R. (2018). Augmented Reality Robot-assisted Radical Prostatectomy: Preliminary Experience. *Urology*, *115*, 184. doi:10.1016/j.urology.2018.01.028 PMID:29548868

Pratt, P., & Arora, A. (2018). Transoral Robotic Surgery: Image Guidance and Augmented Reality. *ORL; Journal for Oto-Rhino-Laryngology and Its Related Specialties*, *80*(3-4), 204–212. doi:10.1159/000489467 PMID:29936505

Quero, G., Lapergola, A., Soler, L., Shahbaz, M., Hostettler, A., Collins, T., Marescaux, J., Mutter, D., Diana, M., & Pessaux, P. (2019). Virtual and Augmented Reality in Oncologic Liver Surgery. *Surgical Oncology Clinics of North America*, *28*(1), 31–44. doi:10.1016/j.soc.2018.08.002 PMID:30414680

Rahman, R., Wood, M. E., Qian, L., Price, C. L., Johnson, A. A., & Osgood, G. M. (2020). Head-Mounted Display Use in Surgery: A Systematic Review. *Surgical Innovation*, *27*(1), 88–100. doi:10.1177/1553350619871787 PMID:31514682

Ropelato, S., Menozzi, M., Michel, D., & Siegrist, M. (2020). Augmented Reality Microsurgery: A Tool for Training Micromanipulations in Ophthalmic Surgery Using Augmented Reality. *Simulation in Healthcare, 15*(2), 122–127.

Rose, A. S., Kim, H., Fuchs, H., & Frahm, J. M. (2019). Development of augmented-reality applications in otolaryngology-head and neck surgery. *The Laryngoscope, 129*(S3, Suppl 3), S1–S11. doi:10.1002/lary.28098 PMID:31260127

Schenkman, N. (2008). Virtual reality training in urology. *The Journal of Urology, 180*(6), 2305–2306. doi:10.1016/j.juro.2008.09.069 PMID:18930286

Shah, J., Mackay, S., Vale, J., & Darzi, A. (2001). Simulation in urology—A role for virtual reality? *BJU International, 88*(7), 661–665. doi:10.1046/j.1464-410X.2001.02320.x PMID:11890232

Shirk, J. D. (2020). RE: 3D Printing, Augmented Reality, and Virtual Reality for the Assessment and Management of Kidney and Prostate Cancer: A Systematic Review. *Urology, 145*, 301. doi:10.1016/j.urology.2020.07.061 PMID:32916192

Siff, L. N., & Mehta, N. (2018). An Interactive Holographic Curriculum for Urogynecologic Surgery. *Obstetrics and Gynecology, 132*(Suppl 1), 27S–32S. doi:10.1097/AOG.0000000000002860 PMID:30247304

Simpfendörfer, T., Baumhauer, M., Müller, M., Gutt, C. N., Meinzer, H. P., Rassweiler, J. J., Guven, S., & Teber, D. (2011). Augmented reality visualization during laparoscopic radical prostatectomy. *Journal of Endourology, 25*(12), 1841–1845. doi:10.1089/end.2010.0724 PMID:21970336

Smigelski, M., Movassaghi, M., & Small, A. (2020). Urology Virtual Education Programs During the COVID-19 Pandemic. *Current Urology Reports, 21*(12), 50. doi:10.100711934-020-01004-y PMID:33090272

Solbiati, L., Gennaro, N., & Muglia, R. (2020). Augmented Reality: From Video Games to Medical Clinical Practice. *Cardiovascular and Interventional Radiology, 43*(10), 1427–1429. doi:10.100700270-020-02575-6 PMID:32632853

Sutherland, J., Belec, J., Sheikh, A., Chepelev, L., Althobaity, W., Chow, B., Mitsouras, D., Christensen, A., Rybicki, F. J., & La Russa, D. J. (2019). Applying Modern Virtual and Augmented Reality Technologies to Medical Images and Models. *Journal of Digital Imaging, 32*(1), 38–53. doi:10.100710278-018-0122-7 PMID:30215180

Sveinsson, B., Koonjoo, N., & Rosen, M. S. (2021). ARmedViewer, an augmented-reality-based fast 3D reslicer for medical image data on mobile devices: A feasibility study. *Computer Methods and Programs in Biomedicine, 200*, 105836. doi:10.1016/j.cmpb.2020.105836 PMID:33250281

Tao, H. S., Lin, J. Y., Luo, W., Chen, R., Zhu, W., Fang, C. H., & Yang, J. (2021). Application of Real-Time Augmented Reality Laparoscopic Navigation in Splenectomy for Massive Splenomegaly. *World Journal of Surgery, 45*(7), 2108–2115. doi:10.100700268-021-06082-8 PMID:33770240

. Teatini, A., Pérez de Frutos, J., Eigl, B., Pelanis, E., Aghayan, D. L., Lai, M., Kumar, R. P., Palomar, R., Edwin, B., & Elle, O. J. (2020). Influence of sampling accuracy on augmented reality for laparoscopic image-guided surgery. *Minimally Invasive Therapy & Allied Technologies*, 1–10. Advance online publication.

Tepper, O. M., Rudy, H. L., Lefkowitz, A., Weimer, K. A., Marks, S. M., Stern, C. S., & Garfein, E. S. (2017). Mixed Reality with HoloLens: Where Virtual Reality Meets Augmented Reality in the Operating Room. *Plastic and Reconstructive Surgery*, *140*(5), 1066–1070. doi:10.1097/PRS.0000000000003802 PMID:29068946

Uppot, R. N., Laguna, B., McCarthy, C. J., De Novi, G., Phelps, A., Siegel, E., & Courtier, J. (2019). Implementing Virtual and Augmented Reality Tools for Radiology Education and Training, Communication, and Clinical Care. *Radiology*, *291*(3), 570–580. doi:10.1148/radiol.2019182210 PMID:30990383

Valdés Olmos, R. A., Vidal-Sicart, S., Giammarile, F., Zaknun, J. J., Van Leeuwen, F. W., & Mariani, G. (2014). The GOSTT concept and hybrid mixed/virtual/augmented reality environment radioguided surgery. *The Quarterly Journal of Nuclear Medicine and Molecular Imaging*, *58*(2), 207–215.

Verhey, J. T., Haglin, J. M., Verhey, E. M., & Hartigan, D. E. (2020). Virtual, augmented, and mixed reality applications in orthopedic surgery. *The International Journal of Medical Robotics + Computer Assisted Surgery*, *16*(2), e2067. PMID:31867864

Viehöfer, A. F., Wirth, S. H., Zimmermann, S. M., Jaberg, L., Dennler, C., Fürnstahl, P., & Farshad, M. (2020). Augmented reality guided osteotomy in hallux Valgus correction. *BMC Musculoskeletal Disorders*, *21*(1), 438. doi:10.118612891-020-03373-4 PMID:32631342

Wake, N., Nussbaum, J. E., Elias, M. I., Nikas, C. V., & Bjurlin, M. A. (2020). 3D Printing, Augmented Reality, and Virtual Reality for the Assessment and Management of Kidney and Prostate Cancer: A Systematic Review. *Urology*, *143*, 20–32. doi:10.1016/j.urology.2020.03.066 PMID:32535076

Yu, F., Song, E., Liu, H., Li, Y., Zhu, J., & Hung, C. C. (2018). An Augmented Reality Endoscope System for Ureter Position Detection. *Journal of Medical Systems*, *42*(8), 138. doi:10.100710916-018-0992-8 PMID:29938379

Zorzal, E. R., Campos Gomes, J. M., Sousa, M., Belchior, P., da Silva, P. G., Figueiredo, N., Lopes, D. S., & Jorge, J. (2020). Laparoscopy with augmented reality adaptations. *Journal of Biomedical Informatics*, *107*, 103463. doi:10.1016/j.jbi.2020.103463 PMID:32562897

KEY TERMS AND DEFINITIONS

Augmented Reality: An improved version of the actual physical world that is attained by the use of digital visual essentials, sound, or additional sensory stimuli provided through technology.

Cystoscopy: A process, where urologist use a cystoscope (a hollow tube equipped with a lens) to inspect the lining of patients' bladder and the tube which carries urine out from urethra.

Surgical Navigation: A system which can permits medical experts or surgeons to exactly track instrument places and then plan the instrument place on the preoperative imaging data.

Urology: A medical study which examines the medicinal and surgical cases and diseases of the patients' urinary tract and reproductive organs of male patients.

Virtual Reality: A computational simulation process in which person can interact within an artificial 3D environment by applying modern electronics devices, like special spectacles with a display or gloves fixed with sensors.

Chapter 9

Emerging Advancement for Augmented Reality (AR) and Virtual Reality (VR) in Dentistry

Anmol Bagaria
CynoDent, India

Sonal Mahilkar
Maitri College of Dentistry and Research Centre, India

Subash C. Sonkar
ⓘ https://orcid.org/0000-0001-7929-3464
Multidisciplinary Research Unit, Maulana Azad Medical College, University of Delhi, New Delhi, India

ABSTRACT

The skill of visual reality has matured, and VR and AR are increasingly being used in educational and surgical settings. The development of virtual reality technologies allows users to mix medical knowledge, medical data, and graphical data. It can provide more precise information, allowing users to increase their safety and reduce their risk. Virtual reality (VR) or augmented reality (AR) simulators that provide direct feedback and objective evaluation could be a useful tool in dental education in the future. Not only has it been applied to education, but it has also been created in therapeutic therapy. The authors believe that in the future VR and AR training and teaching will be extended and used in every aspect of dentistry, enabling students to develop their abilities on their own. In comparison to augmented reality, virtual reality offers a far more immersive experience. It would establish a trusting relationship between patients and doctors based on the experience of the dentists and the use of different hardware and software.

DOI: 10.4018/978-1-7998-8371-5.ch009

OVERVIEW

Dental solutions based on digital technology have made great progress all around the world thanks to advances in information technology (IT). In the future, solutions which are digital in dentistry will become the norm in the professional dental area. Computerized dental solutions are frequently used in both clinical dentistry and dental education due to their quick advancement. Existing dental clinical processes as well as dental education learning approaches will be challenged because of this shift. Clinicians may be able to better address the patients complain area and provide a different treatment as the patient's medical image matures. Over time, the new technology that supported the dental practitioners have been improved.

Image guided therapy (IGT) (Dimaio et al.,2007; Schulz et al.,2012) and image-guided interventions (IGI) technology development (Zadik et al.2006a, 2008b; Sarika et al.2015; Suenagaet al.,2013; Gulati et al.2015) image recognition and tracking system location (Wiles et al.,2004), coordinated computed tomography, position tracker can help to provide much more accurate precision in the surgical area or to learn by estimating the position of the surgical equipment. Therefore, mentioned methodology is also employed in nerve surgery to generate the effect of real-time surgery. Medical imaging developments, such as CT technical developments, a better positioning system will help to reduce surgical errors (Birkfellner et al.,1998), because clarity of the available imaging will affect the entire system (Bhat et al.,2005).

Figure 1. Augmented reality and its use in dentistry.
Joda et al. (2019). Computers in Biology and Medicine 108 (2019) 93–100.

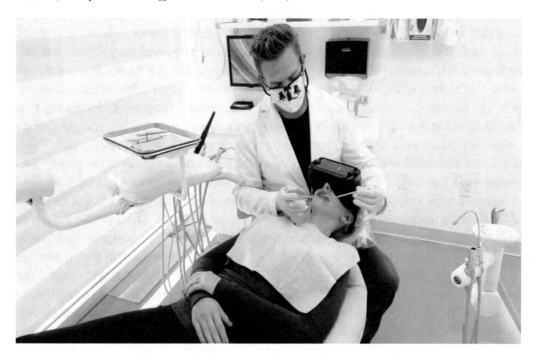

Figure 2.

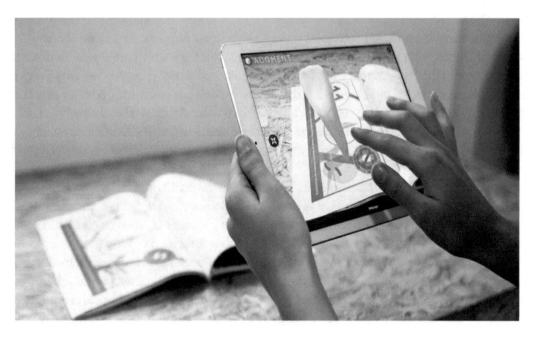

VIRTUAL REALITY VS. AUGMENTED REALITY

Augmented Reality(AR) is an interactive technology that uses computer-animated perceptual information to enhance a real-world experience. In other words, augmented reality (AR) adds virtual content to the real world. In most situations, it involves superimposing supplementary digital data on live or video photographs. VR, on the other hand, relies solely on programmed scenes that are disconnected from reality (Sutherland et al.,2019). Every imaginable mode of experience, primarily visual, aural, and haptic, can be utilized depending on the approach. In addition, there are an increasing number of AR/RV applications in dentistry as a whole and many exciting advances for patients and dental professionals, either separately or in any combination today (Kwon et al., 2018; Joda et al.,2019; Farronato et al., 2019). Users can superimpose virtually produced images onto recordings of the patient in genuine motion using AR/VR software. Any 3D model, such as a prosthetic layout for a potential reconstruction, can be inserted into the individual patient scenario to simulate various, prospective outcomes without the need for invasive work steps ahead of time (Joda & Gallucci, 2015). These digital models can then be inspected in real time and utilized to produce new ones, allowing communication not just with patients to demystify complex treatment stages, but also with dental professionals to improve treatment predictability and efficiency. The options will continue to grow in the future, making dental care more convenient. A noteworthy indication is the use in oral cavity or in connection with other operations of the planning of CBCT-based virtual implants. A potential topic of interest is the area of dental education, which provides intraoral scanners (IOD), projection, and display of the optically detected area in AR glasses, theoretical and practical information for interactive teachings and objective assessments with 24/7 access. The AR/VR motor skills training for tooth preparation improves the autonomous and client learning of students in dentistry. Preliminary research indicates that AR/VR technology provide more meaningful insight (Lee, 2018). Furthermore, tough and sophisticated clinical protocols can be trained in a comprehensive virtual environment without risk or harm to real patients in postgraduate education; further, specialists can keep their skills while training with AR/VR simulations. AR/VR has the potential to completely transform dentistry education in the next several years (Ayoub & Pulijala, 2019; Durham et al., 2019).

VR helps enhance the clinical practice process and dentistry education. Thus, it seems to have extensive application for planning, training, therapeutic treatments, and pain management in dentistry. This technology provides an innovative path for research and development in dentistry. It provides an accurate projection of a radiographic image in a virtual environment like a real-world situation (Joda et al, 2019)

VIRTUAL REALITY IN DENTISTRY: CURRENT AND FUTURE TRENDS

When compared to augmented reality, we found that virtual reality provides a significantly more immersive experience. This is because the technology necessitates a big headpiece that covers the user's eyes and therefore "inserts" them into their own virtual world, where they can interact and engage with their new surroundings as they like. You can, for example, swim with dolphins or immerse yourself or your patients in a graphically vivid instruction, learning experience, or just a plain old-fashioned video game using virtual reality. Indeed, when it comes to the use of virtual reality in dentistry, the benefits are mostly apparent in the improvement of the patient experience. Many practitioners, for example, have already begun to use virtual reality to help alleviate patient anxiety. Virtual reality is not the same as augmented reality. Specifically, it provides virtual information in addition to the environment in which you are immersed (Modern Practice, 2018).

AUGMENTED REALITY IN DENTISTRY: CURRENT AND FUTURE TRENDS

AR gives the user more freedom and eliminates the need for large, heavy pieces of equipment. For example, you can swim with dolphins in virtual reality, but you can watch a dolphin jump out of your business card with augmented reality. You can immerse yourself in a setting where an instructor teaches complex processes in virtual reality, but you can practice procedures yourself in the comfort of your office chair with no pressure in augmented reality. The impact of augmented reality in dentistry is mostly concentrated in the arena of surgery. Dentists can use a simple pop-up screen to rehearse complex operations or check patient vital signs at the touch of a button. It has also proven to be an extremely useful tool for dentists, particularly in terms of continuing education and further training. This is because it provides visual data, which can be incredibly beneficial in terms of rapidly processing and keeping information. When it comes to improving the patient experience, AR can be very effective. In general, during a consultation, a patient is given a treatment plan and a cast of their mouth is taken, which is then sent to a dental lab, where unique replications are created and returned to the office for evaluation. With augmented reality, you can give the patient an immediate visual representation of completed treatments that have been proposed during the consultation (orthodontics, crown and bridgework, implants, and so on), greatly increasing the patient's expectations. The future applications of these technologies are practically limitless. Imagine a world in which practitioners are able to give patients an immediate visual representation of completed treatments that have been proposed during the consultation (orthodontics, crown and bridge, implants, etc). Helping to reduce the length of consultations or repeat visits can only benefit patients, as well as reduce fatigue among practitioners — unless they chose to utilize this down-time to boost patient volume, of course. Obviously overlay of information during dental operations is another possible application. Imagine being able to monitor a larger range of patient data and metrics at the touch of a button on your dental instruments, or absorb information more quickly, which would benefit both practitioners and patients of all ages (Modern Practice, 2018).

Dental training simulators arose from aviation (Helmreich, 1997) and medical technologies (Makransky et al., 2016). DentSimTM, Simodon-t, and IDEA are the top players in this market right now.

1. DentSim™

DentSim™ is a software program that simulates the teeth.

A phantom head, dental instruments, infrared sensors, an overhead infrared camera with a monitor, and two computers are included in the DentSim™ systems. One of the two computers scans the simulated patient's mouth using an infrared sensor. The educational program for evaluating student's work is installed on the second computer. This software is set up to grade student's work for both critical faults and when the student specifically requests it. Students can use the unit to visualize their preparation on a computer screen while also working on plastic teeth. Students can learn autonomously and improve clinical abilities, lowering training expenditures. When compared to traditional preclinical teaching methods, a study by Jasinevicius et al. (2004) found that employing virtual approaches reduced faculty time by fivefold. It has also been shown that when performing and observing tasks rather than being a passive observer, pre-motor and motor neural cortices exhibit significantly enhanced activity, which improves learning outcomes (Horst et al., 2009).

2. Dental Education Assistant on a Per-Individual Basis (IDEA)

The IDEA includes a six-degree-of-freedom stylus attached to a stand (Phantom Omni, SensAble TechnologiesTM, Wilmington, MA, USA) that provides feedback to the holder. This item displays a 3D animated image on the screen that lets the student to practice using tools (such as the Stylus and the Phantom Omni) while receiving haptic input. The simulator calculates and records task time, percentage of desired material removed, and deviation from the allotted drilling task, all of which reflect the level of precision, and displays a score on the screen for each task. Unfortunately, there is currently no literature stating that this grading method has been validated (Gal et al., 2011). Manual DexterityTM, Caries Detection, Oral MedTM, Scaling and Root PlanningTM, and PreDen TouchTM are all available as modules on the current unit. PreDen TouchTM is a cutting-edge device that allows prospective dental students to learn more about dentistry as a profession. In order to improve the learning experience, the company also permits third-party programs to be installed on the device. Root canal obturation, radiography, bridge removal, pain treatment, and more applications are currently accessible. Gal et al. (2011) found that both experienced academics and fifth-year dentistry students thought IDEA simulators may help them learn more effectively. They did say, however, that while the scoring system may use some work, the tactile sense needed to be much improved in order to more accurately resemble the real-world experience.

3. Simodont Dental Trainer

Moog Industrial Group, Amsterdam, manufactures the Simodont Dental Trainer, a haptic 3D Virtual Reality Simulator. ACTA (Academic Centre for Dentistry in Amsterdam) created the Simodont courseware, which is currently being tested at Griffith University's School of Dentistry and Oral Health in Queensland, Australia. Manual dexterity, cariology, crown and bridge exercises, clinical situations, and a whole mouth simulation experience are all included in the Simodont software. Modules for Dental Hygiene/Periodontics and Endodontics are in the works for a future version. These modules include a feature called "The Case Editor," which allows users to scan their own instruments and clinical situations in order to create a new exercise. The Simodont Dental Trainer delivers immediate feedback to the user and allows students to practice in virtual examination environments. Bakr et al. (2014) found a probable advantage in improving manual dexterity in undergraduate dental students after a brief exposure to the Simodont dental trainer. The authors also expressed an optimistic outlook on the usage of haptics to improve learning experiences. Senior dentistry students, in addition to therefore mentioned, valued the educational advantages that the Simodont Dental Trainer could bring. They did agree, however, that virtual simulation should be utilized in conjunction with traditional educational approaches as a supplement (Bakr et al., 2015).

4. Periopsim

PeriopSim is a virtual reality simulator developed by Luciano (2006) that allows students to utilize a variety of animated dental instruments in a haptic environment to visualize, identify, and evaluate caries or periodontal disorders without the requirement for tooth preparation. Students can access this device over the internet, and teachers can upload various dental treatments that can be recorded and replayed by the student at any time. According to Steinberg et al. (2007), the gadget would aid in the development of necessary tactile abilities and should be used in dentistry schools. However, it was discovered that the realism of instrument and oral structure representations, as well as the realism of tactile input, had significant limits that needed to be addressed (Luciano, 2006; Steinberg et al., 2007).

5. Voxel-Man

Another 3D virtual teaching device for surgical procedures is the Voxel-Man simulator, which has been reported to help trainees transfer knowledge from the virtual to the real world. The operator can use animated high and low speed bursts of various shapes controlled by a foot pedal with this device. With the use of a virtual dental mirror, the operator can examine teeth from every angle. Teeth can be magnified and cross-sectional images can be displayed using this device. Microtomography was used to create high-resolution tooth models from actual teeth. Students can get rapid feedback, problem-based learning, and objective performance evaluations with the software. According to Steinberg et al. (2007), students who were exposed to virtual reality software before performing an apicectomy treatment conserved nearby structures such as soft tissue and bone six times better than students who were asked to do the procedure on pig cadavers. Furthermore, following virtual training, the students were allowed to self-assess. Advances in hardware and software technologies may enable for greater virtual reality experience and integration into current schooling.

The addition of elements like virtual water spray, virtual tongue and cheeks for retraction, as well as a larger variety of virtual clinical cases spanning all dental specialties, is a feasible recommendation that could improve virtual reality learning experiences even further.

APPLICATIONS IN ORAL AND MAXILLOFACIAL SURGERY

The oral and maxillofacial regions consist of many surgical and anatomical important structures including canals, foramens, artery, veins, nerves and vessels. The knowledge of craniofacial structures is required for pre-surgical planning. AR technology is well suited for this purpose (Roy et al., 2017). Based on AR principles, the real operative site of a patient is provided with graphic data representation that was extracted and modified from a data source, AR navigation systems have been effectively working (Wang et al., 2017). Previously acquired diagnostic images such as radiographs, computed tomography scans, magnetic resonance imaging scans and angiography can also be good sources of additionally integrated AR information (Meola et al., 2016). AR guidance systems provide real-time intraoperative information with real view of surgical fields (Nijmeh et al.,2005). It is best to offer three-dimensional presentations on the patient's body rather than a separate screen because perception of the real body is more spontaneous and avoids confusion (Meola et al., 2016).

APPLICATION IN DENTAL IMPLANT PLACEMENT

AR technology has been shown to markedly improve implant placement procedures. Dental implant placement method with a graphically superimposed suggested position on the patient was introduced in 1995 (Ploder et al., 1995). AR systems is also helpful in tele planning and surgical navigation of implant placement (Ewers & Schicho, 2009). AR toolkit using head mounted displays (HMD) and marker tracking was described by Kato and Billinghurst (1997). This technique helps in identifying the anatomy of mouth and teeth. It first familiarizes the doctor with the patient's teeth anatomy before implantation in the mouth. Thus, it seems a proper technique as used for the teaching and learning of dental professionals and students. Traditionally, new dentist can feel pressure during the drill. Now using VR technology, the dentist can gain much experience and feel free while performing the actual procedure. This technology can be gainfully used to suggest a treatment plan on the computer screen. There is better communication between the dentist and the patients, which improves patient satisfaction and treatment. This technology creates a highly realistic simulation for the dental patient (Haleem & Javaid, 2019).

APPLICATION IN ORTHODONTICS

AR applications is most widely used in Orthognathic surgery. Wagner et al. (1997) reported augmentation in facial skeleton osteotomy via partial visual immersion using a head-mounted display. The technology helped to visualise the invisible anatomy which offered continuous observation and was very helpful to doctor's for guaranteed successful surgery. Suenaga et al. (2013), reported high accuracy of AR in his study. Different visualization processing are texture maps, surface mesh, wireframes and transparencies. This processing is important for surgeons to obtain accurate 3D views (Wang et al.,2014). Badiali et al. (1976) developed a head-mounted wearable system facilitating augmented surgery and reported that this AR-assisted maxillary repositioning surgery demonstrated only minor errors that were within the acceptable limits. The integrated accurateness of computer-generated imaging was more reliable than that of real-life image alone (Wang et al., 2015).

CONCLUSION

The advantages of AR systems in preoperative planning provide noble and precise outcome predictions. From dental training, surgery and custom orthotics, AR is transforming the very industry that established itself on changing our mouths, while virtual reality is making waves with patients by reducing worries and enhancing comfort. Intraoperative navigation provides surgeons with better chances of achieving good results and for reducing potential risks. As educational tools, AR simulators can offer accentuate opportunities to dental and medical students. Supplementation with other technology can enhance the function of current AR systems such as, Photon emission tomography, near infra-red spectroscopy and the use of dyes, such as indocyanine green have been used with AR systems to identify sentinel nodes and tissue vascularity (Tagaya et al.,2008). Robotics and Haptic force feedback are also promising ways to combine with AR technology.

Together, these two technologies can help increase efficiency, reduction in expenditures and enhance the patient experience in ways.

In conclusion, the AR simulators may become integrated in the future dental practices which can be used for educational purposes as well as enhances clinical skills. In the future AR can become incorporated in the dental training curriculum in various dental divisions so that trainee dentists might be able to improve their clinical skills themselves which would considerably reduce the risk for the procedural errors and will create a safer environment for clinical practices. Similarly, in surgical procedures, accurate data on the medical imaging and tracking system would assist the surgeons to execute the surgical procedures more precisely and accurately.

REFERENCES

Ayoub, A., & Pulijala, Y. (2019). The application of virtual reality and augmented reality in Oral & Maxillofacial Surgery. *BMC Oral Health*, *19*(1), 238. doi:10.118612903-019-0937-8 PMID:31703708

Bhat, S., Shetty, S., & Shenoy, K.K. (2005). Imaging in implantology. *J Indian Prosthodont Soc, 5*, 10-4.

Birkfellner, W., Watzinger, F., Wanschitz, F., Ewers, R., & Bergmann, H. (1998). Calibration of tracking systems in a surgical environment. *IEEE Trans Med Imag, 17*, 737-42.

Dimaio, S., Kapur, T., Cleary, K., Aylward, S., Kazanzides, P., & Vosburgh, K. (2007). Challenges in image-guided therapy system design. *Neuroimage, 37*, S144-51.

Durham, M., Engel, B., Ferrill, T., Halford, J., Singh, T. P., & Gladwell, M. (2019). Digitally augmented learning in implant dentistry. *Oral and Maxillofacial Surgery Clinics of North America*, *31*(3), 387–398. doi:10.1016/j.coms.2019.03.003 PMID:31153725

Ewers, R., & Schicho, K. (2009). Augmented reality telenavigation in cranio maxillofacial oral surgery. *Studies in Health Technology and Informatics*, *150*, 24–25. PMID:19745259

Farronato, M., Maspero, C., Lanteri, V., Fama, A., Ferrati, F., Pettenuzzo, A., & Farronato, D. (2019). Current state of the art in the use of augmented reality in dentistry: A systematic review of the literature. *BMC Oral Health*, *19*(1), 135. doi:10.118612903-019-0808-3 PMID:31286904

Gulati, M., Anand, V., Salaria, S.K., Jain, N., & Gupta, S. (2015). Computerized implant-dentistry: advances toward automation. *J Indian Soc Periodontol, 1*, 5-10.

Joda, T., & Gallucci, G. O. (2015). The virtual patient in dental medicine. *Clinical Oral Implants Research*, *26*(6), 725–726. doi:10.1111/clr.12379 PMID:24665872

Joda, T., Gallucci, G. O., Wismeijer, D., & Zitzmann, N. U. (2019). Augmented and virtual reality in dental medicine: A systematic review. *Computers in Biology and Medicine*, *108*, 93–100. doi:10.1016/j.compbiomed.2019.03.012 PMID:31003184

Kato, H., & Billinghurst, M. (1999). Marker tracking and HMD calibration for a video-based augmented reality conferencing system. In *IWAR '99 Proceedings of 2nd IEEE and ACM International Workshop on Augmented Reality*. IEEE Computer Society. 10.1109/IWAR.1999.803809

Kwon, H. B., Park, Y. S., & Han, J. S. (2018). Augmented reality in dentistry: A current perspective. *Acta Odontologica Scandinavica*, *76*(7), 497–503. doi:10.1080/00016357.2018.1441437 PMID:29465283

Lee, S. H. (2018). Research and development of haptic simulator for dental education using virtual reality and use motion. *Int. J. Adv. Smart Conv.*, *7*, 114–120.

Meola, A., Cutolo, F., Carbone, M., Cagnazzo, F., Ferrari, M., & Ferrari, V. (2016). Augmented reality in neurosurgery: A systematic review. *Neurosurgical Review*, *40*(4), 537–548. doi:10.100710143-016-0732-9 PMID:27154018

Modern Practice. (2018, October 2). *The Future of Dentistry with Augmented and Virtual Reality*. https://blog.net32.com/the-future-of-dentistry-with-augmented-and-virtual-reality/

Nijmeh, A. D., Goodger, N. M., Hawkes, D., Edwards, P. J., & McGurk, M. (2005). Image-guided navigation in oral and maxillofacial surgery. *British Journal of Oral & Maxillofacial Surgery*, *43*(4), 294–302. doi:10.1016/j.bjoms.2004.11.018 PMID:15993282

Ploder, O., Wagner, A., & Enislidis, G. (1995). Computer-assisted intraoperative visualization of dental implants. Augmented reality in medicine. *Der Radiologe*, *35*, 569–572. PMID:8588037

Roy, E., Bakr, M. M., & George, R. (2017). The need for virtual reality simulators in dental education: A review. *The Saudi Dental Journal*, *29*(2), 41–47. doi:10.1016/j.sdentj.2017.02.001 PMID:28490842

Sarika, G., Neelkant, P., Jitender, S., Ravinder, S., & Sanjeev, L. (2015). Oral implant imaging: a review. *Malays J Med Sci, 22*, 7-17.

Schulz, C., Waldeck, S., & Mauer, U. M. (2012). Intraoperative image guidance in neurosurgery: Development, current indications, and future trends. *Radiology Research and Practice*, *2012*, 197364. doi:10.1155/2012/197364 PMID:22655196

Suenaga, H., Tran, H., & Liao, H. (2013). Real-time in situ three dimensional integral videography and surgical navigation using augmented reality: a pilot study. *Int J Oral Sci., 5*, 98–102.

Sutherland, J., Belec, J., Sheikh, A., Chepelev, L., Althobaity, W., Chow, B. J. W., Mitsouras, D., Christensen, A., Rybicki, F. J., & La Russa, D. J. (2019). Applying modern virtual and augmented reality technologies to medical images and models. *Journal of Digital Imaging, 32*(1), 38–53. doi:10.100710278-018-0122-7 PMID:30215180

Tagaya, N., Yamazaki, R., Nakagawa, A., Abe, A., Hamada, K., Kubota, K., & Oyama, T. (2008). Intraoperative identification of sentinel lymph nodes by near-infrared fluorescence imaging in patients with breast cancer. *American Journal of Surgery, 195*(6), 850–853. doi:10.1016/j.amjsurg.2007.02.032 PMID:18353274

Touati, R., Richert, R., Millet, C., Farges, J.C., Sailer, I., & Ducret, M. (2019). Comparison of two innovative strategies using augmented reality for communication in aesthetic dentistry: A pilot study. *Journal of Healthcare Engineering, 6*(24), 5139.

Wagner, A., Rasse, M., Millesi, W., & Ewers, R. (1997). Virtual reality for orthognathic surgery: The augmented reality environment concept. *Journal of Oral and Maxillofacial Surgery, 55*(5), 456–462. doi:10.1016/S0278-2391(97)90689-3 PMID:9146514

Wang, J., Suenaga, H., & Hoshi, K. (2014). Augmented reality navigation with automatic marker-free image registration using 3-D image overlay for dental surgery. *IEEE Transactions on Biomedical Engineering, 61*(4), 1295–1304. doi:10.1109/TBME.2014.2301191 PMID:24658253

Wang, J., Suenaga, H., Liao, H., Hoshi, K., Yang, L., Kobayashi, E., & Sakuma, I. (2015). Real-time computer-generated integral imaging and 3D image calibration for augmented reality surgical navigation. *Computerized Medical Imaging and Graphics, 40*, 147–159. doi:10.1016/j.compmedimag.2014.11.003 PMID:25465067

Wiles, A.D., Thompson, D.G., & Frantz, D.D. (2004). Accuracy assessment and interpretation for optical tracking systems. *Visual Image Guid Proced Displ, 5367*, 421-32.

Zadik, Y., & Levin, L. (2006). Decision making of Hebrew University and Tel Aviv University Dental Schools graduates in every day dentistry-is there a difference? *J Isr Dent Assoc, 4*, 19-23.

Zadik, Y., & Levin, L. (2008). Clinical decision making in restorative dentistry, endodontics, and antibiotic prescription. *J Dent Educ, 72*, 81-6.

Section 4
Mental Intervention

Chapter 10
Virtual Reality Exposure Therapy and Physiological Data Analysis for Treatment of Stress Disorders

Charles V. Trappey
National Yang Ming Chiao Tung University, Taiwan

Amy J. C. Trappey
ID https://orcid.org/0000-0001-7651-7012
National Tsing Hua University, Taiwan

C. M. Chang
Chang Gung Memorial Hospital, Taiwan

M. C. Tsai
Taoyuan General Hospital, Taiwan

Routine R. T. Kuo
National Tsing Hua University, Taiwan

Aislyn P. C. Lin
National Tsing Hua University, Taiwan

ABSTRACT

Anxiety disorders are diagnosed when people become overreactive, disassociated, and feel emotionally unable to control feelings to the extent that their daily lifes are affected. Driving phobia is one of the widespread anxiety disorders in modern society, which cause problematic disruptions of a patient's daily activities. Exposure therapy is an approach gaining popularity for treating patients with stress disorders. Virtual reality (VR) technology allows people to interact with objects and stimuli in an immersive way. The VR for phobic therapy using indirect exposure, which can be safely discontinued or lowed in terms of intensity, is the area of research with literature published and patents granted. This research focuses on reviewing virtual reality exposure therapy (VRET) literature and patents. The chapter also presents the research and development of a novel driving phobia VRET system with the detailed experiments to demonstrate the design, development, implementation, enhancement, and verification of VRET.

DOI: 10.4018/978-1-7998-8371-5.ch010

1. INTRODUCTION

Patients suffering from anxiety disorders have high levels of anxiety and a variety of symptoms, such as inattention, irritability, fatigue, and insomnia. Common types of anxiety disorder include panic disorder (PD), phobia, obsessive-compulsive disorder (OCD), and post-traumatic stress disorder (PTSD) (Gautam et al., 2017). Studies have pointed out that when PTSD is accompanied by other anxiety or comorbid depression, PTSD symptoms are more severe (Spinhoven et al., 2014; Momartin et al., 2004; Hruska et al., 2014). A National Comorbidity survey replication showed that patients with PTSD included about 44% of patients with three or more anxiety diagnoses other than PTSD (Elhai et al., 2008). PTSD also increases the risk of suicidality and functional impairment (Giaconia et al., 1995; Perkonigg et al., 2000).

Motor vehicle accidents (MVA) are the leading cause of medical treated trauma in the United States (US) (Blanchard & Hickling, 2004). In 2018, the number of MVA exceeded 6.7 million and about 2.7 million people were injured during the accidents in the US. Research from the National Institute of Mental Health (NIMH) has shown that 39% of the MVA survivors met DSM-III-R criteria for post-traumatic stress disorder (PTSD). Patients who had PTSD often develop disabling memories and anxiety related to the car accident event. These individuals were more likely to be subjectively distressed by environmental conditions with increased impairment in commuting to work or driving a car for pleasure (Blanchard & Hickling, 1995). The type of PTSD caused by MVAs referred to as driving phobia disorder. Driving phobia is a common disorder and the degree of fear differs significantly between patients. Some patients are only afraid of particular driving situations, while some may break out in a cold sweat when seated in the driver's seat.

System desensitization (SD) refers to slowly exposing patients to the situation that causes neurotic anxiety and psychological relaxation to combat this anxiety to eliminate patients' neurotic anxiety. SD is widely used in clinical psychology, including assisting patients to overcome particular phobias, and the efficacy of SD is recognized. VRET uses the concept of SD to immerse patients in a virtual environment, deepen the sense of presence through visual, sound, and tactile immersion, and create stimuli to make patients feel moderately fearful. Ougrin's research (2011) demonstrated that VRET is as effective as traditional cognitive behavioral therapy (CBT). Some qualitative case studies have initially confirmed the effectiveness of VRET in the treatment of phobias (Beck et al., 2007; Zinzow et al., 2018; Kaussner et al., 2020), and other studies have shown that the efficacy of VRET is even better than that of traditional CBT (Scozzari & Gamberini, 2011).

This research will focus on constructing a new driving phobia VRET system as an example to verify the effectiveness of the treatment. The experiment will provide an immersive experience of driving for subjects, integrating subjects' biodata collection via a control group-based experimental design. The VRET experiment combines comprehensive biodata analysis with the survey analysis between treatment and control group to measure the effectiveness of the system. The chapter is organized in the following sections. In Section 2, the literature of VRET and specific driving phobia treatments are reviewed. Self-measurement surveys related to driving behavior and patents related to VR driving applications are also reviewed. Section 3 describes the methodologies and approaches applied and integrated with this research, including experimental details, fear of driving questionnaire analysis, and real-time physiological data analysis. Section 4 interprets the implications of the experiment. Section 5 summarizes the essential findings and contributions of the research. The analytical results of VRET's effectiveness for treating driving phobia and the future development required in the field are addressed in the final remarks.

2. LITERATURE AND PATENT REVIEWS

Existing mental illnesses, such as post-traumatic stress syndrome, driving phobia, and fear of heights, often inhibit the lives of patients to live and work normally and interact normally with relatives and friends. Cognitive behavioral therapy (CBT) and exposure therapy are used to treat patients' psychological treatment. CBT has two parts: cognitive therapy and behavioral therapy. CBT reduces cognitive anxiety by allowing patients to understand and change the cognition or behavior that will cause anxiety. Hofmann et al., (2012) and Bisson & Andrew (2007) confirmed the efficacy of CBT on mental disorders and demonstrated that CBT can effectively reduce the symptoms of PTSD. Exposure therapy refers to a treatment method that exposes the patient to various stimuli and continuously increases the intensity of the stimulus so that it is gradually tolerated and accepted as normal. Exposure therapy includes imaginary exposure and in vivo exposure. For imaginary exposure, the therapist asks the patient to imagine what they are afraid of, while in vivo exposure causes the patient to face their fears directly. Several studies have confirmed the effectiveness of exposure to PTSD. Bryant et al (1999) devised a study where 45 patients with PTSD were divided into three treatment groups and received long-term exposure (N = 14) a combination of long-term exposure and anxiety control (N = 15) or supportive counseling (N = 16). The results showed that only 14% and 20% of the group members who received long-term exposure and long-term exposure plus anxiety treatment reached PTSD standards after treatment, while 56% of the support counseling group members still had PTSD. These findings indicate that CBT can effectively prevent PTSD, and prolonged exposure may be the most critical factor in the treatment of PTSD. For traditional PTSD treatment, patients are required to imagine their trauma-related situations which patients tend to avoid. The studies have shown that it is difficult to ask patients to clearly imagine the situations they want to avoid, which limits traditional treatment. Virtual reality exposure therapy (VRET) can solve this problem.

Virtual reality devices and bio-signal sensors are used by VRET to customize and control the treatment. A virtual environment simulates three-dimensional space to provide patients with a better sense of presence and provide more direct stimulation to achieve effective exposure therapy while ensuring environmental safety., VRET can be performed in a private space to provide patient privacy (North et al., 1997). The clinician can control environmental characteristics such as difficulty, complexity, and irritation allowing greater scalability and a controllable environment (Romano, 2005).

Several well-known technology companies have invested in the development of virtual reality systems. Facebook acquired Oculus and released Rift and mobile versions of Go called nowQuest. Google launch Daydream; HTC developed Vive; Sony created Playstation VR; and Apple is also researching the developed of virtual reality devices (Miloff et al., 2020). With these powerful hardware and software development resources on the market becoming less expensive, a solid foundation has been laid for the future development of VRET.

The behavioral therapy technique used by VRET to treat phobias usually involves gradually exposing patients to anxiety-producing stimuli (systemic desensitization). Oskam (2005) defined the effectiveness of virtual reality exposure therapy. His research concludes that effective virtual reality exposure therapy must meet three conditions. First, the emotional stimulation ability of the virtual environment must be strong enough to allow users to feel the anxiety. Second, the cognitive existence that people experience in the VRET environment is an important factor. Finally, when the patient returns to the real world, the effect of VRET must be transferrable to the real world.

There have been many studies exploring the effectiveness of VRET. Two meta-analyses in one study examined the efficacy of VRET on social anxiety. The first meta-analysis (Chesham et al., 2018) collected six studies and 233 participants to test whether VRET can reduce social anxiety better than waiting list control conditions. The results showed a significant overall effect size indicating that VRET can effectively reduce social anxiety disorder. The second meta-analysis (Horigome et al., 2020), used seven studies and a total of 340 participants to test whether traditional treatments for social anxiety disorder (including internal or imaginary exposure) can produce more significant effects than VRET. The results show that there is no difference in the effect size between VRET and in vivo or imagined exposure. Our research supports the hypothesis that VRET will be effective in treating social anxiety disorder. Although some studies claim that VRET is an acceptable treatment for SAD patients with significant and long-term efficacy. Another study generally discussed the current effectiveness of VRET for social anxiety disorder (SAD). In existing experiments, dialogs between avatars and patient and virtual audiences, emotional facial expressions, and language interaction with avatars have been studied. The results of these studies show that VRET and traditional ET are equally effective. However, few existing studies have randomized controlled trials (RCT) to study the independent efficacy of VRET in SAD. Most studies have studied RCT that compares VRET with in vivo SAD exposure.

Emmelkamp et al., (2020) explored the effectiveness of VRET in treating dental fear. The first study used a single-blind RCT for 30 randomized patients. The primary outcome anxiety indicators were evaluated before and after the intervention, at one week, three months, and six months follow-up. During the 6-month follow-up, the secondary outcome indicators evaluated included avoidance after the behavior, changes in heart rate and VR experience time, temporal and spatial changes after VRET, and dental treatment acceptance in both cases. Results at the end of VRET and follow-up, the patient's anxiety score was significantly reduced, indicating that VRET is effective in the treatment of dental phobia

A systematic electronic database search following the PRISMA guidelines and conducted two meta-analyses to systematically review the current evidence on the effectiveness of VRET and ARET as treatments for PTSD (Eshuis et al., 2020). The results found 11 studies on the efficacy of VRET on PTSD but no studies on the efficacy of ARET. Most VRET studies are of low quality and have different results. The meta-analysis showed that VRET was better than the waiting list control, and no significant difference was found between VRET and active treatment conditions. Therefore, VRET may be an effective alternative to current treatments, and future research should focus on high-quality RCTs, including information about side effects and adverse events, and increasing the sample size. This research recognizes that there is a gap in the efficacy of ARET, although it may have the potential for the treatment of PTSD.

It is essential to deliver a strong sense of presence to users when immersed in the virtual environment to enhance the VRET system (North & North, 2018). Sheridan (200) claims four influencing factors affect the sense of presence, namely information quantity, sensor position and orientation, change of relative location of objects, and the active imagination in suppressing disbelief. The VR will become more realistic and authentic once these factors being well-managed, and users can better immerse themselves in the virtual environment. The illusion of presence also enhances users' sense of presence, which refers to a psychological phenomenon known as embodiment (Waldrop, 2017). A study reveals that when subjects' virtual avatar is threatened with harm, users' heart rate shifts into fright mode (Slater et al., 2010).

There have been many studies applying VRET to different phobias. For example, to treat acrophobia, Emmelkamp et al. (2002) recruited 33 patients with acrophobia and randomly divided them into two groups for exposure in vivo (N=16) and low-budget VRET (N=17). The results showed that exposure in vivo and low-cost VRET have the same effectiveness and they maintain on the same level during the six-month follow-up, which indicates that VRET can be implemented on a single machine in the current market using relatively inexpensive hardware and software. For fear of flying, Rothbaum et al.'s (2006) research compares the effectiveness of VRET and exposure therapy in vivo in treating fear of flying. A total of 75 participants were randomly assigned to VRET, in vivo or waiting list (25 in each group) and completed the study. Treatment includes four training sessions for anxiety management and six weeks of exposure to virtual aircraft (VRET) or actual aircraft (in vivo) at the airport. The results show that the willingness to fly after treatment, VRET and in vivo are better than the waiting list. Follow-up evaluations performed at 6 and 12 months showed that the treatment effect was maintained. This study supports that VRET is as effective as exposure therapy in vivo for FOF treatment.

Driving is considered an essential skill for individuals living in modern society, a skill that facilitates the maintenance of independence, mobility, enables engagement in crucial activities, and is often the qualification for employment. People who suffered from the psychological impairment of serious motor vehicle accidents account for most patients with driving phobia. Other possible reasons that lead to driving phobia include claustrophobia patients, who may have a panic attack while driving on the highway or in traffic jams. These patients know someone who experienced a terrible car accident or lacked trust in their driving skills (Taylor et al., 2002). Based on the emotional processing theory (Costa et al., 2010), VRET can lead to new and neutral memory structures that, if applied to PTSD patients properly, can diminish old and traumatic memories, such as a bad car crash that often provokes and heightens anxiety. VRET treatment can be provided in a small clinical space providing patient privacy (North et al., 1997). The clinician can control the environmental characteristics that lead to patient embarrassment, complexity, and irritation. The treatment is highly scalable, and the treatment environment's controllability demonstrates the flexibility of the system (Romano, 2005). An increasing number of scholars have conducted research in the VRET domain, especially focusing on driving phobia. One early study used VRET to treat PTSD symptoms as the consequence of a severe motor vehicle accident. Six individuals reported either full or severe subsyndromal PTSD and completed ten sessions of VRET using software designed to create real-time driving scenarios. The results showed significant reductions in post-trauma symptoms involving reexperiencing, avoidance, and emotional numbing, and VRET was successfully applied in the treatment of PTSD following road accidents (Beck et al., 2007). In one VRET plus cognitive-behavioral therapy (CBT) for driving anxiety and aggression pilot study, six U.S. veterans who suffered from MVAs while serving in the military participated in the research. The study was a novel VRET + CBT for patients that integrated the anxiety and anger management components, although the sample size is very small (only six). Each veteran completed eight intervention sessions, as well as six to nine months follow-up assessments. At the end of the experiment, their hyperarousal in driving situations declined by 69%, aggressive driving declined by 29%, and risky driving declined by 21% (Zinzow et al., 2018). In a pilot study adopting VRET, fourteen subjects with severe driving phobia disorders participated in psychotherapeutic, VRET, CBT sessions, and behavioral avoidance tests (BAT) when driving on the road. The treatment design placed the subjects under ten days of therapeutic experiments. After the six to twelve weeks follow-up after experiments, thirteen out of fourteen patients maintained effective treatment results (Kaussner et al., 2020). Although this was a pilot study, the experiment design and procedure provide an excellent reference for future VRET clinical studies. In a previous study, patients received three treatments within ten days. The treatment included four VR driving scenarios. As a result, the patient's anxiety was reduced. The anxiety and avoidance scores began to decline after treatment and were maintained after a seven-month follow-up study (Wald & Taylor, 2000). In one VRET driving phobia pre-test experiment conducted at the Taiwan National Tsing Hua

University (NTHU), 31 subjects participated in a seven-level driving scenario. The clinical design used a pre-test analysis to identify students with driving anxiety, a control group and random assignment. The exposure simulated driving on a country road, a highway, and a mountain road during the day and at night. The level of fear-inducing driving exposure increases with successful completion of lower levels of exposure. The heart rate, respiration rate, skin conductance, and body temperature data were collected to measure the degree of anxiety. The pre-test result examined the effectiveness of the VRET system. The subject's anxiety increases with level progression, verifying that the VRET system design affects the subjects' mental state (Trappey et al., 2020 & 2021).

A self-measurement questionnaire is a research instrument consisting of a series of questions used to measure a subject's anxiety. Many studies apply self-assessment surveys to assess the anxiety level of subjects in specific driving situations. A study used driving behavior questionnaires to conduct surveys at three universities, using the questionnaires to measure which driving situations make drivers feel anxious and uncomfortable. According to factor analysis, this questionnaire includes three dimensions: anxiety-based performance deficits, exaggerated safety/caution behavior, and anxiety-related hostile/aggressive behavior. There are 21 questions in this questionnaire, and each question uses a 7-point Likert scale that ranges from 1 (never) to 7 (always) (Clapp et al., 2011). Another study used a questionnaire to evaluate the avoidance behavior of driving or riding by subjects, which included 20 questions describing driving or riding situations. Each question used a 4-point Likert scale to score avoidance behavior. The 4-point Likert scale ranges from 0 (little or no time to avoid) to 4 (to avoid most or all of the time) (Taylor et al., 2020). Bandura's (2006) research measures anxiety under specific driving situations. The content of the scale includes the driver's confidence in driving in a specific situation and the degree of discomfort. The study used a questionnaire to investigate subjects' subjective feelings when driving under seven different conditions, including neighborhood blocks, residential areas, downtown streets, main arterial roads, freeways, major city roads, and mountain roads.

Among the patents related to VRET collected through Derwent Innovation, most patents are from large international companies. This research analyzes the patents applied by these large companies as a reference for the development of the system without infringement. Among the patents collected, the most numerous patents came from two companies: Magic Leap and LG Electronics. Magic Leap (2017) is an American augmented reality company. Its patents cover the shape and structure of mixed reality equipment, system methods, and waveguide display principles and use advanced optical display technology to construct a virtual image generation system (. LG Electronics (2016) is a South Korean company whose business scope includes household appliances, electronics, communication technology, and chemistry. In some of LG's patents, the user's emotions are identified by measuring the user's heart rate, skin temperature, breathing volume, and blood pressure. LG patents focus on VR headsets and VR display image quality. In terms of improving the image quality and speed of virtual reality display, LG proposes a display device with multiple data lines, multiple gate lines, and multiple pixels arranged in a matrix where the data lines and the gate lines intersect. By controlling the display, the driver shifts the gate signals, minimizing data while reducing user fatigue to improve the virtual reality display image quality and speed (LG Display Co Ltd., 2019). Another academic institution, Korean University, also has many patents related to VRET. In their research, they focused on making the system automatically adapt to the users. The Korean University and Business Research Foundation Korea (2020) measure the pressure and load level of PTSD patients through electroencephalography (EEG) and heart rate variability (HRV) and automatically adjusts the exposure intensity based on the patient's response. Through such an adaptive system, the treatment effect can be effectively improved. Another company, Blaubit Co.

Ltd. (2019), provides appropriate treatment content based on the patient's mental state. They developed a pressure disorder detection system for VRET panic attacks, which analyzes the patient's behavioral data to detect the panic level of the patient and provide corresponding treatment. Qingdao Saibo Kaier Information Technology Co. (2016) filed a patent on a VRET system which combines head-mounted display, sound effects, and physiological feedback. The system has high safety, significant effect, strong controllability, and short treatment time, which significantly improves the applicability of VRET.

The interpretation of physiological signals is very important for the development and verification of the VRET system. The human body's physiological signals are responses that humans cannot control allowing emotional responses to be captured using signal sensing devices. The human body's mental state becomes tense during anxiety, anger, tension, and stress. Using physiological equipment, medical professionals can directly observe the stress state. Physiological feedback, such as muscle tightness, heart rate, skin conductance, or skin temperature, can be used as a measure of the state of the subject by the VRET system. Shu, Xie, and others (2018) provide a comprehensive review of emotion recognition based on physiological signals, including emotion models, emotion induction methods, published emotional physiological data sets, and feature classifiers. The most commonly used physiological feedback is the heart rate. Herumurt's study (2019) treated a patients' public speaking anxiety. The study simulates the scene of a speech on stage and projects the audiences off stage. The system measures the heart rate of the subject to determine the difficulty level from different audience responses. If the patient's heart rate is very high, then the subject is very anxious and the audience will doze off and be inattentive, making the subject less anxious. On the other hand, if the subject's heart rate is not high, which represents a lack of anxiety, the system creates a group of attentive listeners and increase the difficulty of the speech. Dingli and Bondin, (2019) used heart rate to help define emotions as joy or anger. The study classifies the measurement of emotions as going well or poorly and then adjust the level of difficulty over time to improve the classification.

Another physiological feedback is skin resistance and skin conductance. Studies have confirmed that blood oxygen is the least effective among the many physiological feedbacks for measuring emotions, while blood volume and skin response are the most effective (Trivedi, 2018). One study recruited 22 non-fear participants and 36 people who fear flying to participate in the VRET experiment (Wieder-hold et al., 2002). During the treatment, heart rate, skin resistance, and skin temperature were used as physiological indicators to record the physiological trends of the participants. As a result, the fearers and non-fearers showed a significant difference in skin resistance, and as the treatment progressed, the skin resistance of the fearers also tended to approach the non-fearers, showing that the skin resistance can effectively reflect human anxiety.

The concepts of convolution and machine learning have been applied to physiological data analysis. In Jacob Kritikos's research (2019), he used skin resistance to measure emotion combined with continuous deconvolution analysis (CDA) to disassemble data to optimize the analysis results. Another study (Hinkle et al., 2019) used a 3x3 matrix to define the level of arousal, dividing the physiological data every 10 seconds as input for machine learning classification. The research results show that feature extraction is a critical step in the classification process, and SVM can achieve improve sentiment classification. Another study combined VRET with psychological stress detection and collected physiological signals of 30 participants, including blood volume pressure (BVP), galvanic skin response (GSR), and skin temperature (Salehi et al., 2020). The psychological stress test used the subjective unit of distress scale (SUDS) and divides anxiety into four levels: low, mild, moderate, and high. The SVM classifier achieves an accuracy higher than 80%. In the study of Kim and Jo (2018), a physiological model for identifying human emotions was introduced called the Deep Physiological Affect Network. The model is based on a convolutional long short-term memory (ConvLSTM) network and a new loss function based on time margins. The model uses public data and EEG signals to classify the problem and significantly improves the recognition rate of the latest technology. Yin, Zhao, and others (2017) believe that conventional deep sentiment classifiers are too simplified in feature extraction. They proposed a multiple fusion layer classifier consisting of stacked autoencoders (MESAE) to recognize emotions. Each SAE consists of three hidden layers to filter noise in physiological features and derive stable data Another deep learning model is used to achieve SAE integration. According to different feature extraction methods, the physiological features are divided into several subsets, and each subset is coded separately by SAE. According to the SAE abstract derived from the combination of physiological modalities, six sets of codes are created, which are then input into the three-layer network based on adjacent graphs for feature fusion. Fusion features are used to identify binary arousal or valence. DEAP is used to verify that MESAE improves accuracy.

The Technical Function Matrix (TFM) is an effective method of analyzing patents. For a specific patent or technology, the patent or technology and the corresponding function are analyzed in a two-dimensional table to form a matrix-type statistical table. This two-dimensional table visually explains the distribution of patents, allowing users to understand the strategic position of a particular patented technology, the position that competitors have already occupied, and the R&D strategy that they should adopt, and discover the key strategic points in the industry (Jhuang, Sun, etc., 2017). The technology of this research is defined using the Themescape Map function provided by Derwent Innovation. Themescape Map analyzes and interprets the patent search results in depictions of key themes. Our research defined six leading technologies from the Themescape Map figure: vehicle simulation, virtual reality-related technology, PTSD diagnosis, bio-signal analysis, health systems, and artificial intelligence (self-adaptive systems). As for functions, four typical VR applications are defined here, namely entertainment, VRET, driving training, and healthcare.

All 428 patents collected were analyzed using TFM, and the analysis results are shown in Table 1. It can be seen from the results that VR driving-related patents are concentrated in vehicle simulation (T01) and VR-related technology (T02) with the function of driving training (F03). Our research belongs to the category of PTSD diagnosis (T03) in terms of technology. The function is related to VRET (F02) and driving training (F03). It can be seen from Table 1 that the existing patents for PTSD diagnosis (T03) and VRET (F02) are far fewer than those for PTSD diagnosis (T03) and driving training (F03). Therefore, according to the results of TFM analysis, PTSD diagnosis combined with VRET has promising development potential.

Table 1. Technology function matrix

			Function			
			F01	**F02**	**F03**	**F04**
			Entertainment	**VRET**	**Driving training**	**Healthcare application**
Technology	T01	Vehicle simulation	14	6	92	12
	T02	VR-related technology	42	61	178	26
	T03	PTSD diagnosis	1	18	10	8
	T04	Bio-signal analysis	7	16	33	26
	T05	Health system	3	5	8	23
	T06	Artificial intelligence	7	15	39	5

3. VR ENABLED DRIVING PHOBIA TREATMENT: METHODOLOGIES AND PROCEDURE

In this research, the integrated VRET system with the biological data sensing module for driving phobia treatment is presented. Thirty subjects were recruited to conduct the VRET experiment for the effectiveness test of the proposed system. Section 3.1 introduces the filtering and screening process to select 30 subjects among 130 subjects who have answered the prior experiment survey. Section 3.2 demonstrates the 4-level scenario design of the VRET immersive system. Section 3.3 introduces the system architecture and experiment flow of the proposed experiment. During the experiment, subjects' multi-biofeedback data were collected and the physiological data analysis is presented in section 3.4. Section 3.5 introduces the development of self-adaptive VRET design, which aims for subject's emotional recognition used for dynamically configuring the ET parameters. Section 3.6 discusses the treatment effectiveness of the VRET design through the post-treatment survey review.

Figure 1. Subject selection flow chart.

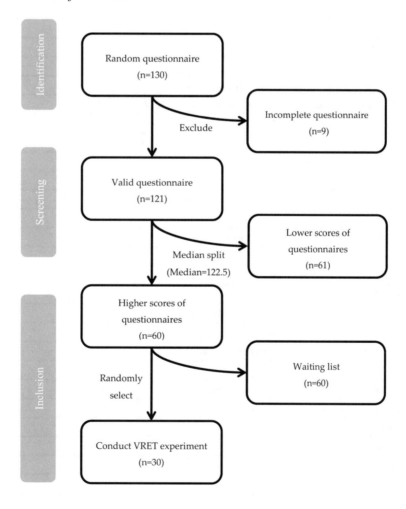

3.1 Subject Selection: Pre-treatment Phobia (Psychological) Survey to select Subjects to Undergo VRET

Table 2. Self-measurement driving behavior survey.

Q1	I get lost while driving
Q2	When other people's driving behaviors cause me anxiety, I will yell at them
Q3	I will slow down when passing the intersection, even if the traffic light is green
Q4	I accidentally drive too close to the far lane line when I drive
Q5	I will forget to adjust my speed
Q6	When other people's driving behaviors cause anxiety, I will express my anxiety to them
Q7	I keep a large distance from the vehicle in front
Q8	I often forget my destination
Q9	When other people's driving behaviors cause anxiety, I will gesture to them
Q10	I need to maintain a constant speed to calm down while driving
Q11	I try to stay away from other vehicles
Q12	I am not sure which lane I should drive in
Q13	I slap the steering wheel when I feel anxious
Q14	I will slow down until I feel at ease
Q15	When other people's driving behaviors cause anxiety, I will blow my car horn
Q16	I will find a way to let other drivers know that their driving behavior caused anxiety
Q17	When the weather is bad, I will drive more carefully than other vehicles on the road
Q18	I curse at others while driving
Q19	I am not used to entering the main road
Q20	I will avoid trips, errands, and activities that require driving
Q21	To avoid driving, I walk, ride a bicycle, or find an alternative such as a bus
Q22	I avoid driving through busy intersections
Q23	There are sections of the road that I avoid in fear of traffic jams
Q24	I am afraid of encountering traffic jams when I drive
Q25	I will avoid driving because of bad weather (for example: fog, rain, snow)
Q26	I avoid driving at night
Q27	I will avoid alternative modes of transportation because of bad weather
Q28	I avoid alternative modes of transportation at night
Q29	When I ride in a car or bus when not driving, I'm afraid of encountering traffic jams
Q30	I avoid riding on the highway
Q31	I will avoid trips and errands that require transportation in a vehicle
Q32	I will take the bus or MRT to somewhere to avoid driving by myself
Q33	I am afraid to drive in a residential area
Q34	I am afraid to drive in the suburbs
Q35	I am afraid to drive into the city
Q36	I am afraid to drive on the highway
Q37	I am afraid to drive through tunnels
Q38	I am afraid to drive on mountain roads
Q39	I am afraid to drive across the bridge

The subject's filtering and screening process for this study is presented in Figure 1. A self-measurement driving behavior survey, which refers to three academic studies concerning driving behavior measurements (Clapp et al., 2011; Taylor et al., 2020; Bandura, 2006), is rated on a 7-point Likert scale. The questions Q1~Q19 were adapted from and refer to the behavior-rating scales for anxious driving behavior (Clapp et al., 2011). Questions Q20~Q32 refer to a driving and riding avoidance scale (DRAS), a promising measure of anxiety-related avoidance research (Taylor et al., 2020). Finally, questions Q33~Q39 refer to a self-efficacy survey that focuses on driving in specific situations (Bandura, 2006). Our questionnaire for the self-measurement of driving behavior incorporates these published and validated questions (Table 2). Possession with a valid driver's license and aged between 20 and 60 years old are the criteria in prerequisite screening for qualified subjects to fill out the survey. Drivers in this age range are considered mature drivers and drivers with sufficient driving experience. While drivers younger than 20 years of age are considered inexperienced and drivers over 60 years of age demonstrated higher rates of accident and fatality involvement, as reported by the previous research (Duke et al., 2010). Recruiting subjects between the ages of twenty to sixty years old in order to minimize age factors affecting the VRET experiment outcome. Subjects who had experienced severe car accident injuries has been removed to minimize subjects from having panic attacks during the experiment. A total of 130 randomly selected subjects have filled out the driving behavior questionnaire, and 9 were excluded due to incomplete answers. The 121 valid subjects were median-split into two groups based on their questionnaire score: 60 subjects belong to high-fear of driving and 61 subjects belong to low-fear of driving. Afterward, 30 subjects were randomly drawn from the high-fear driving group to participate in the VRET experiment as the treatment group (TG). Furthermore, 61 subjects with low or no fear of driving fear were assigned to the control group (CG) for VRET effectiveness comparison without participating in the VRET clinical experiment. The 30 randomly selected subjects as the TG conduct the VRET experiment (sample size of 30) provide the appropriate sample size required for experiment validity (Hogg & Tanis, 2013).

3.2 Driving Phobia VRET Therapy Design - Levels 0~4

The VRET system includes a pre-experiment practice level and four realistic virtual environments for the actual implementation of scenarios (Figure 2, 5-level scenery descriptions) and Figure 3 (scenery snapshots). To provide subjects with a fully immersive driving experience, an integrated traffic system was incorporated into every level with traffic signals at crossways and several vehicles driving near or passing the subject's vehicle. Some patients are extremely fearful of car crashes and collision events in VR which leads to motion sickness. The system has integrated an anticollision function to prevent subjects from crashing into other vehicles, buildings, or the roadside. At each treatment level, subjects drive for five minutes and are asked if they wish to advance to a higher level if the immersive driving environment is no longer challenging or fear-inducing. Each level has a unique virtual surrounding and scenery for treatment purposes. The details of the five levels (0~4) are described as follows:

Level 0: The pre-experiment practice session. Driving on a straight wide road with no vehicles drive near subjects and the speed limit is set at 50 km/hr.

Level 1: Driving in the city road with intersections during the daytime, the speed limit is set at 50 km/hr.

Level 2: Driving through a highway tunnel during the daytime, the speed limit is set at 110 km/hr. Subjects will be asked to increase speed if lower than 80 km/hr.

Level 3: Driving across a cross-bay bridge and a tall bridge, the speed limit is set at 50 km/hr.

Level 4: Driving on a slope mountain road at night, the speed limit is set at 50 km/hr.

Figure 2. The five-level driving scenarios.

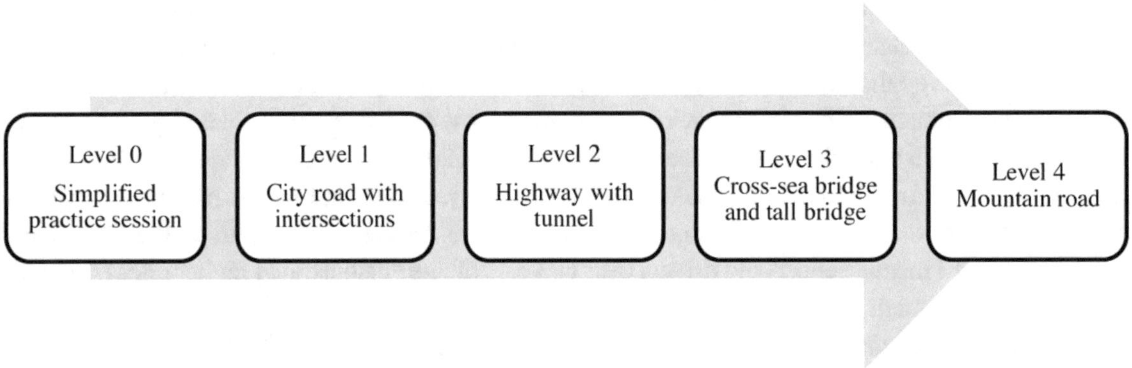

| Level 0
Simplified
practice session | Level 1
City road with
intersections | Level 2
Highway with
tunnel | Level 3
Cross-sea bridge
and tall bridge | Level 4
Mountain road |

Figure 3. Sample road conditions for levels 0~4 scenario designs.

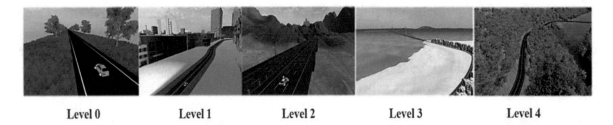

Level 0 Level 1 Level 2 Level 3 Level 4

3.3 System Framework of VRET

Figure 4 presents the system architecture of the proposed VRET, which is a refined version of an earlier research design (Trappey et al., 2020). The five-level exposure therapy (ET) scenario module was designed based on systematic desensitization, which provides a baseline for scene construction. The VR environment module contains a system development engine and a VR software development kit. The VR user interface module provides an immersive experience for subjects. Subjects' physiological feedback and system parameter data are collected within the data collection module. The database management vault records experimental data; these data were used for outcome evaluation and system refinement.

The hardware of the VRET system includes the VR HMD headset (HTC, VIVE Pro; Taipei, Taiwan), the steering wheel with joystick and pedals (Guillemot Co., Thrustmeter T300 RS GT; Carentoir, France), and biological signal sensors (Thought Technology Ltd., ProComp Infiniti; Montreal, Canada). The software components include the development engine (Unity Technologies, Unity; San Francisco (HQ), CA, USA) and the VR platform (Valve Corp., SteamVR; Bellevue, WA, USA). For data storage and management, SQLite (SQLite.org) is used as DBMS, and BioGraph Infinite software is used to record and visualize the biodata. Please refer to our previous research for the software and hardware configuration and description (Trappey et al., 2020).

Figure 4. The driving phobia VRET system framework.

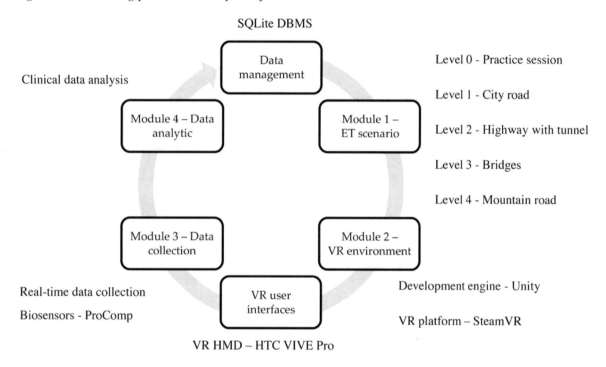

Figure 5 provides a detailed overview of the experiment flow. The experiment procedure can be divided into two parts. In the first part of the experiment, the treatment begins with an introduction by the psychotherapist. An instructional short film is shown to the subjects to introduce the experiment and provides introductions about the experimental objective, method, procedure, expected risk, equipment usage, and relevant disclaimer information. Subjects are equipped with IoT sensors that measure their biodata, including temperature, respiration, heart rate, and skin conductance. While watching the film and after signing the disclaimer, subjects' biodata is collected to establish a baseline-state biofeedback. The subjects start their VR driving simulation and their biofeedback data are collected using biosensors. Subjects practice at level 0 until they were familiar with the VR environment and then advanced to level 1 and level 2. When the subject finish level 2, the first part of the experiment ends, and they take a one-week break before continuing the second part. During the second part, subjects are equipped with biosensors and start from level 0 again. After getting used to the VR environment, the subject will advance to level 3 and level 4. When both parts of immersive treatment are finished, subjects are asked to complete the post-treatment questionnaire to measure the subject's mental state after the VRET treatments. If a subject experiences panic, vertigo, or motion sickness during the experiment, an emergency stop can be triggered to stop the experiment session.

Figure 5. The driving phobia VRET experiment flow.

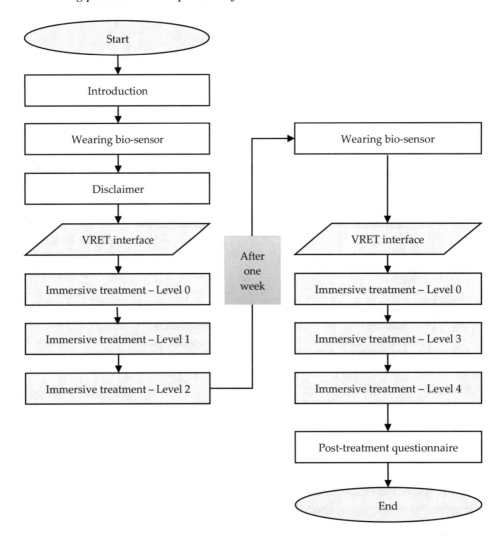

3.4 Real-Time Physiological and Experiment Data Collection and Analysis

The subjects' biofeedback data, including skin conductance, body temperature, respiration, and heart rate, were collected while experimenting with each session to assess changes over the VRET sessions. Base heart rate and base respiration rate differ between individuals, reducing reliability to compare mean biofeedback values between different sessions. The data were standardized before comparison. Comparisons of the maximum and mean value difference biofeedback were used to standardize the heart rate and respiration rate. The magnitude of the subjects' heart rate and respiration rate remained stable between different experimental scenarios and affected the intensity of the stimulus. For driving anxiety, emotion plays a vital role in maximum and mean value differences for biofeedback. Greater value differences indicate a more robust anxiety response.

While performing data analysis, a 99 percentile data level was used to collect each session's maximum biofeedback value to avoid outliers and changes within VRET sessions for the four driving scenarios

(Figure 6). The value of mean and maximum biofeedback differences progressively increased over sessions, with the exceptions occurring in skin conductance differences observed in level 4 and respiration differences observed in level 3. As a whole, the subjects' anxiety arousal became stronger over sessions, indicating subjects were more anxious driving across long bridges and on mountain roads.

Although we were unable to perform a pairwise comparison with our previous experiment, we observed an improvement with the enhanced immersive environment in the second experiment (Trappey et al., 2021). The mean and maximum biofeedback differences collected from the current experiment are higher than those collected from the first experiment. The data show that subjects participating in the current experiment received increased intensity from a more realistic driving anxiety scenario. However, we have no evidence that VRET with a more robust anxiety-provoking scenario design will enhance the effectiveness of the treatment, the improved design with increased visual immersion induced a higher feeling of presence and improved driving performance on the part of the subject. VRET environments that increase the subjects' anxiety are more effective for driving training and exposure therapy (Stevens & Kincaid, 2015).

Figure 6. (a) Mean and maximum skin conductance differences; (b) mean and maximum body temperature differences; (c) mean and maximum respiration differences; (d) mean and maximum heart rate differences.

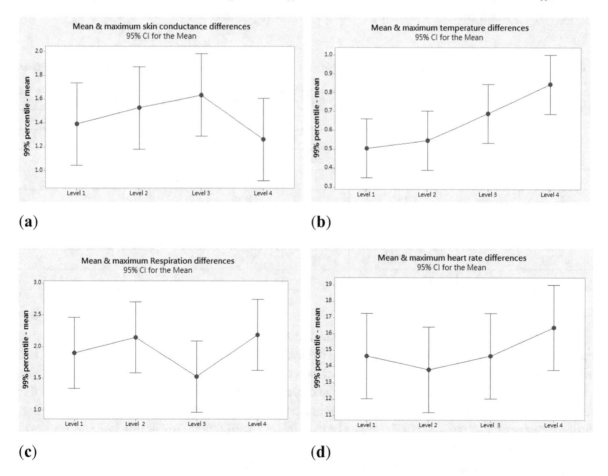

(a)

(b)

(c)

(d)

Heart rate variability (HRV) was analyzed and can be grouped under time-domain methods and frequency-domain methods. Time-domain methods are based on inter-beat interval analysis, the commonly used methods including standard deviation of NN intervals (SDNN), root mean square of successive differences (RMSSD), the standard deviation of successive differences (SDSD), the number of pairs of successive NN intervals that differ by more than 50 ms (NN50), and the proportion of NN50 (pNN50). Due to the short experiment length of this research, SDNN and pNN50 have been selected as time-domain methods. The fast Fourier transform (FFT) is a widely used algorithm for the calculation of frequency-domain methods, and the NN intervals are divided into three kinds of frequency range – high frequency (HF, 0.15 Hz to 0.4 Hz), low frequency (LF, 0.04 Hz to 0.15 Hz), and ultralow frequency (ULF, ≤ 0.04 Hz). HF is directly correlated to the sympathetic nervous system, which could be influenced by the subject's emotions, such as fear and nervousness, so HF has been selected as the frequency-domain method (Shaffer & Ginsberg, 2017).

Two kinds of HRV comparisons have been conducted in this research – HRV data in normal circumstances versus HRV during the experiment and the comparisons between the current experiment and previous experiment. The first comparison focuses on examining whether subjects become much nervous during the experiment, and the second experiment compares which experiment design could provide stronger anxiety arousal to the subjects. The one-way ANOVA of HRV methods is presented in Tables 3 and 4; the mean and standard deviation of SDNN, HF, and pNN50 of each group are presented in Table 5; the result comparisons using *t*-test are present in Table 6 and 7.

Table 3. One-way ANOVA of HRV methods in normal circumstances versus HRV during the experiment

		SS	DF	MS	*F*	Significance
SDNN	Factor	3356	1	3355.7	14.55	0
	Error	13375	58	230.6		
	Total	16731	59			
HF	Factor	128	1	128.5	0.02	0.88
	Error	321547	58	5543.9		
	Total	321675	59			
pNN50	Factor	244.8	1	244.79	6.33	0.015
	Error	2241.4	58	38.64		
	Total	2486.2	59			

According to ANOVA results, time-domain methods (SDNN, pNN50) show a significant difference between different groups, while the frequency-domain method shows no significant difference. This may be caused by insufficient sample size, short experiment length, or incorrect data collection. Thus, in the following *t*-tests, we will focus on SDNN and pNN50 results interpretation. Table 6 indicates that subject's SDNN and pNN50 data in normal circumstances is significantly higher than their HRV data during the experiment; reduced HRV represents that subject's heart rate control ability become less sensitive, it indicates that subject is nervous, so we could conclude that subjects become much nervous during the experiment. Although Table 7 indicates no significant difference in HRV data between current and previous experiments, the decreasing trends in HRV data could be observed in the current experiment. In summary, there exists substantial evidence that the system refinement is effective that the current VRET design yields stronger anxiety.

Table 4. One-way ANOVA of HRV comparisons between current experiment and previous experiment

		SS	DF	MS	F	Significance
	Factor	644.9	1	644.9	3.59	0.063
SDNN	Error	10769.4	60	179.5		
	Total	11414.3	61			
	Factor	2	1	1.8	0	0.988
HF	Error	499492	60	8324.87		
	Total	499494	61			
	Factor	74.48	1	74.48	1.66	0.203
pNN50	Error	2692.64	60	44.88		
	Total	2767.13	61			

Table 5. Descriptive statistics for HRV methods between groups

		Mean	SD
	Normal	65.3	16.5
SDNN	Current	50.4	13.7
	Previous	56.8	13.1
	Normal	74.8	70.3
HF	Current	77.7	78.4
	Previous	77	102
	Normal	10.79	6.82
pNN50	Current	6.75	5.54
	Previous	8.95	7.62

Table 6. HRV data in normal circumstances versus HRV during the experiment

	t-Value	Significance
SDNN	3.81	<0.001
HF	-0.15	0.88
pNN50	2.52	0.015

Table 7. HRV data comparisons between current experiment and previous experiment

	t-Value	Significance
SDNN	-1.89	0.063
HF	0.01	0.988
pNN50	-1.3	0.198

3.5 Self-Adaptive VRET System Design

Machine learning approaches for recognizing emotion can use feedback data measures to adjust the experimental output to match phobia patients' anxiety state. In this research, feature vectors extracted from multiple physiological data, including heart rate, skin conductance, and body temperature, are used for constructing a stress recognition system based on a support vector machine (SVM) classifier. The intelligent system will interpret a subjects' anxiety state based on physiological feedback data collected in the previous level, and the details of the immersive environment in the following level are adjusted to provide subjects to the appropriate stimulus intensity.

3.5.1 Self-Adaptive Design Flow

The flowchart of the self-adaptive system is presented in Figure 7. Levels 2, 3, and 4 were divided into two levels - an easy stage and a normal stage. The low difficulty level 1 has a lower speed limit, an additional traffic lane, and lower traffic density than normal difficulty levels and does not have a normal stage. At the beginning of the experiment, each subject will start at level 1. After subjects' finish level 1, the program's self-adaptive design will determine the anxiety level based on physiological feedback and adjust the difficulty of the following level - subjects with high anxiety will advance to level 2 (easy stage, where subjects with low anxiety will then advance to level 2 normal. The self-adaptive design is activated after subjects finish levels 2 and 3 to determine the practical difficulty in levels 3 and 4.

Figure 7. The self-adaptive design flow.

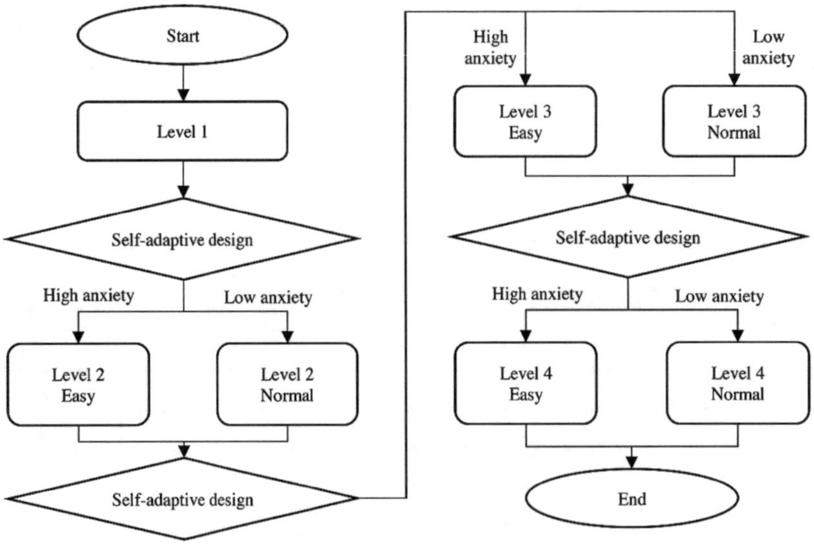

3.5.2 Self-Adaptive Design Algorithm

SVM is a supervised machine learning algorithm that can be used for classification problems. Assume that we have a set of vector data with N features; each data is labeled with one of two classes and can be plotted in N-dimensional space. These data are differentiated into two classes using a linear classifier by finding an appropriate (n-1)-dimensional hyperplane that segregates two classes on different sides. There exist several hyperplanes that can differentiate these data, and our goal is to find the best hyperplane to segregate classes with maximum margin, where the margin represents the distance between the hyperplane and the nearest data point. The larger the margin, the much more accurate the classification could be. The only data points affecting the margin are those closest to the hyperplane, and these data points are called support vectors. The main objective of the SVM is to find the maximum margin hyperplane (MMH) based on support vectors; when new vector data without a class label are added to the dataset, the SVM can classify them into the proper class.

During the self-adaptive VRET system designing phase, a publicly available reference dataset of physiological signals is used for SVM training and testing. Soleymani et al. (2011) conducted emotion recognition and implicit tagging research, and the experimental data collected from the experiment could be assessed from the MAHNOB-HCI-Tagging database. This database contains various physiological signals, including EEG, ECG, skin conductance response, respiration amplitude, and skin temperature data collected from 30 participants. Each participant has to watch 20 video clips and then reporting their respectively experienced arousal and valence levels on a nine-point scale using Self-Assessment Manikin (SAM) (Bradley & Lang, 1994).

The physiological signals feature extraction and training label generation of this research has referred to Ali et al. (2018). Eight features extracted from ECG (mean, standard deviation, SDNN, pNN50), skin conductance response (mean, standard deviation), and skin temperature data (mean, standard deviation) assessed from the MAHNOB-HCI-Tagging database have been selected as training data. Arousal and valence levels are used to generate training labels. The valence scale of (1–5) was mapped to Low-Valance and (6–9) to High-Valance. The arousal scale of (1–5) was mapped to Low-Arousal and (6–9) to High-Arousal. Fear is an emotion related to Low-Valance and High-Arousal, so data with these two scales will be labeled High anxiety, and otherwise labeled Low anxiety. 70% of the dataset is randomly selected as a training set, and the remaining dataset is placed into a test set.

After the training data and training labels are prepared a suitable SVM kernel is used to transform a low-dimensional input space into a higher-dimensional space. The Radial basis function (RBF) algorithm is defined by Equation (1):

$$K\left(x, x'\right) = \exp\left(-\gamma x - x'^2\right) \tag{1}$$

Where $K\left(x, x'\right)$ is the product between two vectors x and x' which ranges between 0 to 1; γ is kernel coefficient which ranges from 0 to 1, a higher value of γ will perfectly fit the training dataset but also causes over-fitting, we will assign γ=0.01 here; and $\left\| x - x' \right\|^2$ is the squared Euclidean distance between x and x'.

3.6 Post-treatment Psychological Survey - Treatment Effectiveness of VRET

Before the experiment, the difference between the average scores of TG and CG driving behavior questionnaires was measured using *t*-tests. The results showed a significant difference between the two groups of data (95% confidence interval = (51.7, 66.12); p-value = 0.000). The treatment group for VRET filled out the same driving behavior questionnaire after completing the treatment. If the score of the TG drops close to the CG score level after receiving VRET, then the subjects are behaving more like drivers who do not experience fear as measured in the control group. Table 8 shows the statistical results of the questionnaire, including the TG pre-treatment questionnaire score (TG pre), TG post-treatment questionnaire score (TG post), and CG questionnaire score (CG), and calculate the average value and standard for each topic Poor (SD). Analyzed by one-way ANOVA test, there are no significant differences on SDs of all survey questions between TG pre, TG post, and CG.

To compare three mean scores (i.e., TG pre, TG post, and CG) for all the 39 questions, a one-way ANOVA test was applied. Pairwise comparisons of 95% confidence interval (CI) of three groups show significant differences between the means of the scores. Figure 8 shows the result of Fisher's least significant difference test for multiple comparisons to examine the means for different groups. The results of multiple comparisons show significant differences between all pairs (i.e., TG pre vs. TG post, TG pre vs. CG score, TG post vs. CG score). The analysis of variance test also shows that VRET reduces the distress of the TG during driving, even if the reduction of fear (after TG) is not reduced to the same level as the control group. In summary, this experiment demonstrates with high confidence that the driving phobia VRET system can effectively reduce the subjects' anxiety and avoidance of driving.

Figure 8. One-way ANOVA interval plot of TG pre, TG post, and CG score.

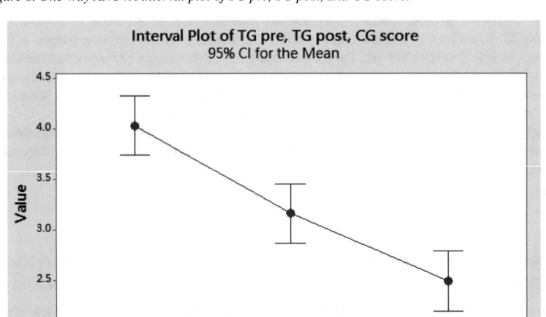

Table 8. Driving behavior survey comparisons—means and standard deviations (SDs).

	TG Pre		TG Post		CG	
	Mean	SD	Mean	SD	Mean	SD
Q1	4.3	1.79	3.2	1.57	3.2	1.67
Q2	3.8	1.93	4.4	1.54	3.1	1.79
Q3	5.3	1.27	2.1	1.33	4.1	1.48
Q4	4.5	1.67	2.5	1.66	2.8	1.53
Q5	3.9	1.46	3.9	1.59	2.4	1.24
Q6	4.3	1.74	5	1.71	2.5	1.33
Q7	4.9	1.21	3	1.08	3.5	1.42
Q8	2.5	1.45	2.1	1.13	1.3	0.6
Q9	3.4	1.99	4.3	1.81	1.9	1.26
Q10	4.6	1.2	2.6	1.63	2.5	1.61
Q11	5.3	1.06	2.7	1.27	3.9	1.68
Q12	3.8	1.61	5.3	1.53	1.8	1.03
Q13	2.4	1.48	2.4	1.45	1.4	0.7
Q14	4.7	1.54	3.9	1.87	2.9	1.7
Q15	3.2	1.76	3.2	1.73	3	1.81
Q16	3.4	1.75	4.4	1.49	2.5	1.61
Q17	5.9	0.86	2.1	1.31	5	1.61
Q18	3.2	1.57	2.5	1.79	2.9	1.83
Q19	4.3	1.35	3.9	1.31	2	1.2
Q20	4	1.62	3.4	1.69	1.7	1.32
Q21	3.8	1.88	3.2	1.79	1.9	1.25
Q22	4.1	1.92	4.3	1.62	2.3	1.54
Q23	4.9	1.44	4.5	1.65	3.8	1.84
Q24	5.5	1.07	4.6	1.7	3	1.46
Q25	5	1.53	4.4	1.82	2.6	1.57
Q26	4.1	1.56	3.8	1.7	2.1	1.19
Q27	2.8	1.6	2.3	1.47	2.4	1.52
Q28	2.5	1.48	1.7	0.96	1.9	1.06
Q29	3.6	1.66	3	1.99	2.6	1.77
Q30	2.2	1.29	2	1.36	1.5	0.72
Q31	2.5	1.6	1.8	1.21	1.7	1.12
Q32	4.7	1.72	3.9	1.62	2.9	1.83
Q33	3.8	1.65	2	1.17	1.7	0.89
Q34	3	1.22	1.9	1.01	1.5	0.68
Q35	4.5	1.4	2.2	1.03	2	1.46
Q36	4.6	1.64	3	1.48	2.6	0.94
Q37	4.3	1.39	2.3	1.04	2	0.77
Q38	5.7	1.36	3.3	1.28	2.5	1.36
Q39	4	1.66	2.1	1.07	1.6	0.74

Since this questionnaire consists of two different types of parts, one part comes from the American Psychological Association and the other comes from other international organizations. We further analyze the results of each part using a single analysis of variance test and Fisher's least significant difference model (used for multiple comparisons). First, for anxious driving behavior and anxiety-related avoidance problems (Q1~Q32), the results of the analysis of variance showed that the questionnaire score after TG treatment was significantly reduced, although the results were still higher than the CG questionnaire score. Secondly, according to driving-related problems in a specific environment (Q33~Q39), there is no significant difference between the scores after TG treatment and the CG scores. In this regard, we further carried out a non-parametric test, the Mann–Whitney test, to determine whether the medians of the two groups are different, to avoid excessive inferences caused by the small number of questions (only seven questions). The results showed no significant difference between late TG and CG (95% CI = (-0.2999, 1.0001); p-value = 0.1599). VRET reduces the subjects' anxiety toward driving and helps subjects adapt to a specific driving environment.

4. EXPERIMENT RESULTS AND IMPLICATIONS

A positive result of the driving phobia experiment verifies that there is no significant difference between the TG's post-treatment scores and CG scores for Q33~Q39, i.e., the questions related to driving in specific conditions as designed in our VRET scenario design. This result was not discovered in the previous study. The research leads to a new hypothesis that the driving phobia treatments are more effective when specific driving fear conditions or environments (e.g., darkness, high speed, bad weather, etc.) are designed into the VRET scenarios. Our current VRET sessions are constructed using four road scenarios, and the subjects are aware that the experimental design is based on the scene changes during the experiment. Our original VRET design focused on observing the subjects' biofeedback changes over different driving environments. More design changes were implemented to improve the realism of the experience of virtual driving. The driving environment changes, such as traffic jams or bad weather, which is often linked to anxiety-related avoidance behavior, can be considered for future VRET scenario designs. The driving behavior survey results support that participating in VRET therapy will help people become increasingly comfortable with specific driving environments. Future scenarios will be tested and analyzed statistically, considering traffic events, traffic lights, bad weather, and the endurance of the treatment effect. In comparison to our preliminary VRET design, the latest VRET platform is proven to be more realistic with scenarios that are more anxiety-provoking and more effective in reducing distress through exposure.

5. CONCLUSION

Virtual reality uses computer simulation to generate three-dimensional virtual reality scenes. Through head-mounted displays and other related configurations, it provides visual, auditory, and even tactile simulations, allowing users to feel like they are in the environment. This feature provides a novel way to treat anxiety in an immersive environment. The subjects are exposed to the virtual environment of traumatic stimulation, and the degree of traumatic stimulation is gradually strengthened in multiple levels and scenarios, which is in line with the principle of desensitization of the system. The advantage of VRET is that it reduces the patient's risk of physical injury and solves the problem of avoiding fear in traditional exposure therapy. Furthermore, the intensity and duration of exposure can be adjusted, and treatment can be terminated immediately to stop panic attacks. VRET can be used for more flexible treatment times and allows patients to repeat specific scenarios until they eliminate their fear. The device's design allows doctors to better monitor the patient's physical and mental condition during ET treatment.

This study reviewed various situations of stress disorder and the corresponding traditional exposure therapy and advanced VRET methods. The research focuses on driving phobias that are common and have a severe negative impact on life. Patent analysis shows that VR has an excellent opportunity for the treatment of driving phobias. Following the psychotherapy model, this experiment constructed various fear inducing driving scenes in the VR environment, recruited subjects, and compared their fear before and after receiving VRET. At the same time, the physiological data of the subjects when they use VR is collected to analyze their emotional arousal. In the initial driving fear scale, 121 subjects were divided into two groups according to a median split: one group had a higher degree of fear of driving, and the other group had a lower degree of fear of driving. The *t*-test showed that the two groups had significant differences in fear of driving situations. Among 60 subjects with a high degree of driving fear, 30 were randomly selected as TGs to participate in the VRET experiment. The experiment included driving in 4 scenarios, collecting real-time physiological data, and filling out the driving fear scale again after completing VRET. According to the self-assessed driving fear scale, VRET effectively improved the participants' fear of driving. Their fear is reduced to the same level as CG subjects (that is, there is no significant difference between their anxious driving and anxiety-related avoidance behavior). In short, the results of the research demonstrate that VRET is of great help for phobia treatment, providing new treatment methods that are different from the traditional ones. Although significant progress has been made in the treatment of VRET in this study, driving phobia and other PTSD are still far from achieving satisfactory treatment results.

REFERENCES

Ali, M., Al Machot, F., Haj Mosa, A., Jdeed, M., Al Machot, E., & Kyamakya, K. (2018). A globally generalized emotion recognition system involving different physiological signals. *Sensors (Basel)*, *18*(6), 1905. doi:10.339018061905 PMID:29891829

Bandura, A. (2006). Guide for constructing self-efficacy scales. *Self-Efficacy Beliefs of Adolescents*, *5*(1), 307-337.

Beck, J. G., Palyo, S. A., Winer, E. H., Schwagler, B. E., & Ang, E. J. (2007). Virtual reality exposure therapy for PTSD symptoms after a road accident: An uncontrolled case series. *Behavior Therapy*, *38*(1), 39–48. doi:10.1016/j.beth.2006.04.001 PMID:17292693

Bisson, J., & Andrew, M. (2007). Psychological treatment of post-traumatic stress disorder (PTSD). *Cochrane Database of Systematic Reviews*, 3. PMID:17636720

Blanchard, E. B., & Hickling, E. J. (2004). *After the crash: Psychological assessment and treatment of survivors of motor vehicle accidents*. American Psychological Association. doi:10.1037/10676-000

Blanchard, E. B., Hickling, E. J., Taylor, A. E., & Loos, W. (1995). Psychiatric morbidity associated with motor vehicle accidents. *The Journal of Nervous and Mental Disease, 183*(8), 495–504. doi:10.1097/00005053-199508000-00001 PMID:7643060

Blaubit Co Ltd. (2019). *Stress Disorder Detection System for Use in Panic Attack Treatment Has Display Section to Display Analyzed Behavioral Data So Virtual Reality (VR) Content Information Outputted by Information Management Department Can Be Revealed to Patient. KR2019061826A.* KPO.

Blei, D. M., Ng, A. Y., & Jordan, M. I. (2003). Latent dirichlet allocation. *The Journal of Machine Learning Research, 3*, 993-1022.

Bradley, M. M., & Lang, P. J. (1994). Measuring emotion: The self-assessment manikin and the semantic differential. *Journal of Behavior Therapy and Experimental Psychiatry, 25*(1), 49–59. doi:10.1016/0005-7916(94)90063-9 PMID:7962581

Bryant, R. A., Sackville, T., Dang, S. T., Moulds, M., & Guthrie, R. (1999). Treating acute stress disorder: An evaluation of cognitive behavior therapy and supportive counseling techniques. *The American Journal of Psychiatry, 156*(11), 1780–1786. PMID:10553743

Chesham, R. K., Malouff, J. M., & Schutte, N. S. (2018). Meta-analysis of the efficacy of virtual reality exposure therapy for social anxiety. *Behaviour Change, 35*(3), 152–166. doi:10.1017/bec.2018.15

Clapp, J. D., Olsen, S. A., Beck, J. G., Palyo, S. A., Grant, D. M., Gudmundsdottir, B., & Marques, L. (2011). The driving behavior survey: Scale construction and validation. *Journal of Anxiety Disorders, 25*(1), 96–105. doi:10.1016/j.janxdis.2010.08.008 PMID:20832988

Costa, R. T. D., Carvalho, M. R. D., & Nardi, A. E. (2010). Virtual reality exposure therapy in the treatment of driving phobia. *Psicologia: Teoria e Pesquisa (Brasília), 26*(1), 131–137. doi:10.1590/S0102-37722010000100015

Dingli, A., & Bondin, L. (2019, August). Realtime Adaptive Virtual Reality for Pain Reduction. In *2019 IEEE Conference on Games (CoG)* (pp. 1-4). IEEE. 10.1109/CIG.2019.8848119

Duke, J., Guest, M., & Boggess, M. (2010). Age-related safety in professional heavy vehicle drivers: A literature review. *Accident; Analysis and Prevention, 42*(2), 364–371. doi:10.1016/j.aap.2009.09.026 PMID:20159055

Elhai, J. D., Grubaugh, A. L., Kashdan, T. B., & Frueh, B. C. (2008). Empirical examination of a proposed refinement to DSM-IV post-traumatic stress disorder symptom criteria using the National Comorbidity Survey Replication data. *The Journal of Clinical Psychiatry, 69*(4), 597–602. doi:10.4088/JCP.v69n0411 PMID:18294026

Emmelkamp, P. M., Krijn, M., Hulsbosch, A. M., De Vries, S., Schuemie, M. J., & van der Mast, C. A. (2002). Virtual reality treatment versus exposure in vivo: A comparative evaluation in acrophobia. *Behaviour Research and Therapy, 40*(5), 509–516. doi:10.1016/S0005-7967(01)00023-7 PMID:12038644

Emmelkamp, P. M., Meyerbröker, K., & Morina, N. (2020). Virtual reality therapy in social anxiety disorder. *Current Psychiatry Reports, 22*(7), 1–9. doi:10.100711920-020-01156-1 PMID:32405657

Eshuis, L. V., van Gelderen, M. J., van Zuiden, M., Nijdam, M. J., Vermetten, E., Olff, M., & Bakker, A. (2020). Efficacy of immersive PTSD treatments: A systematic review of virtual and augmented reality exposure therapy and a meta-analysis of virtual reality exposure therapy. *Journal of Psychiatric Research*. Advance online publication. doi:10.1016/j.jpsychires.2020.11.030 PMID:33248674

Gautam, S., Jain, A., Gautam, M., Vahia, V. N., & Gautam, A. (2017). Clinical practice guidelines for the management of generalised anxiety disorder (GAD) and panic disorder (PD). *Indian Journal of Psychiatry, 59*(5), S67. doi:10.4103/0019-5545.196975 PMID:28216786

Giaconia, R. M., Reinherz, H. Z., Silverman, A. B., Pakiz, B., Frost, A. K., & Cohen, E. (1995). Traumas and post-traumatic stress disorder in a community population of older adolescents. *Journal of the American Academy of Child and Adolescent Psychiatry, 34*(10), 1369–1380. doi:10.1097/00004583-199510000-00023 PMID:7592275

Gujjar, K. R., van Wijk, A., Kumar, R., & de Jongh, A. (2019). Efficacy of virtual reality exposure therapy for the treatment of dental phobia in adults: A randomized controlled trial. *Journal of Anxiety Disorders, 62*, 100–108. doi:10.1016/j.janxdis.2018.12.001 PMID:30717830

Herumurti, D., Yuniarti, A., Rimawan, P., & Yunanto, A. A. (2019, July). Overcoming glossophobia based on virtual reality and heart rate sensors. In *2019 IEEE International Conference on Industry 4.0, Artificial Intelligence, and Communications Technology (IAICT)* (pp. 139-144). IEEE. 10.1109/ICIAICT.2019.8784846

Hinkle, L., Khoshhal, K., & Metsis, V. (2019, June). Physiological Measurement for Emotion Recognition in Virtual Reality. In *2019 2nd International Conference on Data Intelligence and Security (ICDIS)* (pp. 136-143). IEEE. 10.1109/ICDIS.2019.00028

Hofmann, S. G., Asnaani, A., Vonk, I. J., Sawyer, A. T., & Fang, A. (2012). The efficacy of cognitive behavioral therapy: A review of meta-analyses. *Cognitive Therapy and Research, 36*(5), 427–440. doi:10.100710608-012-9476-1 PMID:23459093

Hogg, R. V., Tanis, E. A., & Zimmerman, D. L. (2013). *Probability and statistical inference* (9th ed.). Pearson Education.

Horigome, T., Kurokawa, S., Sawada, K., Kudo, S., Shiga, K., Mimura, M., & Kishimoto, T. (2020). Virtual reality exposure therapy for social anxiety disorder: A systematic review and meta-analysis. *Psychological Medicine, 50*(15), 2487–2497. doi:10.1017/S0033291720003785 PMID:33070784

Hruska, B., Irish, L. A., Pacella, M. L., Sledjeski, E. M., & Delahanty, D. L. (2014). PTSD symptom severity and psychiatric comorbidity in recent motor vehicle accident victims: A latent class analysis. *Journal of Anxiety Disorders, 28*(7), 644–649. doi:10.1016/j.janxdis.2014.06.009 PMID:25124501

Jhuang, A. C., Sun, J. J., Trappey, A. J., Trappey, C. V., & Govindarajan, U. H. (2017, April). Computer supported technology function matrix construction for patent data analytics. In *2017 IEEE 21st International Conference on Computer Supported Cooperative Work in Design (CSCWD)* (pp. 457-462). IEEE. 10.1109/CSCWD.2017.8066737

Kaussner, Y., Kuraszkiewicz, A. M., Schoch, S., Markel, P., Hoffmann, S., Baur-Streubel, R., Kenntner-Mabiala, R., & Pauli, P. (2020). Treating patients with driving phobia by virtual reality exposure therapy–a pilot study. *PLoS One*, *15*(1), e0226937. doi:10.1371/journal.pone.0226937 PMID:31910205

Kim, B. H., & Jo, S. (2018). Deep physiological affect network for the recognition of human emotions. *IEEE Transactions on Affective Computing*, *11*(2), 230–243. doi:10.1109/TAFFC.2018.2790939

Korea University Research and Business Foundation. (2020). *Virtual Reality-Based Exposure Treatment Method for Patients with Post-traumatic Stress Disorder (PTSD) Involves Adjusting Exposure Intensity of Content According to Stress Index. KR2170379B1*. KPO.

Kritikos, J., Tzannetos, G., Zoitaki, C., Poulopoulou, S., & Koutsouris, D. (2019, March). Anxiety detection from Electrodermal Activity Sensor with movement & interaction during Virtual Reality Simulation. In *2019 9th International IEEE/EMBS Conference on Neural Engineering (NER)* (pp. 571-576). IEEE. 10.1109/NER.2019.8717170

LG Display Co Ltd. (2019). *Display Device for a Virtual Reality Device Used in Military, Architecture, Tourism, Movies, Multimedia or Gaming, Comprises a Display Panel Having Multiple Data Lines, Multiple Gate Lines and Multiple Pixels Arranged in a Matrix. DE102017129795A1*. DPMA.

LG Electronics Inc. (2016). *Wearable Mobile Terminal e.g., Handheld Terminal, for User, Has Controller for Controlling Processor to Transmit Signal for Notifying Emotional State of First User to External Devices in Response to Identified State Corresponding to State. US20160381534A1*. USPTO.

MacQueen, J. (1967, June). Some methods for classification and analysis of multivariate observations. In *Proceedings of the fifth Berkeley symposium on mathematical statistics and probability* (*Vol. 1*, No. 14, pp. 281-297). Academic Press.

Magic Leap Inc. (2017). *Augmented and Virtual Reality Display Systems and Methods for Determining Optical Prescriptions by Imaging Retina. US20170000343A1*. USPTO.

Miloff, A., Lindner, P., & Carlbring, P. (2020). The future of virtual reality therapy for phobias: Beyond simple exposures. *Clinical Psychology in Europe*, *2*(2), e2913. doi:10.32872/cpe.v2i2.2913

Momartin, S., Silove, D., Manicavasagar, V., & Steel, Z. (2004). Comorbidity of PTSD and depression: Associations with trauma exposure, symptom severity and functional impairment in Bosnian refugees resettled in Australia. *Journal of Affective Disorders*, *80*(2-3), 231–238. doi:10.1016/S0165-0327(03)00131-9 PMID:15207936

North, M. M., & North, S. M. (2018). The sense of presence exploration in virtual reality therapy. *J. UCS*, *24*(2), 72–84.

North, M. M., North, S. M., & Coble, J. R. (1997). Virtual reality therapy: An effective treatment for psychological disorders. *Studies in Health Technology and Informatics*, 59–70. PMID:10175343

Oskam, P. (2005). *Virtual reality exposure therapy (VRET) effectiveness and improvement*. In 2nd Twente University Student Conference on IT, Enschede, The Netherlands.

Ougrin, D. (2011). Efficacy of exposure versus cognitive therapy in anxiety disorders: Systematic review and meta-analysis. *BMC Psychiatry*, *11*(1), 1–13. doi:10.1186/1471-244X-11-200 PMID:22185596

Perkonigg, A., Kessler, R. C., Storz, S., & Wittchen, H. U. (2000). Traumatic events and post-traumatic stress disorder in the community: Prevalence, risk factors and comorbidity. *Acta Psychiatrica Scandinavica, 101*(1), 46–59. doi:10.1034/j.1600-0447.2000.101001046.x PMID:10674950

Qingdao Cybercare Information Technology Co Ltd. (2016). *Driving Virtual Reality Post-Traumatic Stress Disorder Treatment System, has Display Displayed Virtual Scene, which is Matched with User Physiological Data, Vibrator Fixed with Controller, and Physiological Data Output Sent to Controller. CN103405239B.* CNIPA.

Romano, D. M. (2005). Virtual reality therapy. *Developmental Medicine and Child Neurology, 47*(9), 580–580. doi:10.1111/j.1469-8749.2005.tb01206.x PMID:16138662

Rothbaum, B. O., Anderson, P., Zimand, E., Hodges, L., Lang, D., & Wilson, J. (2006). Virtual reality exposure therapy and standard (in vivo) exposure therapy in the treatment of fear of flying. *Behavior Therapy, 37*(1), 80–90. doi:10.1016/j.beth.2005.04.004 PMID:16942963

Salehi, E., Mehrabi, M., Fatehi, F., & Salehi, A. (2020). Virtual Reality Therapy for Social Phobia: A Scoping Review. *Studies in Health Technology and Informatics, 270*(06), 2020. PMID:32570476

Scozzari, S., & Gamberini, L. (2011). Virtual reality as a tool for cognitive behavioral therapy: a review. *Virtual reality in psychotherapy, rehabilitation, and assessment*, 63-108.

Shaffer, F., & Ginsberg, J. P. (2017). An overview of heart rate variability metrics and norms. *Frontiers in Public Health, 5*, 258. doi:10.3389/fpubh.2017.00258 PMID:29034226

Sheridan, T. B. (2000, October). Interaction, imagination and immersion some research needs. In *Proceedings of the ACM symposium on Virtual reality software and technology* (pp. 1-7). 10.1145/502390.502392

Shu, L., Xie, J., Yang, M., Li, Z., Li, Z., Liao, D., Xu, X., & Yang, X. (2018). A review of emotion recognition using physiological signals. *Sensors (Basel), 18*(7), 2074. doi:10.339018072074 PMID:29958457

Slater, M., Spanlang, B., Sanchez-Vives, M. V., & Blanke, O. (2010). First person experience of body transfer in virtual reality. *PLoS One, 5*(5), e10564. doi:10.1371/journal.pone.0010564 PMID:20485681

Soleymani, M., Lichtenauer, J., Pun, T., & Pantic, M. (2011). A multimodal database for affect recognition and implicit tagging. *IEEE Transactions on Affective Computing, 3*(1), 42–55. doi:10.1109/T-AFFC.2011.25

Spinhoven, P., Penninx, B. W., Van Hemert, A. M., De Rooij, M., & Elzinga, B. M. (2014). Comorbidity of PTSD in anxiety and depressive disorders: Prevalence and shared risk factors. *Child Abuse & Neglect, 38*(8), 1320–1330. doi:10.1016/j.chiabu.2014.01.017 PMID:24629482

Stevens, J. A., & Kincaid, J. P. (2015). The relationship between presence and performance in virtual simulation training. *Open Journal of Modelling and Simulation, 3*(02), 41–48. doi:10.4236/ojmsi.2015.32005

Taylor, J., Deane, F., & Podd, J. (2002). Driving-related fear: A review. *Clinical Psychology Review, 22*(5), 631–645. doi:10.1016/S0272-7358(01)00114-3 PMID:12113199

Taylor, J. E., Sullman, M. J., & Stephens, A. N. (2018). Measuring anxiety-related avoidance with the Driving and Riding Avoidance Scale (DRAS). *European Journal of Psychological Assessment.*

Trappey, A. J. C., Trappey, C. V., Chang, C. M., Kuo, R. R. T., & Lin, A. P. C. (2021). Virtual reality exposure therapy for driving phobia disorder (2): System refinement and verification. *Applied Sciences (Basel, Switzerland)*, *11*(1), 347. doi:10.3390/app11010347

Trappey, A. J. C., Trappey, C. V., Chang, C. M., Kuo, R. R. T., Lin, A. P. C., & Nieh, C. H. (2020). Virtual reality exposure therapy for driving phobia disorder: System design and development. *Applied Sciences (Basel, Switzerland)*, *10*(14), 4860. doi:10.3390/app10144860

Trivedi, P. G. (2018). *Human Emotion Recognition from Physiological Biosignals*. Academic Press.

Wald, J., & Taylor, S. (2000). Efficacy of virtual reality exposure therapy to treat driving phobia: A case report. *Journal of Behavior Therapy and Experimental Psychiatry*, *31*(3-4), 249–257. doi:10.1016/S0005-7916(01)00009-X PMID:11494960

Waldrop, M. M. (2017). News feature: Virtual reality therapy set for a real renaissance. *Proceedings of the National Academy of Sciences of the United States of America*, *114*(39), 10295–10299. doi:10.1073/pnas.1715133114 PMID:28951492

Wiederhold, B. K., Jang, D. P., Kim, S. I., & Wiederhold, M. D. (2002). Physiological monitoring as an objective tool in virtual reality therapy. *Cyberpsychology & Behavior*, *5*(1), 77–82. doi:10.1089/109493102753685908 PMID:11990977

Yin, Z., Zhao, M., Wang, Y., Yang, J., & Zhang, J. (2017). Recognition of emotions using multimodal physiological signals and an ensemble deep learning model. *Computer Methods and Programs in Biomedicine*, *140*, 93–110. doi:10.1016/j.cmpb.2016.12.005 PMID:28254094

Zinzow, H. M., Brooks, J. O., Rosopa, P. J., Jeffirs, S., Jenkins, C., Seeanner, J., McKeeman, A., & Hodges, L. F. (2018). Virtual reality and cognitive-behavioral therapy for driving anxiety and aggression in veterans: A pilot study. *Cognitive and Behavioral Practice*, *25*(2), 296–309. doi:10.1016/j.cbpra.2017.09.002

Chapter 11
Evidence–Based Virtual Reality Use for Mental Health Conditions

Jagrika Bajaj
Touchkin eServices Private Limited., India

Aparna Sahu
https://orcid.org/0000-0002-7383-7675
Turiyan Psyneuronics Private Limited., India

ABSTRACT

The advancements in immersive technologies have impacted various sectors, with mental healthcare being one of them. The subsequent interaction between immersive technologies, particularly virtual reality and mental health, has created interesting effects that call for a closer look. This chapter intends to provide a comprehensive picture of mental health conditions, namely anxiety and related disorders, post-traumatic stress disorder, and major depressive disorder, as tackled by VR-based therapy. The focus is on its effectiveness and how the results compare to the traditional modes of treatment in terms of efficacy. The impact of user experience towards this approach of intervention and the importance of ethical consideration when VR intersects with the field of mental health are addressed.

INTRODUCTION

Global burden of disease (GBD) research provides the prevalence of various diseases, their risk factors and the debilitating effect it has on the population (Institute for Health Metrics and Evaluation (IHME), 2020). The GBD 2019 report provides the descriptive epidemiology from 204 countries and territories through the use of Disability-adjusted life years (DALYs) from 1990-2019 (Vos, et al., 2020). Though there has been improvement in global health, mental health concerns such as anxiety and depression have remained the top concerns. The ongoing global health (COVID-19) crisis has contributed to an increase in the pooled estimates of various mental health concerns compared to prior results (Nochaiwong, et al.,

DOI: 10.4018/978-1-7998-8371-5.ch011

2021). This has made it essential to deliver safe services to customers through alternative means from different sectors in a way that gives them the experience. In such situations, immersive technology has garnered attention.

Virtual reality (VR) therapy for psychiatric disorders have been evaluated, however, its impact is different across different disorders owing to the evolving nature of VR technology (Cieślik, et al., 2020). The mental health disorders emphasised in relation to VR as given below are: Anxiety-related disorders, posttraumatic stress disorder (PTSD) and Major depressive disorder.

Anxiety-Related Disorders

According to the Diagnostic and Statistical Manual – 5th edition (DSM-5; American Psychiatric Association, 2013), Anxiety disorders include various disorders characterised by excessive fear and anxiety and related behavioural disturbances. The various disorders in this category differ in terms of the associated cognitive ideations and the situations and objects that elicit the feared, anxious or avoidant response in individuals. Anxiety, in general, is an emotional state characterised by an excess feeling of tension, increased occurrence of worrying thoughts, and this state of mind is accompanied by physical symptoms such as increased blood pressure. Most often in daily life, feeling mildly anxious helps one to handle situations. However, uncertain times and sudden changes in lifestyle and routine potentially add stress. When the duration and severity of this feeling is disproportionate to the triggers that cause it, they result in anxiety disorders.

Amid a worldwide pandemic, stress and anxiety are reported to be exacerbated (Salari, et al., 2020). Exposure therapy is a technique of behavioural therapy used for the treatment of anxiety disorder. The premise is that repeated exposure to fearful stimuli in a safe environment can help deal with stressful responses better. Depending on how the stimuli are presented to the individual, exposure therapy can be imaginal (vividly imagining the feared stimuli), in-vivo exposure (facing the fearful object/situation in real life), and interoceptive exposure (through eliciting safe yet fearful sensation). VR exposure (exposure to fearful stimuli in a virtual environment) has also been examined because of its ability to mimic the real world or create imagined realities that lend its usage in the therapeutic setup. One of the first controlled studies by Rothbaum et al. (1995b) found promising results for improving the fear of heights experienced by the VR graded exposure treatment group compared to the waitlist condition. Since exposure therapy works differently in each anxiety disorder, VR environments are presented differently. Studies and supporting evidence for the explanation for the VR effect for particular disorders are tabulated (see Table 1). For this purpose, only studies with randomised controlled trials in the past decade or so have been considered.

Virtual reality exposure therapy (VRET) combined with CBT are usually used for Social anxiety disorder (SAD); however, results from randomised controlled trials do not provide a clear picture regarding the effectiveness of VRET for social anxiety disorders (Anderson et al. 2013; Bouchard et al., 2017; Kampmann et al., 2016). This is perhaps due to study differences in terms of participant characteristics, specific aspects of social anxiety disorder, VR equipment, virtual scenarios and delivery of VR sessions. The superiority of In vivo exposure to standalone CBT in the study by Kampmann et al. (2016) can be due to the presentation of different scenarios to the VRET condition and In vivo condition. A recent review points towards no difference in efficacy between VRET and traditional treatment of CBT, yet more data is required to support the effectiveness of VRET as a standalone treatment (Emmelkamp, et al., 2020).

Table 1. Anxiety disorders and their VR findings

Name of Anxiety Disorder	Definition of Disorder	Supportive Findings of VR	Unsupportive Findings of VR	Final Comments
Social anxiety disorder (SAD)	Marked by the presence of intense fear and anxiety in a social setting where an individual can be scrutinised by others	--Bouchard et al. (2017): VRET combined with CBT more effective than In-vivo exposure combined with CBT at post-treatment for social anxiety disorder - Anderson et al. (2013): VRET to be as equally effective as exposure group therapy for social anxiety disorder - Emmelkamp et al. (2020): No difference in efficacy between VRET and traditional treatment of CBT	- Kampmann et al., (2016): In vivo exposure therapy was superior to standalone VRET.	-There is inconsistency in the targetted aspect of Social anxiety disorder (Public speaking only, broad social situations) - VR equipment used, VR scenarios
Specific Phobias	Presence of fear relating to a specific object or a situation	-Triscari et al. (2015): CBT with systematic desensitisation (CBT-SD), with eye movement desensitisation (CBT-EMDR) and with VRET (CBT-VRET) all were equally effective. -Freeman et al. (2018): VRET better than Usual care - Donker et al. (2019): Large significant reduction in the acrophobia symptoms even when participants used self-guided app-based VR cognitive therapy. - Chou et al., (2021): VR based technology for treating acrophobia with VR coach delivered psychotherapy to be the most effective treatment.	- Michaliszyn et al. (2010): greater improvement in in-vivo exposure as compared to VRET for Spider phobia	- Different types of specific phobias have different effectiveness -Different number of VR sessions and different VR scenarios used
Panic disorder	Experiencing recurring sudden panic attacks (sudden, unreasonable feeling of fear and anxiety that are accompanied by physical symptoms)	- Pelissolo et al. (2012): VRET is equally effective as CBT	- Meyerbroeker et al. (2013): CBT combined with in vivo was more effective than CBT combined with Virtual reality.	-Different number of sessions and protocols across studies
Agoraphobia	Fear and anxiety of the fear related to real or imagined exposure to situations such as open spaces, enclosed spaces, public transportation, being in a crowd and/or being outside of the home alone.	- Malbos et al. (2012): VRET alone and VRET with CBT are equally effective - Meyerbroeker et al. (2013): CBT combined with VR and CBT combined with in vivo exposure were both effective.	Studies not available	-VR based interventions are effective

Research evidence for specific phobias has pointed to the effectiveness of VR based interventions in reducing the symptoms experienced by the individual. Dysfunctional beliefs and perceived self-efficacy have been found as the best predictors of change (Côté & Bouchard, 2009). These results were replicated in the study by Tardif et al. (2019).

In the case of panic disorder, the recent controlled randomised trials were unable to provide a clear picture. The study designs had various multicomponent therapeutic techniques (e.g., interoceptive techniques, relaxation exercises, presence of homework); therefore, measuring the specific effect of VRET could have been difficult. There were no randomised control trial design studies for agoraphobia that provided unsupportive evidence for the use of VRET. A recent metanalysis of randomised control trial found non-significant effect sizes when comparing VR condition with In vivo exposure condition for agoraphobia, thus furthering the point that VRET is as effective as in vivo for reduction of symptoms for agoraphobia (Wechsler et al., 2019).

Carl et al. (2018), in their review of metanalysis for the efficacy of Virtual Reality exposure therapy (VRET) for treatment of anxiety-related disorders, found a large effect size for VRET vs waitlist control situation but a nonsignificant effect size when it was comparing VRET with in vivo exposure situation. These results point to the finding that VRET did not show significant differences in efficacy compared to in vivo treatment.

VR offers an advantage to this therapeutic technique by allowing for the presentation of fearful stimuli to participants in a safe environment, thus allowing them to practice before venturing out into the real world. Moreover, there is a chance that the virtual scenes can be altered, providing greater flexibility and control to participants to withdraw participation or repeat the module (Botella, et al., 2017). Moreover, Jerdan et al. (2018), in their critical review, raised the need for having accessible products delivering VR based interventions. To this extent, Lindner et al. (2019), in their randomised controlled trial, found a significant decrease in self-reported public speaking anxiety in participants even with the use of off the shelf VR hardware and software for this study. This shows promise for more efficient results when used in the clinical setting and paves the way for disseminating cost-effective VR based interventions for anxiety.

Attitudes of clinicians regarding VR and VRET is worth noting. Lindner et al. (2019), in their cross-sectional survey, assessed the attitudes of cognitive behaviour therapists and found that they had an overall positive attitude towards VRET. They also believed the applications of VR to be broader (e.g., Mood disorders, neuropsychiatric disorders, eating disorders, gambling disorder, and substance use disorders) than just being limited to the treatment of anxiety conditions. Similar results were seen by Bouchard et al. (2017) where they found that conducting CBT with in-virtuo exposure (VRET) was more practical for therapists as compared to in vivo exposure. These benefits give an edge to the VR based intervention; however, more research is required to check for its continued advantages compared to the traditional in vivo exposure treatment.

Post-Traumatic Stress Disorder (PTSD)

PTSD involves extreme distress and impairment in daily functioning experienced by individuals after traumatic incidents, such as direct exposure to the traumatic event, from witnessing and even from being exposed to the details of the traumatic event (DSM-5; American Psychiatric Association, 2013). It is accompanied by changes in reactivity, altered arousal of the individual, by the presence of intrusive and involuntary recollection of the event that causes distress to the individual and is almost always related to active avoidance of the triggering stimuli.

The American Psychological Association (2017) recommend interventions such as Cognitive Behavioral Therapy (CBT), Cognitive Therapy (CT), Prolonged Exposure (PE) and Cognitive Processing Therapy (CPT). PE works on the premise that emotional engagement during exposure to traumatic thoughts, feelings and situations through multiple senses can help an individual learn a better manner of coping. It involves psychoeducation, breathing training, imaginal exposure through recounting of the traumatic memory in some manner, along with in vivo exposure to the situations that were being avoided. CPT is based on the premise that after a traumatic event, individuals try and make sense of what happened, they form cognitive distortions about themselves, the world and others. It includes psychoeducation, emphasis on maladaptive thinking patterns and exploration of the traumatic incidents conceptualisation by the individual. For the treatment of PTSD, positive outcomes have been seen in CPT, PE therapy and the cognitive model of PTSD. Exposure to a traumatic event is a common element among PE and cognitive models (Beidel, et al., 2019). The component of exposure in these interventions has created space to see how VR can help in this area. VR systems like BraveMind and Virtual Iraq/Afghanistan was funded by the research division of the United States of America's armed forces to treat PTSD in veterans. The Virtual Iraq/Afghanistan system is composed of four scenarios which are based on the initial Virtual Iraq prototype that laid the groundwork for its feasibility. This system was then upgraded and expanded and was known as the BraveMind system that includes various scenarios that a therapist can alter depending on the requirement of the individual and help them by exposing them to safer and controlled situations (Rizzo & Shilling, 2017).

A recent feasibility study compared pre and post-treatment scores for PTSD due to military sexual trauma and showed a significant reduction following VR intervention that used the modified BraveMind system (Loucks, et al., 2019). This modification allowed for the addition of military sexual trauma related features and scenario that aligned with the user's trauma narrative. It included exposing them to contextual cues about the incident (time of day, starting location, surrounding sounds) in a safer manner and laid a supportive groundwork for usage of VR interventions for PTSD from such personal trauma. However, some studies have shown that using VR based interventions is as effective as an active control condition (McLay et al., 2010) and even effective for active service members (Reger, et al., 2011). Reger et al., (2016) found that there was a significant reduction in PTSD symptoms in both VRET Virtual Iraq system and PE. Moreover, both conditions showed a significant reduction as compared to the waitlist condition. Due to varied symptoms associated with PTSD, different studies have targeted different aspects of PTSD and measured the results. Beidel et al. (2019) compared VRET Virtual Iraq/Afghanistan system combined with Trauma Management Therapy and VRET combined with psychoeducation as a control condition to study their effectiveness in the treatment of PTSD. It was found that PTSD scores reduced significantly in both conditions. Moreover, pairing VRET with other therapies yielded better outcomes in bringing about changes in other domains of PTSD.

Reger et al. (2019) built upon the results of their previous study and tried to assess the emotional engagement component and its role in VRET Virtual Iraq/Afghanistan system. The premise was that since there would be a greater emotional engagement in the VRET condition, owing to the activation trauma relevant stimuli through multiple senses, it would yield better results for treatment of PTSD as compared to the PE condition. The component of emotional engagement was assessed through the Subjective unit of distress (SUDs). It was found that though there was a reduction in SUDs over time in both conditions, there was no significant difference in SUDs reduction over time for the VRET or the PE condition. Thus, VRET did not manage to increase the emotional engagement above and beyond the PE condition. This may be due to the VR system used for the purpose of this study, that has not been updated since its release in 2009. On the other hand, Katz et al. (2020) targetted the increased emotional reactivity component of PTSD. They compared the change in physiological reactivity among active-duty soldiers in two treatment conditions: VRET Virtual Iraq/Afghanistan system, PE and a waitlist group that served as a control condition. They wanted to determine if the arousal of the individual responded to the treatment. Consistent with the previous results of Reger et al. (2016, 2019), Katz et al. (2020) found that physiological reactivity decreased in both treatment conditions from pre-treatment measurement to post-treatment outcomes. However, unlike the results from Reger et al. (2016), in this study, only the VRET condition differed significantly from the waitlist condition. This study was only able to establish the equal effectiveness of VRET and PE both in the treatment of PTSD. Norr et al. (2018) also provided valuable insight through their study, which employed the use of Virtual Iraq/Afghanistan system and showed that younger individuals, those not on medication, with minimal suicide risk and with greater arousal symptoms, were predictors for greater reduction in symptoms of PTSD. In conclusion, VR based interventions have shown to be as effective as the traditional active based ones. At the same time, VR based interventions have not been able to show their effect above and beyond the traditional active controls.

Major Depressive Disorder

Depression (Major depressive disorder) is a mood disorder characterised by a persistent feeling of sadness and loss of interest or pleasure in activities (anhedonia) (DSM-5; American Psychiatric Association, 2013). The specifiers of depression allow one to learn more about the disorder, prognosis, and treatment that would work (Kessing & Bukh, 2017). Depression negatively impacts the way an individual thinks, feels, and acts, with impairment seen in daily functioning.

While antidepressant medications are prescribed to deal with the core features of depression - mood and interest, less emphasis is laid on the associated features presented in depression (Kennedy, 2008). However, a recent meta-analysis based on four-decade of outcome research on depression reported that all psychotherapies are equally as effective as pharmacotherapies, and both combined are better than any one approach alone (Cuijpers, 2017). Among psychotherapies, CBT aims to change the unhelpful ways of thinking, feeling and acting through various techniques, and has often been considered as the gold standard for treatment (Cuijpers et al., 2020; David, et al., 2018) and found to be effective in reducing symptoms of depression (Cuijpers, et al., 2016).

Positive outcomes are reported for treating mild to moderate depression using CBT techniques via the internet (Arjadi, et al., 2018; Health Quality Ontario, 2019), smartphones (Lukas, et al., 2021), and games (Fleming, et al., 2011). In recent times, VR based therapy and techniques for depression have been attempted. With depression owing to the diverse symptomology and presentation of symptoms, facets of CBT, like psychoeducation, behavioural activation, physical activity, social skill training, cognitive restructuring and positive affect through virtual scenarios, are tailored so that they can be delivered through the VR medium (Lindner, et al., 2019).

Psychoeducation. Psychoeducation is the process of imparting knowledge to individual and family members about their psychological distress to aid in the treatment process and outcomes. In a VR setup, one is conversing with a virtual character who imparts knowledge about mental health. VRight, a novel VR software, works on this premise and enables interaction between the individual and a digital character to increase awareness (Migoya-Borja et al., 2020). Moreover, through the immersive nature of VR, one can experience the things to be learned. Also, this offers an avenue where an individual could first experience the learning outcomes that are to be learned, which can even be tailored to their situation through VR (Lindner, Hamilton, Miloff, & Carlbring, 2019). A strong association between psychoeducation and better prognosis (Tursi, et al., 2013), greater levels of overall satisfaction (Migoya-

Borja et al., 2020), and an overall reduction in depression symptoms (Kim et al., 2020) were reported in patients with depression.

Behavioural activation and Physical activity. Behavioural activation is an evidence-based technique that decreases depressive symptoms through engagement in activities that provide pleasure or mastery to individuals. A case study that measured the effectiveness of VR to deliver behavioural activation intervention found a significant decrease in the depression score for the participant (Paul, et al., 2020). Physical activity as a behavioural intervention helps in alleviating the symptoms of depression. Kandola et al. (2019), in their review, assessed mechanisms responsible for the antidepressant effect of physical activity, in particular, exercise, and found its ability to bring about change in inflammation, neuroplasticity, oxidative stress and the endocrine system. In the VR setup, the physical exercise consists of the stationary treadmill or bicycle with a headset that takes the user into different immersive scenarios. For the effect of VR based exercises on the psychological outcome of depression, Zeng et al. (2018), in their review, found that several studies showed an improvement in depression-related measures among the varied population. However, Monteiro-Junior et al. (2017) found no significant difference in depression scores between the experimental group and control group of institutionalised older adults when compared on selected virtual activities on the Nintendo Wii system.

Though most of the studies were effective, there was insufficient support for using VR-based exercises as a standalone treatment. Another systematic review that assessed VR-based exercises' physiological and psychological effects also found promising results (Qian, et al., 2020). Of the selected literature for this review, three of the four studies found a positive impact of VR exercises in reducing depression tendencies among the participants. However, such results are not consistent. In a systematic review and metanalysis, Wu et al. (2021) found that though VRCBT (Virtual reality cognitive behavioural therapy) was better than the waitlist group, the effectiveness of VRCBT was similar to that of standard CBT in treating depression. Similar results were found in a clinical pilot study by Gamito et al. (2010), where they assessed the effectiveness of Virtual reality exposure therapy (VRET) on war veterans suffering from posttraumatic stress and the impact it would have on the symptoms of depression and anxiety. The study found a statistical reduction in the symptoms of reduction in the VRET group compared to the control group and the waitlist condition. Indeed, VR based exercises can offer a great avenue for treatment; however, the effect is not above and beyond the traditional treatment methods.

Social skill training. Social skill training includes interventions that help an individual gain a better understanding of social behaviour. In a real-life setting, such interventions consist of the individual practising the social skill they find difficult with the therapist. Social skill training within the VR setup provides an avenue for individuals to try out social interaction in spaces at a pace they are comfortable with. Dehn et al. (2017) compared cognitive training consisting of grocery shopping for an individual with depression in a computerised environment and VR environment. The VR environment used the Octavis system that displayed the everyday scenario on eight 26" LCD touch screens. Though results indicated a significant decrease in depressive symptoms across both groups, there was no difference between groups. Moreover, the decrease in depression scores was independent of the cognitive training task measures. These results were not replicated in another study. Gamito et al. (2018) studied the effect of cognitive-based virtual reality exercises on elderly individuals in a pre-post treatment design; however, there was no improvement seen on the depression scores of the individual.

Cognitive restructuring. Cognitive restructuring is a group of techniques that help individuals recognise their faulty thinking patterns and is an important part of CBT for depression. A VR setup allows an individual to experience the scenarios where they are exposed to negative thoughts about themselves, the world or the future. It allows the individual to situationally emerge themselves in the scenario and experience the situation. Since they have control, they can pause at any time and discuss the thoughts that the situation elicits. Another way this can be done is through activities that an individual has trouble with and practice till they feel comfortable (Lindner, et al., 2019). A recent network meta-analysis by Ciharova et al. (2021) found cognitive restructuring and behavioural activation alone or their combination with CBT to be effective in treating adult depression. Since in cognitive restructuring, negative cognitions are restructured, arousal plays a role. Bolinski, et al., (2021), in their experimental study, worked on this premise and found that there was greater physiological arousal in the VR condition than the imaginal condition. The VR condition consisted of a VR application called Lunchroom Zondag (English: Lunchroom Sunday) that allowed the participant to be involved in different VR scenarios that elicit negative automatic thoughts and give them a chance to rework them.

Positive scenarios. A characteristic of depression is negative thinking patterns. In a VR setup, positive scenarios can be experienced by the individual rather than just thinking about them. In a study, Dainer-Best et al. (2018) used positive images relating to self for individuals with depression for two weeks and found a reduction in the depressive symptoms for the treatment group compared to the control group. In the VR scenario, targeting the symptom of anhedonia (loss of pleasure), which is a risk factor to suicide in depression, Chen et al. (2021), in their pilot study, exposed the participants to positive scenarios through a VR environment. The scenarios were selected from the Oculus library. They found a significant reduction in symptoms of anhedonia and depression for the participants.

In summary, a metanalysis of VR interventions for depression found VR therapies to be more effective than controls with a moderate to high effect size. On the other hand, on comparing VR based interventions with active control, the results were non-significant (Fodor, et al., 2018). This can be due to the fact that there has been a dearth of literature on depression in the VR framework (Freeman, et al., 2017). This depicts that VR intervention for depression shows promise but more studies need to be conducted before results can be generalised.

Overall, despite the popularity of VR for the improvement of mental health, rigorous scientific investigation demonstrating the need for VR in mental health treatment is required (Frewen, et al., 2020). Methodological differences in VR based studies plague the mental health scenario (Riva, 2002). This affects the generalizability and the replicability of the results obtained. The technical advancements being made over time also make it difficult to ascertain whether the effect of VR being observed is due to the treatment effect or due to the improved technology.

USER IN VR: PRESENCE AND PREFERENCE

VR use in therapy hinges on the user interaction with the VR environment. For this purpose, it is essential that the user is able to feel like a part of the VR scenario. The user involvement in the VR platform is measured by the concept of presence, which is an individual's experience when in the VR environment is the psychological sense of 'being' in the virtual environment (Slater & Wilbur, 1997). Visual realism is one of the factors that influence the presence an individual feels in the virtual environment. Slater et al., (2009) studied if the realness of the virtual environment influenced the sense of presence felt by the user. They found that the group immersed in a more real VR environment felt significantly greater presence than the active control group. Moreover, there was a significant difference from the baseline in terms of the physiological response experienced group exposed to a more realistic environment. Riches, et al., (2019) expanded on the factor that affected the presence of an individual in the VR environment through their qualitative study. Some of the common themes that emerged were emotions about self and others, thoughts about self and others, physiological reactions experienced, the behaviour of the avatars, the level of interactivity with the environment, and environmental characteristics. These findings are of essence as they would not only guide the future development of VR scenarios but also give insight to a therapist about how the engagement in the scenarios can be manipulated.

Preference in the VR scenario also plays an integral part. Colour temperature preference plays a role in user engagement in the VR space. Siess and Wölfel (2018) found that gender plays a role in the colour temperature preference for immersive scenarios wherein females preferred colder tones in immersive scenarios as compared to computer screens, while men had an identical colour preference in both. Apart from gender, the time of the day the VR environment is viewed, as well as the season, has an effect on the user. These results are important as these factors can work as confounding variables when measuring a VR scenario's effect on an individual. The choice and preference of the scenario effects the level of physiological response elicited. In the context of natural scenarios, in an exploratory study by Tsutsumi, et al., (2017), the effect of the preference of a scenario on the relaxation was evaluated by comparing two groups of users, those who had a strong preference for the video of the sea, and those who did not have a preference for the video (sea or forest). They found that there was a quicker decrease in the heart rate when participants viewed their preferred video of the sea. In terms of their arousal level, while viewing the preferred video of the sea, their arousal was maintained, and this facilitated a feeling of relaxation. The sea preference group also reported a significant decrease in the tension anxiety subscale of the Profile of Mood States (POMS) scale after viewing the sea video. In another study by Anderson et al. (2017), VR scenes were presented, and their effect was studied for reducing stress and improving the moods of individuals. The study consisted of 3 VR scenes: 2 natural scenes (beach scene and a scene from Ireland) and a control scene (empty indoor classroom). In terms of evaluation of the natural scenes based on individual preference, there was no difference in objective physiological measures (electrodermal activity and heart rate variability). However, on a subjective level, the choice of the scene mattered. The first preference video reduced more negative affect in participants as compared to their second preference, implicating that the choice of scenario plays a role in the experience of relaxation for participants. Understanding the preference is essential in the therapeutic setup as this knowledge can help us make the VR scenario and sessions more individualised so that the best results can occur.

MOVING FORWARD: ETHICAL CONSIDERATIONS

The introduction of VR in the therapeutic setup requires evaluation of how it measures against the ethical standard that has been guiding the work in this field so far. Therapy within the digital space improves user accessibility, however, it also poses a few ethical hurdles that must be resolved for the safe dissemination of online services. The American Psychological Association (APA) has given Ethical Principles of Psychologists and Code of Conduct that applies to a psychologist's role in the scientific, educational and professional area. These ethics cover activities taking place in-person as well as through postal, telephone, internet and other electronic transmissions (American Psychological Association, 2017). These principles, though aspirational, have guided psychologists to maintain an ethical standard in their research and praxis. Evaluating VR through this lens allows us a unique perspective to direct the advancements in the field. A brief about the general principles is given below:

Beneficence and Nonmaleficence. This principle strives and guides psychologists to carry out the work in a manner that is beneficial to those whom they interact with on a professional level and at the same time not cause them harm.

Fidelity and responsibility. This principle inspires and guides psychologists to maintain relationships of trust, accountability and ethical consideration relating to their work and that of their colleagues in order to work in the best of interest.

Integrity. This principle strives and encourages psychologists to be honest and transparent in their practice. They stay away from dishonest, malicious, fraudulent practices and subterfuge. In cases where manipulation is present, it is ethically justified, and the advantages outweigh the harm. There are four conditions under which deception can be used: when the value of the study justifies the deception; a nondeceptive alterative is not available; when pain or emotional distress is anticipated, deception is not used; deception is disclosed to the participants as early as it can be.

Justice. This principle recognises that all persons are entitled to the advancements made in psychology and are equally privileged to attain the services offered by the professional within this field.

Respect for people's rights and dignity. This principle recognises the right of individuals to privacy and confidentiality and respects the dignity and worth of all persons. Psychologists are aware of the vulnerabilities of some groups of individuals and strive to avoid their own personal biases towards any person based on their age, gender, gender identity, race, ethnicity, culture, national origin, religion, sexual orientation, disability, language, and socioeconomic status, and consider these factors when working with members of such groups.

Keeping these principles in mind, various aspects and usage of VR in the therapeutic setup are evaluated with respect to the role they serve and the points where steps need to be taken to adhere to these principles. One of the major issues that arise when we consider the use of VR for online therapy is the potential negative effects of being immersed in the virtual environment like cybersickness or VR sickness. Cybersickness is defined as a group of symptoms that produce discomfort and malaise because of VR exposure (Stanney, et al., 1997) and includes unpleasant physiological symptoms like nausea and dizziness. Yildirim (2020), in their study, investigated if cybersickness was experienced by individuals while using state of the art VR equipment and compared it to the effects felt while using the desktop display. The study found more severe cybersickness while using the state-of-the-art equipment as compared to the desktop display condition. Seeing this aspect from the principle of beneficence and non-maleficence makes us strive to ensure that no harm comes to the individual while in the VR environment and the need to have strategies to mitigate the effects of cybersickness. There have been studies that have investigated approaches to decrease cybersickness through the reduction in the field of view (Chang, et al., 2013), through rotational blurring (Budhiraja, et al, 2017), by using static rest frames in the virtual environment (Cao, et al., 2018). Also, having the individual habituated to the simulator condition has been shown to decrease cybersickness (Nader & Kruszewski, 2013; Reinhard, et al., 2017).

Furthermore, due to the individual differences, VR sickness on various users are reported (Howard & Van Zandt, 2021). Individual factors such as motion sickness susceptibility, gender, real-world experience, technological experience and knowledge, presence of a neurological disorder, and presence of relevant phobia are significantly related to VR sickness. This brings to light the importance of the principle of respect for people's right and dignity. Furthermore, this depicts how some groups of individuals are more susceptible to VR sickness. Therefore, it comes with an urgency to address and evaluate the potential advantages and disadvantages of utilising this avenue for an optimum experience and a need to have relevant strategies in place to safeguard the interest of every individual.

Another point to reflect on is the effects of immersion in VR space that linger on in an individual. Research has pointed to a negative relation between presence (subjective psychological experience of being in the VR environment) and the symptoms of cybersickness (Weech, et al., 2019). While presence in the VR environment is a desirable outcome, it could become a matter of concern. When coupled with exposure therapy, this immersion in the VR environment allows the therapist to help the individual overcome their fear. At the same time, there are instances when immersion in the VR environment has caused behavioural changes. The Proteus Effect is one such example where the individual behaves in a manner that is expected of them based on the avatar they have in the VR space (Yee & Bailenson, 2007). Szpak et al. (2019) went beyond the measurement of cybersickness through self-reported questionnaires and studied the effect of VR on an individual through visual and cognitive assessments after participants. For the visual measurement, researchers measured the accommodation (adjustment of eyes muscle to form a clear image) and vergence (rotation of the eyes in order to form a single image). Essentially, in a VR setup, the accommodation typically occurs at the screen level, while vergence occurs at the depth depicted by the VR scene. They found that the VR group differed significantly from the control group in terms of visual measures of accommodation after VR exposure. On the cognitive front, the VR group was slower in decision making. The after-effects of VR exposure can have a negative impact on the day to day activities that user resumes after sessions. Although these effects did not meet the criteria for a clinical diagnosis, such after-effects warrant that more in-depth analysis and study be conducted to garner a greater understanding of what is at play.

While virtual scenarios can increase the presence felt by the individual, they can also increase the risk for depersonalisation and derealisation. Aardema et al. (2010) in their study assessed the effect of VR on the dissociative experiences of the participants and found a significant increase in the dissociative symptoms after VR exposure. Though not a concern for everyone, these results urge us to delve deeper into how this can affect the vulnerable population.

ETHICS RELATED TO VR DATA

Data security is another crucial aspect that needs scrutiny. This concern lines with the principle of respect for people's dignity and rights. Using an online platform brings the need to use encrypted communication to further protect the privacy and client confidentiality, emphasising regular checks on software and hardware. There is a security risk of virtual reality technology where personal data that may be collected is deployed to vying markets for profits (Spiegel, 2018). With the integration of such technologies with the therapeutic setup, more sensitive and personalised data can be collected. If necessary precautions are not maintained, this threatens the privacy of the client through the potential loss of personally identifiable information.

It is well acknowledged that the constant use of digital technology leads to the digital footprint (O'Brolchain, et al., 2016), and with VR use, kinematic footprint, a term that represents how body movements via VR are recorded by motion sensors which can identify an individual (Madary, 2017). Any datum that is collected using technologies that can be hooked to the online systems invariably is under watch and threatens privacy. O'Brolchain et al. (2016) refer to threat to informational privacy, information related to a person's thoughts, actions, other records associated with them. More importantly, other metrics that are collected via the VR system that could include but is not limited to eye movements, emotions (O'Brolchain, et al., 2016), and even facial expressions and posture (Bailenson, 2018).

It is indeed a conundrum when it comes to using technology. While on the one hand, there are numerous uses for the benefit of mankind, on the other, these technologies can be vulnerable and hence can be misused. Several researchers and companies that create these technologies enforce the collection of data to improve user experience and deliver better versions to the user. Furthermore, the use of VR type technologies for vulnerable populations such as those with mental health concerns and young children have been time and again brought up in discussions and policy formulations (e.g., Madary & Metzinger, 2016).

That said, it is possible to deal with data privacy issues in the mental health sector.

The greatest advantage of using VR in therapy has been its reachability, especially in times when it has been challenging for patients to show up at a clinic or when clients are travelling and are unable to be present for in-person sessions. Given VR therapies are likely to stay around for some time, some general rules that have been proposed by Slater et al. (2020) for immersive technologies can be implemented. These include the amount of time spent with the technology, setting a limit on the amount of personal data collected and shared with third parties, and having legal formalities in place in order to safeguard an individual's right to privacy. Madary and Metzinger (2016) have proposed various guidelines for VR use in the research sphere; however, they can also be applied in the clinical set-up. These include informed consent for participating in a VR based therapy and providing the effects/risks that VR could induce on the individual. The criteria used by APA to assess treatment guidelines include evaluating them based on how an intervention is compared to no intervention or an alternative intervention and also taking into account the generalisability and the feasibility of the intervention (American Psychological Association, 2002).

In terms of VR use for therapy, Madary and Metzinger (2016) also recommend the presence of a licensed therapist/clinical practitioner who is administering the therapy to patients. Parsons (2021) recommends that clinicians follow the Health Information Portability and Accountability Act (HIPAA) guidelines for using immersive technologies as a form of therapy. HIPAA offers rules and regulations regarding appropriate means of safeguarding patients' medical records and their privacy. Furthermore, Parsons (2021) also recommends using third-party cloud storage that stores patient data using authentication information that is accessible to the clinician only. In this way, the medical data and therapy data are disconnected from one another in the sense that they are in two different databases and hence would be less likely to encounter potential data leaks and misuse.

Online data are vulnerable to getting hacked for the stealing of personal information. Hence, if VR data is being transmitted via the internet, great care is required, so the data do not get into the wrong hands. In this regard, safe internet security is required. Furthermore, countries have already established laws (e.g., the General Data Protection Regulation (GDPR)) that ensure safe and secure data transmission. An interesting technology has been proposed by Proniewska et al. (2021) to access data remotely by medical practitioners. They recommend remote authentication by means of using a QR/barcode assigned to a patient, and this is validated by a medical doctor who then enters the password to gain access to patient data via holographic technology (i.e., hololens, a mixed reality technique). This way, the practitioner's eyes are the authentication points through the hololens, which is a smart way to ensure that no unauthorised individual can access sensitive patient data. A similar idea can be implemented for VR based data to ensure the safety of the data.

VR is on the way to becoming an affordable avenue owing to its technological advancements; however, it can arguably create a digital divide between individuals who can and cannot avail of this service. A digital divide refers to the gap between demographics that have access to modern information and communication technology and those who do not (Selwyn, 2004). With VR equipment and integration into therapy, there is a possibility that such services may not be equally available to every individual, creating a VR divide (Rizzo, et al., 2002). This would not be in line with the principle of Justice that strives to provide the advancement being made in the field to everyone equally.

In summary, some essential things to be considered by when adopting VR in the mental health setup are:

- The lack of information about VR's utility in the therapeutic setup persists. Hence, providing individuals with relevant information about the use of VR, detailing the advantages/risks of VR therapy, and obtaining informed consent is important.
- The concerns of data security can be handled by adhering to the HIPPA guidelines that ensure the safety of the medical records and personal information, employing strategies like using third-party cloud storage that can only be accessed by a clinician, using data encryption, regular security testing and being mindful of insider threats (ensuring policies around how much information each person working within an organisation can have) and having protocols in place in case of negligence.
- Ensuring data privacy for safer collection, usage, and transportation can be handled by being compliant with the GDPR.
- Evaluating treatment guidelines for new interventions by taking into account its effectiveness as compared to alternatives and assessing the feasibility and generalisability of the intervention.

CONCLUSION

VR offers the unique advantage of presenting virtual environments for users to practice and learn before stepping out into the real world. VR's reachability allows the user to be part of the therapy process, especially when being at therapy in person is challenging. Moreover, catering to the user's preferences offers flexibility towards different ways VR can be integrated into therapy. Thus, the integration of VR in the therapeutic setup has offered new avenues to explore, has provided alternatives to drawbacks in existing therapies, and has extended add-ons unique to the VR setup to current therapies. The role and advantages of VR have been explored to a greater extent for some conditions, more so than the other (such as, anxiety); yet, collectively, the results have shown its efficacy to be at least at par with traditional approaches. From the ethics perspective, many measures are in place for safer dissemination of services of VR based therapies and endeavours to ensure confidentiality of data continues till date. VR's use in the mental health space holds promise given its inherent features, which, if put to use in a methodologically sound manner, can validate its use.

REFERENCES

Aardema, F., O'Connor, K., Côté, S., & Taillon, A. (2010). Virtual Reality Induces Dissociation and Lowers Sense of Presence in Objective Reality. *Cyberpsychology, Behavior, and Social Networking*, *13*(4), 429–435. doi:10.1089/cyber.2009.0164 PMID:20712501

American Psychological Association. (2002). Criteria for Evaluating Treatment Guidelines. *The American Psychologist*, *57*(12), 1052–1059. doi:10.1037/0003-066X.57.12.1052 PMID:12617064

American Psychological Association. (2013, July 31). *Guidelines for the Practice of Telepsychology*. Retrieved from https://www.apa.org/practice/guidelines/telepsychology

American Psychological Association. (2017). *Clinical Practical Guideline for the Treatment of PTSD*. Retrieved from American Psychological Association: https://www.apa.org/ptsd-guideline

American Psychological Association. (2017). *Ethical principles of psychologists and code of conduct (2002, amended effective June 1, 2010, and January 1, 2017)*. Retrieved from http://www.apa.org/ethics/code/index.html

Anderson, A. P., Mayer, M. D., Fellows, A. M., Cowan, D. R., Hegel, M. T., & Buckey, J. C. (2017, June). Relaxation with Immersive Natural Scenes Presented Using Virtual Reality. *Aerospace Medicine and Human Performance*, *88*(6), 520–526. doi:10.3357/AMHP.4747.2017 PMID:28539139

Anderson, P. L., Price, M., Edwards, S. M., Obasaju, M. A., Schmertz, S. K., Zimand, E., & Calamaras, M. R. (2013). Virtual reality exposure therapy for social anxiety disorder: A randomized controlled trial. *Journal of Consulting and Clinical Psychology*, *81*(5), 751–760. doi:10.1037/a0033559 PMID:23796315

Arjadi, R., Nauta, M. H., Scholte, W. F., Hollon, S. D., Chowdhary, N., Suryani, A. O., Uiterwaal, C. S. P. M., & Bockting, C. L. (2018). Internet-based behavioural activation with lay counsellor support versus online minimal psychoeducation without support for treatment of depression: A randomised controlled trial in Indonesia. *The Lancet. Psychiatry*, *5*(9), 707–716. doi:10.1016/S2215-0366(18)30223-2 PMID:30006262

Bailenson, J. (2018). Protecting Nonverbal Data Tracked in Virtual Reality. *JAMA Pediatrics*, *172*(10), 905–906. doi:10.1001/jamapediatrics.2018.1909 PMID:30083770

Beidel, D. C., Frueh, B. C., Neer, S. M., Bowers, C. A., Trachik, B., Uhde, T. W., & Grubaugh, A. (2019). Trauma management therapy with virtual-reality augmented exposure therapy for combat-related PTSD: A randomized controlled trial. *Journal of Anxiety Disorders*, *61*, 64–74. doi:10.1016/j.janxdis.2017.08.005 PMID:28865911

Bolinski, F., Etzelmüller, A., Witte, N. A., Beurden, C., Debard, G., Bonroy, B., ... Kleiboer, A. (2021). Physiological and self-reported arousal in virtual reality versus face-to-face emotional activation and cognitive restructuring in university students: A crossover experimental study using wearable monitoring. *Behaviour Research and Therapy*, *142*, 103877. doi:10.1016/j.brat.2021.103877 PMID:34029860

Botella, C., Fernández-Álvarez, J., Guillén, V., García-Palacios, A., & Baños, R. (2017). Recent Progress in Virtual Reality Exposure Therapy for Phobias: A Systematic Review. *Current Psychiatry Reports*, *19*(42), 1–13. doi:10.100711920-017-0788-4 PMID:28540594

Bouchard, S., Dumoulin, S., Robillard, G., Guitard, T., Klinger, É., Forget, H., Loranger, C., & Roucaut, F. X. (2017). Virtual reality compared with in vivo exposure in the treatment of social anxiety disorder: A three-arm randomised controlled trial. *The British Journal of Psychiatry*, *210*(4), 276–283. doi:10.1192/bjp.bp.116.184234 PMID:27979818

Budhiraja, P., Miller, M. R., Modi, A. K., & Forsyth, D. (2017). Rotation Blurring: Use of Artificial Blurring to Reduce Cybersickness in Virtual Reality First Person Shooters. *arXiv 2017*, arXiv:1710.02599

Cao, Z., Jerald, J., & Kopper, R. (2018). Visually-Induced Motion Sickness Reduction via Static and Dynamic Rest Frames. In *2018 IEEE Conference on Virtual Reality and 3D User Interfaces (VR)* (pp. 105-112). IEEE. 10.1109/VR.2018.8446210

Carl, E., Stein, A. T., Levihn-Coon, A., Pogue, J. R., Rothbaum, B., Emmelkamp, P., ... Powers, M. B. (2018). Virtual reality exposure therapy for anxiety and related disorders: A meta-analysis of randomized controlled trials. *Journal of Anxiety Disorders*. Advance online publication. doi:10.1016/j.janxdis.2018.08.003 PMID:30287083

Chang, E., Hwang, I., Jeon, H., Chun, Y., Kim, H., & Park, C. (2013). Effects of rest frames on cybersickness and oscillatory brain activity. In *Proceedings of the 2013 International Winter Workshop on Brain-Computer Interface (BCI)* (pp. 62–64). IEEE. 10.1109/IWW-BCI.2013.6506631

Chen, A., Jacobsen, K. H., Deshmukh, A. A., & Cantor, S. B. (2015). The evolution of the disability-adjusted life year (DALY). *Socio-Economic Planning Sciences*, *49*, 10–15. doi:10.1016/j.seps.2014.12.002

Chen, K., Barnes-Horowitz, N., Treanor, M., Sun, M., Young, K. S., & Craske, M. G. (2021). Virtual Reality Reward Training for Anhedonia: A Pilot Study. *Frontiers in Psychology*, *11*, 613617. doi:10.3389/fpsyg.2020.613617 PMID:33488482

Chou, P.-H., Tseng, P.-T., Wu, Y.-C., Chang, J. P.-C., Tu, Y.-K., Stubbs, B., ... Sui, K.-P. (2021). Efficacy and acceptability of different interventions for acrophobia: A network meta-analysis of randomised controlled trials. *Journal of Affective Disorders*, *282*, 786–794. doi:10.1016/j.jad.2020.12.172 PMID:33601719

Cieślik, B., Mazurek, J., Rutkowskic, S., Kiper, P., Turolla, A., & Szczepańska-Gierachae, J. (2020). Virtual reality in psychiatric disorders: A systematic review of reviews. *Complementary Therapies in Medicine*, *52*, 102480. doi:10.1016/j.ctim.2020.102480 PMID:32951730

Ciharova, M., Furukawa, T. A., Efthimiou, O., Karyotaki, E., Miguel, C., Noma, H., Cipriani, A., Riper, H., & Cuijpers, P. (2021). Cognitive restructuring, behavioral activation and cognitive-behavioral therapy in the treatment of adult depression: A network meta-analysis. *Journal of Consulting and Clinical Psychology*, *89*(6), 563–574. doi:10.1037/ccp0000654 PMID:34264703

Côté, S., & Bouchard, S. (2009). Cognitive mechanisms underlying virtual reality exposure. *Cyberpsychology & Behavior*, *12*(2), 121–129. doi:10.1089/cpb.2008.0008 PMID:19250009

Cuijpers, P. (2017). Four Decades of Outcome Research on Psychotherapies for Adult Depression: An Overview of a Series of Meta-Analyses. *Canadian Psychology*, *58*(1), 7–19. doi:10.1037/cap0000096

Cuijpers, P., Cristea, I. A., Karyotaki, E., Reijnders, M., & Huibers, M. J. (2016). How effective are cognitive behavior therapies for major depression and anxiety disorders? A meta-analytic update of the evidence. *World Psychiatry; Official Journal of the World Psychiatric Association (WPA)*, *15*(3), 245–258. doi:10.1002/wps.20346 PMID:27717254

Cuijpers, P., Noma, H., Karyotaki, E., Vinkers, C. H., Cipriani, A., & Furukawa, T. A. (2020, February). A network meta-analysis of the effects of psychotherapies, pharmacotherapies and their combination in the treatment of adult depression. *World Psychiatry; Official Journal of the World Psychiatric Association (WPA)*, *19*(1), 92–107. doi:10.1002/wps.20701 PMID:31922679

Dainer-Best, J., Shumake, J. D., & Beevers, C. G. (2018). Positive Imagery Training Increases Positive Self-Referent Cognition in Depression. *Behaviour Research and Therapy*, *111*, 72–83. doi:10.1016/j.brat.2018.09.010 PMID:30321746

David, D., Cristea, I., & Hofmann, S. G. (2018, January). Why Cognitive Behavioral Therapy is the Current Gold Standard of psychotherapy. *Frontiers in Psychiatry*, *9*, 4. doi:10.3389/fpsyt.2018.00004 PMID:29434552

Dehn, L. B., Kate, L. M. P., Botsch, M., Driessen, M., & Beblo, T. (2017). Training in a comprehensive everyday-like virtual reality environment compared to computerized cognitive training for patients with depression. *Computers in Human Behavior*, *79*, 40–52. doi:10.1016/j.chb.2017.10.019

Donker, T., Cornelisz, I., Klaveren, C., Straten, A., Carlbring, P., Cuijpers, P., & Gelder, J.-L. (2019). Effectiveness of Self-guided App-Based Virtual Reality Cognitive Behavior Therapy for Acrophobia: A Randomized Clinical Trial. *JAMA Psychiatry*, *76*(7), 682–690. doi:10.1001/jamapsychiatry.2019.0219 PMID:30892564

Emmelkamp, P. M., Meyerbröker, K., & Morina, N. (2020). Virtual Reality Therapy in Social Anxiety Disorder. *Current Psychiatry Reports*, *22*(7), 32. doi:10.100711920-020-01156-1 PMID:32405657

Fleming, T., Dixon, R., Frampton, C., & Merry, S. (2011). A Pragmatic Randomised Controlled Trial of computerised CBT (SPARX) for symptoms of depression among adolescents excluded from mainstream education. *Behavioural and Cognitive Psychotherapy*, *40*(5), 529–541. doi:10.1017/S1352465811000695 PMID:22137185

Fodor, L. A., Coteț, C. D., Cuijpers, P., Szamoskozi, Ș., David, D., & Cristea, I. A. (2018). The effectiveness of virtual reality based interventions for symptoms of anxiety and depression: A meta-analysis. *Scientific Reports*, *8*(1), 10323. Advance online publication. doi:10.103841598-018-28113-6 PMID:29985400

Freeman, D., Haselton, P., Freeman, J., Spanlang, B., Kishore, S., Albery, E., Denne, M., Brown, P., Slater, M., & Nickless, A. (2018). Automated psychological therapy using immersive virtual reality for treatment of fear of heights: A single-blind, parallel-group, randomised controlled trial. *Psychiatry*, *5*(8), 625–632. doi:10.1016/S2215-0366(18)30226-8 PMID:30007519

Freeman, D., Reeve, S., Robinson, A., Ehlers, A., Clark, D., Spanlang, B., & Slater, M. (2017). Virtual reality in the assessment, understanding, and treatment of mental health disorders. *Psychological Medicine*, *47*(14), 2393–2400. doi:10.1017/S003329171700040X PMID:28325167

Gamito, P., Oliveira, J., Morais, D., Coelho, C., Santos, N., Alves, C., Galamba, A., Soeiro, M., Yerra, M., French, H., Talmers, L., Gomes, T., & Brito, R. (2018). Cognitive Stimulation of Elderly Individuals with Instrumental Virtual Reality-Based Activities of Daily Life: Pre-Post Treatment Study. *Cyberpsychology, Behavior, and Social Networking*, *22*(1), 69–75. doi:10.1089/cyber.2017.0679 PMID:30040477

Gamito, P., Oliveira, J., Rosa, P., Morais, D., Duarte, N., Oliveira, S., & Saraiva, T. (2010). PTSD Elderly War Veterans: A Clinical Controlled Pilot Study. *Cyberpsychology, Behavior, and Social Networking*, *13*(1), 43–48. doi:10.1089/cyber.2009.0237 PMID:20528292

Health Quality Ontario. (2019). Internet-Delivered Cognitive Behavioural Therapy for Major Depression and Anxiety Disorders: A Health Technology Assessment. *Ontario Health Technology Assessment Series*, *19*(6), 1–199. PMID:30873251

Howard, M., & Van Zandt, E. (2021). A meta-analysis of the virtual reality problem: Unequal effects of virtual reality sickness across individual differences. *Virtual Reality (Waltham Cross)*, *25*(4), 1221–1246. Advance online publication. doi:10.100710055-021-00524-3

Institute for Health Metrics and Evaluation (IHME). (2020). Retrieved 2021, from Health Data: http://www.healthdata.org/gbd/about

Jerdan, S. W., Grindle, M., Woerden, H. C., & Boulos, M. N. (2018). Head-Mounted Virtual Reality and Mental Health: Critical Review of Current Research. *JMIR Serious Games*, *6*(3), e14. doi:10.2196/games.9226 PMID:29980500

Kampmann, I. L., Emmelkamp, P. M., Hartanto, D., Brinkman, W.-P., Zijlstra, B. J., & Morina, N. (2016). Exposure to Virtual Social Interactions in the Treatment of Social Anxiety Disorder: A Randomized Controlled Trial. *Behaviour Research and Therapy*, *77*, 147–156. doi:10.1016/j.brat.2015.12.016 PMID:26752328

Kandola, A., Ashdown-Franks, G., Hendrikse, J., Sabiston, C. M., & Stubbs, B. (2019). Physical activity and depression: Towards understanding the antidepressant mechanisms of physical activity. *Neuroscience and Biobehavioral Reviews*, *107*, 525–539. doi:10.1016/j.neubiorev.2019.09.040 PMID:31586447

Katz, A. C., Norr, A. M., Buck, B., Fantelli, E., Edwards-Stewart, A., Koenen-Woods, P., Zetocha, K., Smolenski, D. J., Holloway, K., Rothbaum, B. O., Difede, J. A., Rizzo, A., Skopp, N., Mishkind, M., Gahm, G., Reger, G. M., & Andrasik, F. (2020). Changes in physiological reactivity in response to the trauma memory during prolonged exposure and virtual reality exposure therapy for posttraumatic stress disorder. *Psychological Trauma: Theory, Research, Practice, and Policy*, *12*(7), 756–764. doi:10.1037/tra0000567 PMID:32338946

Kennedy, S. H. (2008). Core symptoms of major depressive disorder: Relevance to diagnosis and treatment. *Dialogues in Clinical Neuroscience*, *10*(3), 271–277. doi:10.31887/DCNS.2008.10.3hkennedy PMID:18979940

Kessing, L. V., & Bukh, J. D. (2017). The clinical relevance of qualitatively distinct subtypes of depression. *World Psychiatry; Official Journal of the World Psychiatric Association (WPA)*, *16*(3), 318–319. doi:10.1002/wps.20461 PMID:28941112

Kim, M., Choi, S.-W., Moon, S., Park, H.-I., Hwang, H., Kim, M.-K., & Seok, J.-H. (2020). Treatment Effect of Psychoeducation and Training Program Using Virtual Reality Technique in the Patients with Depressive Symptoms. *Journal of Korean Neuropsychiatric Association*, *59*(1), 51–60. doi:10.4306/jknpa.2020.59.1.51

Lindner, P., Hamilton, W., Miloff, A., & Carlbring, P. (2019). How to Treat Depression With Low-Intensity Virtual Reality Interventions: Perspectives on Translating Cognitive Behavioral Techniques Into the Virtual Reality Modality and How to Make Anti-Depressive Use of Virtual Reality–Unique Experiences. *Frontiers in Psychiatry*, *10*, 792. doi:10.3389/fpsyt.2019.00792 PMID:31736809

Lindner, P., Miloff, A., Fagernäs, S., Andersen, J., Sigeman, M., Andersson, G., Furmark, T., & Carlbring, P. (2019). Therapist-led and self-led one-session virtual reality exposure therapy for public speaking anxiety with consumer hardware and software: A randomized controlled trial. *Journal of Anxiety Disorders*, *61*, 45–54. doi:10.1016/j.janxdis.2018.07.003 PMID:30054173

Lindner, P., Miloff, A., Zetterlund, E., Reuterskiöld, L., Andersson, G., & Carlbring, P. (2019). Attitudes Toward and Familiarity With Virtual Reality Therapy Among Practicing Cognitive Behavior Therapists: A Cross-Sectional Survey Study in the Era of Consumer VR Platforms. *Frontiers in Psychology*, *10*, 176. doi:10.3389/fpsyg.2019.00176 PMID:30800086

Loucks, L., Yasinski, C., Norrholm, S. D., Maples-Keller, J., Post, L., Zwiebach, L., ... Rothbauma, B. O. (2019). You can do that?!: Feasibility of virtual reality exposure therapy in the treatment of PTSD due to military sexual trauma. *Journal of Anxiety Disorders*, *61*, 55–63. doi:10.1016/j.janxdis.2018.06.004 PMID:30005843

Lukas, C. A., Eskofier, B., & Berking, M. (2021). A Gamified Smartphone-Based Intervention for Depression: Randomized Controlled Pilot Trial. *JMIR Mental Health*, *8*(7), e16643. doi:10.2196/16643 PMID:34283037

Madary, M. (2017). The Ethics of Virtual Reality: Risks and Recommendations. In Wirklichkeit(en): Gegenwart neu wahrnehmen - Zukunft kreativ gestalten (pp. 49-55). De Gruyter. doi:10.1515/9783110543711-008

Madary, M., & Metzinger, T. (2016). Real virtuality: A code of ethical conduct: Recommendations for good scientific practice and the consumers of VR technology. *Frontiers in Robotics and AI*, *3*. Advance online publication. doi:10.3389/frobt.2016.00003

Malbos, E., Rapee, R. M., & Kavakli, M. (2012). A controlled study of agoraphobia and the independent effect of virtual reality exposure therapy. *The Australian and New Zealand Journal of Psychiatry*, *47*(2), 160–168. doi:10.1177/0004867412453626 PMID:22790176

McLay, R. N., McBrien, C., Wiederhold, M. D., & Wiederhold, B. K. (2010). Exposure Therapy with and without Virtual Reality to Treat PTSD while in the Combat Theater: A Parallel Case Series. *Cyberpsychology, Behavior, and Social Networking*, *13*(1), 37–42. doi:10.1089/cyber.2009.0346 PMID:20528291

Meyerbroeker, K., Morina, N., Kerkhof, G., & Emmelkamp, P. (2013). Virtual Reality Exposure Therapy Does Not Provide Any Additional Value in Agoraphobic Patients: A Randomized Controlled Trial. *Psychotherapy and Psychosomatics*, *82*(3), 170–176. doi:10.1159/000342715 PMID:23548832

Michaliszyn, D., Marchand, A., Bouchard, S., Martel, M.-O., & Poirier-Bisson, J. (2010). A Randomized, Controlled Clinical Trial of In Virtuo and In Vivo Exposure for Spider Phobia. *Cyberpsychology, Behavior, and Social Networking*, *13*(6), 689–695. doi:10.1089/cyber.2009.0277 PMID:21142994

Migoya-Borja, M., Delgado-Gómez, D., Carmona-Camacho, R., Porras-Segovia, A., López-Moriñigo, J.-D., Sánchez-Alonso, M., Albarracín García, L., Guerra, N., Barrigón, M. L., Alegría, M., & Baca-García, E. (2020). Feasibility of a Virtual Reality-Based Psychoeducational Tool (VRight) for Depressive Patients. *Cyberpsychology, Behavior, and Social Networking, 23*(4), 246–252. doi:10.1089/cyber.2019.0497 PMID:32207997

Monteiro-Junior, R. S., Figueiredo, L. F., Maciel-Pinheiro, P., Abud, E. L., Engedal, K., Barca, M. L., Nascimento, O. J. M., Laks, J., & Deslandes, A. C. (2017). Virtual reality–based physical exercise with exergames (PhysEx) improves mental and physical health of institutionalized older adults. *Journal of the American Medical Directors Association, 18*(5), 454–e1. doi:10.1016/j.jamda.2017.01.001 PMID:28238675

Nader, M., & Kruszewski, M. (2013). Wykorzystanie zaawansowanych symulatorów jazdy w badaniach zachowania i umiejętności kierowców. *Prace naukowe Politechniki Warszawskiej*, 321-331.

Nochaiwong, S., Ruengorn, C., Thavorn, K., Hutton, B., Awiphan, R., Phosuya, C., Ruanta, Y., Wongpakaran, N., & Wongpakaran, T. (2021). Global prevalence of mental health issues among the general population during the coronavirus disease-2019 pandemic: A systematic review and meta-analysis. *Scientific Reports, 11*(1), 10173. doi:10.103841598-021-89700-8 PMID:33986414

Norr, A. M., Smolenski, D. J., Katz, A. C., Rizzo, A. A., Rothbaum, B. O., Difede, J., ... Regera, G. M. (2018). Virtual Reality Exposure vs. Prolonged Exposure for PTSD: Which Treatment for Whom? *Depression and Anxiety, 35*(6), 523–529. doi:10.1002/da.22751 PMID:29734488

O'Brolcháin, F., Jacquemard, T., Monaghan, D., O'Connor, N., Novitzky, P., & Gordijn, B. (2016). The Convergence of Virtual Reality and Social Networks: Threats to Privacy and Autonomy. *Science and Engineering Ethics, 22*(1), 1–29. doi:10.100711948-014-9621-1 PMID:25552240

Parsons, T. D. (2021). Ethical challenges of using virtual environments in the assessment and treatments of psychopathological disorders. *Journal of Clinical Medicine, 10*(3), 378. doi:10.3390/jcm10030378 PMID:33498255

Paul, M., Bullock, K., & Bailenson, J. (2020). Virtual Reality Behavioral Activation as an Intervention for Major Depressive Disorder: Case Report. *JMIR Mental Health, 7*(11), e24331. doi:10.2196/24331 PMID:33031046

Pelissolo, A., Zaoui, M., Aguayo, G., Yao, S. N., Roche, S., & Ecochard, R. (2012). Virtual reality exposure therapy versus cognitive behavior therapy for panic disorder with agoraphobia: A randomized comparison study. *Journal of Cyber Therapy and Rehabilitation, 5*(1), 35–43.

Proniewska, K., Pregowska, A., Dolega-Dlegowski, D., & Dudek, D. (2021). Immersive technologies as a solution for general data protection regulation in Europe and impact on the COVID-19 pandemic. *Cardiology Journal, 28*(1), 23–33. doi:10.5603/CJ.a2020.0102 PMID:32789838

Qian, J., McDonough, D. J., & Gao, Z. (2020). The Effectiveness of Virtual Reality Exercise on Individual's Physiological, Psychological and Rehabilitative Outcomes: A Systematic Review. *International Journal of Environmental Research and Public Health, 17*(11), 4133. doi:10.3390/ijerph17114133 PMID:32531906

Reger, G. M., Holloway, K. M., Candy, C., Rothbaum, B. O., Difede, J., Rizzo, A. A., & Gahm, G. A. (2011). Effectiveness of Virtual Reality Exposure Therapy for Active Duty Soldiers in a Military Mental Health Clinic. *Journal of Traumatic Stress*, *24*(1), 93–96. doi:10.1002/jts.20574 PMID:21294166

Reger, G. M., Koenen-Woods, P., Zetocha, K., Smolenski, D. J., Holloway, K. M., Rothbaum, B. O., Difede, J. A., Rizzo, A. A., Edwards-Stewart, A., Skopp, N. A., Mishkind, M., Reger, M. A., & Gahm, G. A. (2016). Randomized Controlled Trial of Prolonged Exposure Using Imaginal Exposure vs. Virtual Reality Exposure in Active Duty Soldiers With Deployment-Related Posttraumatic Stress Disorder (PTSD). *Journal of Consulting and Clinical Psychology*, *84*(11), 946–959. doi:10.1037/ccp0000134 PMID:27606699

Reger, G. M., Smolenski, D., Norr, A., Katz, A., Buck, B., & Rothbaum, B. O. (2019). Does Virtual Reality Increase Emotional Engagement During Exposure for PTSD? Subjective Distress During Prolonged and Virtual Reality Exposure Therapy. *Journal of Anxiety Disorders*, *61*, 75–81. doi:10.1016/j.janxdis.2018.06.001 PMID:29935999

Reinhard, R., Rutrecht, H. M., Hengstenberg, P., Tutulmaz, E., Geissler, B., Hecht, H., & Muttray, A. (2017). The best way to assess visually induced motion sickness in a fixed-base driving simulator. *Transportation Research Part F: Traffic Psychology and Behaviour*, *48*, 74–88. doi:10.1016/j.trf.2017.05.005

Riches, S., Elghany, S., Garety, P., Rus-Calafell, M., & Valmaggia, L. (2019). Factors Affecting Sense of Presence in a Virtual Reality Social Environment: A Qualitative Study. *Cyberpsychology, Behavior, and Social Networking*, *22*(4), 288–292. doi:10.1089/cyber.2018.0128 PMID:30802148

Rizzo, A., Schultheis, M. T., & Rothbaum, B. O. (2002). Ethical issues for the use of virtual reality in the psychological sciences. In Ethical issues in clinical neuropsychology (pp. 243-280). Swets & Zeitlinge.

Rizzo, A. S., & Shilling, R. (2017). Clinical Virtual Reality tools to advance the prevention, assessment, and treatment of PTSD. *European Journal of Psychotraumatology*, *8*(sup5), 1414560. doi:10.1080/20008198.2017.1414560 PMID:29372007

Rothbaum, B., Hodges, L., Kooper, R., Opdyke, D., Williford, J., & North, M. (1995b). Effectiveness of computer-generated (virtual reality) graded exposure in the treatment of acrophobia. *The American Journal of Psychiatry*, *152*(4), 626–628. doi:10.1176/ajp.152.4.626 PMID:7694917

Salari, N., Hosseinian-Far, A., Jalali, R., Vaisi-Raygani, A., Rasoulpoor, S., Mohammadi, M., Rasoulpoor, S., & Khaledi-Paveh, B. (2020). Prevalence of stress, anxiety, depression among the general population during the COVID-19 pandemic: A systematic review and meta-analysis. *Globalization and Health*, *16*(57), 57. Advance online publication. doi:10.118612992-020-00589-w PMID:32631403

Selwyn, N. (2004). Reconsidering Political and Popular Understandings of the Digital Divide. *New Media & Society*, *6*(3), 341–362. doi:10.1177/1461444804042519

Siess, A., & Wölfel, M. (2018). User color temperature preferences in immersive virtual realities. *Computers & Graphics*, *81*, 20–31. doi:10.1016/j.cag.2019.03.018

Slater, M., Khanna, P., Mortensen, J., & Yu, I. (2009). Visual Realism Enhances Realistic Response in an Immersive Virtual Environment. *IEEE Computer Graphics and Applications*, *29*(3), 76–84. doi:10.1109/MCG.2009.55 PMID:19642617

Slater, M., & Wilbur, S. (1997). framework for immersive virtual environments (FIVE): Speculations on the role of presence in virtual environments. *Presence (Cambridge, Mass.), 6*(6), 603–616. doi:10.1162/pres.1997.6.6.603

Spiegel, J. S. (2018). The Ethics of Virtual Reality Technology: Social Hazards and Public Policy Recommendations. *Science and Engineering Ethics, 24*(5), 1537–1550. doi:10.100711948-017-9979-y PMID:28942536

Stanney, K. M., Kennedy, R. S., & Drexler, J. M. (1997). Cybersickness is Not Simulator Sickness. *Proceedings of the Human Factors and Ergonomics Society Annual Meeting, 41*(2), 1138–1142. doi:10.1177/107118139704100292

Szpak, A., Michalski, S. C., Saredakis, D., Chen, C. S., & Loetscher, T. (2019). Beyond feeling sick: The visual and cognitive aftereffects of virtual reality. *IEEE Access: Practical Innovations, Open Solutions, 7*, 130883–130892. doi:10.1109/ACCESS.2019.2940073

Tardif, N., Therrien, C.-É., & Bouchard, S. (2019). Re-Examining Psychological Mechanisms Underlying Virtual Reality-Based Exposure for Spider Phobia. *Cyberpsychology, Behavior, and Social Networking, 22*(1), 29–35. doi:10.1089/cyber.2017.0711 PMID:30256675

Triscari, M. T., Faraci, P., Catalisano, D., D'Angelo, V., & Urso, V. (2015). Effectiveness of cognitive behavioral therapy integrated with systematic desensitization, cognitive behavioral therapy combined with eye movement desensitization and reprocessing therapy, and cognitive behavioral therapy combined with virtual reality expo. *Neuropsychiatric Disease and Treatment, 11*, 2591–2598. doi:10.2147/NDT.S93401 PMID:26504391

Tsutsumi, M., Nogaki, H., Shimizu, Y., Stone, T. E., & Kobayashi, T. (2017, May). Individual reactions to viewing preferred video representations of the natural environment: A comparison of mental and physical reactions. *Japan Journal of Nursing Science, 14*(1), 3–12. doi:10.1111/jjns.12131 PMID:27160351

Tursi, M. F., Baes, C., Camacho, F. R., Tofoli, S. M., & Juruena, M. F. (2013). Effectiveness of psycho-education for depression: A systematic review. *The Australian and New Zealand Journal of Psychiatry, 47*(11), 1019–1031. doi:10.1177/0004867413491154 PMID:23739312

Vos, T., Lim, S. S., Abbafati, C., Abbas, K. M., Abbasi, M., Abbasifard, M., Abbasi-Kangevari, M., Abbastabar, H., Abd-Allah, F., Abdelalim, A., Abdollahi, M., Abdollahpour, I., Abolhassani, H., Aboyans, V., Abrams, E. M., Abreu, L. G., Abrigo, M. R. M., Abu-Raddad, L. J., Abushouk, A. I., ... Murray, C. J. (2020). Global burden of 369 diseases and injuries in 204 countries and territories, 1990–2019: A systematic analysis for the Global Burden of Disease Study 2019. *Lancet, 396*(10258), 1204–1222. doi:10.1016/S0140-6736(20)30925-9 PMID:33069326

Wechsler, T. F., Kümpers, F., & Mühlberger, A. (2019). Inferiority or Even Superiority of Virtual Reality Exposure Therapy in Phobias? A Systematic Review and Quantitative Meta-Analysis on Randomized Controlled Trials Specifically Comparing the Efficacy of Virtual Reality Exposure to Gold Standard in vivo Exp. *Frontiers in Psychology, 10*, 1758. Advance online publication. doi:10.3389/fpsyg.2019.01758 PMID:31551840

Weech, S., Kenny, S., & Barnett-Cowan, M. (2019). Presence and Cybersickness in Virtual Reality Are Negatively Related: A Review. *Frontiers in Psychology*, *10*, 158. Advance online publication. doi:10.3389/fpsyg.2019.00158 PMID:30778320

Wu, J., Sun, Y., Zhang, G., Zhou, Z., & Ren, Z. (2021). Virtual Reality-Assisted Cognitive Behavioral Therapy for Anxiety Disorders: A Systematic Review and Meta-Analysis. *Frontiers in Psychiatry*, *12*, 575094. doi:10.3389/fpsyt.2021.575094 PMID:34366904

Yee, N., & Bailenson, J. (2007). The proteus effect. The effect of transformed self-representation on behavior. *Human Communication Research*, *33*(3), 271–290. doi:10.1111/j.1468-2958.2007.00299.x

Yildirim, C. (2020). Don't make me sick: Investigating the incidence of cybersickness in commercial virtual reality headsets. *Virtual Reality (Waltham Cross)*, *24*(2), 231–239. doi:10.100710055-019-00401-0

Zeng, N., Pope, Z., Lee, J. E., & Gao, Z. (2018). Virtual Reality Exercise for Anxiety and Depression: A Preliminary Review of Current Research in an Emerging Field. *Journal of Clinical Medicine*, *7*(3), 42. doi:10.3390/jcm7030042 PMID:29510528

Chapter 12
Evidence–Based Immersive Technology Use in Cognitive Assessments and Cognition–Based Interventions

Aparna Sahu

https://orcid.org/0000-0002-7383-7675
Turiyan Psyneuronics Private Limited, India

Jagrika Bajaj
Touchkin eServices Private Limited, India

ABSTRACT

The merging of immersive technologies and cognition has been around for a while. However, it is only in the last decade or so that immersive technologies' contributions in the areas of cognitive assessments and interventions have gathered recognition. This chapter covers findings from published research in cognition-based assessments and interventions using the immersive technologies of virtual reality (VR) and augmented reality (AR). The role of immersive technologies in cognition is critically evaluated to inform all its stakeholders about its potential for use in the future.

LEARNING OBJECTIVES

1. Readers will briefly learn about the psychometric requirements for cognitive tests
2. Readers will be acquainted with the latest trends in the use of immersive technologies for cognition-based assessments and interventions
3. The chapter will facilitate a critical discussion for the adoption of immersive technologies for cognition based assessments and interventions

DOI: 10.4018/978-1-7998-8371-5.ch012

1. INTRODUCTION

… What if Sherlock Holmes of the famous BBC series 'Sherlock' had not used the mind palace technique to recall objects of a scene? That he did, earned him the added advantage of piecing the puzzle of the crime.

The mind palace, also known as the method of loci and was described in Roman rhetorical treatise (Cicero, 55BCE/2001), is a memory technique that involves a vivid imagination of a path with salient landmarks and adding the required objects that need to be recalled later. This technique sets itself apart from the others in that it involves a visual map that one can navigate on and imagine objects at specific points in the mind's eye. Probably the technique's reliance on visual stimuli and a graphic environment affords an advantage in recalling memories in detail. Moreover, with immersive technologies, facilitating the virtual environment as in the case of virtual reality or working within a real environment as in the case of augmented reality are now available choices for the user.

The chapter covers a brief overview of the process in which cognitive tests are created, and current advancements, and feasibility in adapting traditional cognitive tests and interventions with immersive technologies.

2. COGNITIVE ASSESSMENTS

Eminent researchers and academics from the fields of cognitive psychology, neuroscience, experimental psychology, and philosophy were asked for their understanding of cognition in the scheme of their training and speciality and their evolved understanding (Bayne et al., 2019). They had different perspectives; nevertheless, a more refined understanding of cognition emerged when their viewpoints were put together. Cognition represents the scientific basis of behaviour and is driven by neural processes which are shaped by environmental variables. As it now stands, it continues to be understood as a broad term for processes of attention, learning, memory, perception, decision-making, language, categorisation, and mental and motor control.

Cognitive testing encompasses assessments for attention (sustaining concentration over a period of time, or being able to attend to information in the midst of noise or distractors), executive functioning (problem-solving skills, ability to inhibit a response), short term memory or working memory (the ability to hold on to information for a short period of time, and/or manipulate it), long term memory (memory about/ for events in one's life, recalling meaning of words, or definitions of concepts), prospective memory (remembering an intention which needs to be carried out in the future), visuospatial abilities (the ability to navigate in space, find locations), and language (ability to express and comprehend in one's language of choice).

2.1 Psychometric Rigour for Tests

Cognitive testing, like many other assessments in a scientific discipline, needs to undergo rigorous psychometric evaluation before they are released for use. In their recent review, Jin, Pilozzi, and Huang (2020) summarise some pivotal requirements for cognitive testing. These include measures for sensitivity and specificity to differentiate performances between patient and healthy controls, items and their progressive levels of difficulty and performances which are independent of someone administering the

test. Additionally, psychometric properties of standardisation, reliability, and validity are required to be established for assessments. A short overview of these is presented here.
To Note…

- Cognitive testing and neuropsychological testing may be used interchangeably or together as a single expression;
- Neuropsychological assessment in its pure sense incorporates assessment of cognition (hence, *neuro*) as well as behaviours, mood, personality (hence, *psyche*)

At the outset, tests need to be standardised. Standardisation involves a) consistency in following test procedures of administration across participants, scoring of responses, and interpretation of the scores, and b) creation of benchmarks which involves norms or normative data from a group of individuals who form the standard against which one's performance can be compared (Urbina, 2014).

Measurement based instruments in psychology account for the actual performance (or score) accompanied with some error. In keeping with this, tests keep room for variation in test performance. The concept of reliability emanates from such testing events. Reliability refers to consistency in one's performance, i.e., if one were to take the same test at different times or different locations or attempt a test with equivalent items, the score would be more or less the same (Anastasi, 1976). Indeed, it is likely that one would not obtain the same score throughout; hence some room for variation is permitted. Reasons for not obtaining similar scores at different testing times may not necessarily be due to the test characteristic but might be related to the test taker; these could include lack of motivation, fatigue, and noises in the environment during testing. There are several types of reliability that one can test for, depending on the nature of the test. Some of them which have been referred to in the context of immersive technologies are test-rest and internal consistency reliability. Test-retest reliability refers to a test being administered on two different occasions separated by time on the same individual to check how much inconsistency there is in the two performances due to time (Urbina, 2014). Internal consistency reliability refers to the extent to which items in a test consistently measure the same construct. In other words, when a particular test is administered, the responses to the test items are consistent with each other (Anastasi, 1976).

Validity, on the other hand, broadly deals with how well a test measures what it is meant to measure (Anastasi, 1976; Strauss, Shermann, & Spreen, 2006). There are various types of validity which deal with specific aspects of the test. Construct validity is the extent to which a test measures the construct (psychological /cognitive concept, trait, entity). For example, a memory test would successfully and predominantly measure memory; however, it would not measure visuo-spatial abilities significantly. Convergent validity is considered to be a type of construct validity in that it checks if a test performance is related to the performance of other tests' that measure a similar concept. Divergent validity of a test, on the other hand, would show no association with another test. For instance, the association between memory and a visuo-spatial test would be non-significant, confirming that no items are overlapping between the two constructs. Tests also measure for ecological validity, which refers to how closely the test measurement and the result reflects real-life performance (Chaytor & Schmitter-Edgecombe, 2003; Wasserman & Bracken, 2003).

3. COGNITIVE ASSESSMENTS USING IMMERSIVE TECHNOLOGIES

Cognitive assessments had primarily emerged from the clinical world in order to assess cognitive deficits in neurological and psychiatric patients. They can be dated to as far back as the 19th century, which involved clinicians making a scientific inquiry about why patients presented with specific deficits. These inquiries eventually resulted in the creation of diagnostic tests to assess levels of cognitive deficits (e.g., Eling, 2019). Paper-pencil and smart device-based testing (laptops and tablets) are the two modalities of cognitive testing that have dominated the scene. However, since the late '90s, VR was being experimented with, with a primary goal to improve precision in testing (Rizzo, 1998) and eventually to improve its ecological validity (Parsons, Carlew, Magtoto, & Stonecipher, 2015). Indeed, several studies using immersive technologies have fulfilled these requirements for some cognitive functions, namely attention, executive function, and memory and psychometric characteristics based on studies performed on both healthy controls and patients presenting with different neurological conditions.

3.1 Attention

Attention is the ability to maintain a steady level of concentration on a particular task that could be continuous or repetitive in nature. For instance, the continuous performance test (CPT) is a test of sustained attention, wherein the participant views a series of stimuli (letters or numbers or symbols) which are presented continuously at a particular pace for a set period of time; participants are instructed to respond only to a particular target stimulus while avoiding the other distractor stimuli (Rosvold, Mirsky, Sarason, Bransome, & Beck, 1956). As seen in figure 1, a series of numbers are shown on the screen, one per second, and the target number is 6, at which the participant needs to react (by pressing a key on the keyboard).

In the VR setup, Climent et al. (2021), collected normative data and conducted reliability testing for their VR task called Nesplora Aquarium. The task is similar to the CPT, which involves watching an aquarium in the VR setting, and the participant needs to press a button when they see the target (a fish type) or hear the name of the target (fish name). Norms are based on a large sample across age and sex groups for several parameters such as correct scores, omission errors (missing out on the target stimulus), commissions errors (false alarms), reaction time for correct responses and commissions, errors based on the sensory modality (visual and auditory), and even motor activity as measured by head movements to check for potential motor hyperactivity.

The advantage of running a CPT in VR enables the researcher/ clinician to obtain many more metrics that could be considered for diagnosis and/or studying attention ability from a research perspective. Furthermore, a classic CPT is considered to be boring (E.g., Raz, Bar-Haim, Sadeh, & Dan, 2014), which could additionally affect one's performance. However, the same task, when presented in a VR environment as done by Climent et al., could control boredom and measure sustained attention in a more realistic manner.

Figure 1.

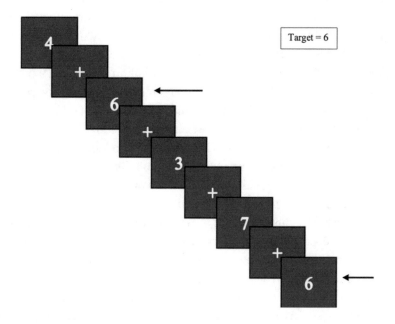

3.2 Executive Function

Executive function is a unique ability that defines an individual's existence. It predominantly includes motivation, planning, purposive acts, decision making, and effective performance (Lezak, Howieson, Bigler, & Tranel, 2012). Consider a real-life instance; one plans to prepare a meal for their friends who are to visit that evening. Given there are no ingredients at home, it is then likely that one would prepare a list of things to buy, visit the grocery store, purchase the required items from the store, i.e., go directly to the shelves with those items and not get distracted by the other fascinating products, choose items among the many available brands of the same ingredient, complete the purchase by paying the cashier, head back home in time and not socialise with a friend who one runs into at the store so as to prepare the meal prior to the meet-up. This instance covers several aspects of executive function. These include one's motivation to socialise with guests; the intention to prepare a meal, realising that ingredients are out of stock and hence heading to pick them from the grocery store, also keeping in mind the time factor of reaching back in time to finish all preparation before the friends arrive, one's planning ability, decision making, and awareness are at play.

Figure 2.

YELLOW   GREEN   BLUE   **YELLOW**   GREEN   RED   **BLUE**   RED

There are several cognitive tests that allow for testing these abilities. For instance, the famous Stroop task measures a host of cognitive abilities such as selective attention, inhibiting responses, and managing response conflict (Stroop, 1935). The Stroop task uses stimuli in a way that can be in conflict with each other. As seen in figure 2, the colour-word inconsistency measures response inhibition, which is part of executive functions. Here, the participant is supposed to inhibit saying the word and respond to the colour in which the word is written. The written word and it's colour, if not congruent with each other, will most likely create dissonance and will reflect in the form of errors and increased response times.

On the VR front, some fantastic variations have been brought about to the classic Stroop task. This is backed by a strong rationale to program it in VR to make it more ecologically valid. While Stroop is one such task which successfully measures response inhibition, its representation in real life is far more complex than was thought to be. In the real world, there are many more distractors in the environment which are taken into account when we are indulging in some cognitive task. In this regard, then, the virtual apartment Stroop task (Parsons & Barnett, 2018), which is adapted from the original Stroop task but also makes room for incorporating distractors, which is more representative of the real-world. The scene involves an apartment with a window, furniture pieces, a television – flat screen, which shows words in different colours. A female voice calls out the colour names (auditory stimulus). If the auditory colour name matched the colour of the word, the participant is supposed to click the mouse or else refrain from making a response. Given the virtual environment of an apartment, distractors were in the form of sounds from outside the window, or a virtual being walking around the apartment, a phone kept on the table, ringing, to name a few.

This task attained convergent validity based on its comparison with the paper-pencil and computerised versions (correlation coefficients of 0.22 and 0.29, respectively), and divergent validity with a memory test. The distinguishing aspect of this test, though are several; in addition to recording accuracies, errors, and reaction times, with the additional component of distractors during the test, one also obtains metrics for how performances differ with and without distractors. As an extension of this work, Parsons and Barnett (2018) have tested for age effects on VR based Stroop task and found older adults performed more poorly than the younger adults, more so during the distractor presentation.

The Multiple Errands test is another classic test that measures executive function (MET: Shallice & Burgess, 1991), which involves a real-world assessment of planning and hence possesses high ecological validity. There are a series of instructions that need to be followed specific to time and place, in keeping with the rules of the test. For instance, the participant is taken to a mall and is asked to purchase specific items within 15 minutes while also following rules such as not entering the same shop more than once and spending as little as possible. In a preliminary study, the Virtual MET has been validated with healthy controls and stroke patients to show that the task is correlated with other experimental paradigms that measure executive function (Raspelli et al., 2011). Another VR version of the MET was tested on patients with acquired brain injury and healthy matched controls, which found a clear distinction in the performance, further demonstrating the use of such tasks on patients with brain injury, and its ability to detect subtle deficits in executive function which went undetected on other paper-pencil based tasks (Jansari et al., 2014).

In another study that could have practical relevance, Giglioli, Vidal, and Raya (2019) compared the performance of VR and AR on a cooking task with the underlying cognitive construct of executive functioning. The idea is to complete the cooking tasks in a particular time frame by avoiding burning (i.e., the item was on fire for more time than it should be), or cooling the item (by switching off the stove or removing the food from the hot pan). Furthermore, this task had challenges, in that, the simplest level the participant had to cook three foods in 2 minutes in one cooker, and the most challenging level required cooking of 5 foods in two cookers in 5 minutes as well as setting the table. Once the foods were cooked, they had to be transferred into a dish, and the stove also had to be switched off. Total time for cooking the foods and performance parameters of burning and cooling times were recorded. In comparison to VR, AR based cooking task took more time, and participants reported a greater sense of presence in the VR task than in the AR, despite the latter.

Highlights of using VR for cognitive assessments

- High ecological validity ~ testing environment is similar to real-life settings
- Greater opportunity for standardisation
- Multi-sensory modalities capture responses and reactions in real-time
- Acquired data is rich and, if analysed from an analytics perspective, can help in creating strong models for predicting the course of the condition or potential of a person meeting the criteria for a degenerative condition

3.3 Memory

Memory is the ability to remember by means of rehearsing the information which comes through sensory modalities, storing it, and retrieving it at a later point (Crowder, 1976) which can have personal relevance (Tulving & Craik, 2000). In typical memory paradigms, two processes are assessed, a) recall – wherein the participant brings back from memory the stored information, and, b) recognition – wherein the participant identifies the piece of information out of a set of information presented to them (Sternberg, 1967, 1969). For instance, in a laboratory set-up, you are presented with a list of 20 words to be read out one at a time and asked to recall the words in any order after the presentation, which is also referred to as immediate recall; this represents one trial. Some paradigms incorporate one or several trials to facilitate the learning of this set of information. The participant is tested for delayed recall of this information; as the word suggests, the delay from the last presentation of the list of words to recalling the information at a later point (could be 15 minutes or 30 minutes or even after a day), tests for recall as a function of time. In the same paradigm, a recognition trial would present a set of words, ones which were presented during the encoding phase, and new words, and the participant is required to identify only the presented ones.

Memory processes can also be classified into retrospective and prospective. In the former, one recalls information from the past, e.g., recalling the name of the president of the country you are a citizen of; recalling what you had for breakfast the previous day; recalling a personal event from your life which had a strong impact on you. Prospective memory, on the other hand, requires one to remember intentions in the future, e.g., remembering a doctor's appointment after two days; remembering to give a message to your colleague when they get into the office.

In the VR world, several studies have been performed to test its use for memory. The rationale for implementing this testing on VR is to meet the ecological validity criteria. In the real world, we use memory processing for multiple purposes, such as remembering (or even writing down) grocery lists, remembering people's names and faces, their professions, life story (if applicable), and recalling these pieces of information in social situations, for example. Remembering important events, dates, episodes of our lives add value to our existence. All these similar experiences and processes can be captured naturally in the VR world.

Ouellet et al. (2018) created and tested their memory paradigm called the virtual shop (La boutique virtuelle) to test individuals' memories for a list of items to be purchased from the shop. Participants navigated within the shop, and the interactivity was so immersive that they were able to lift objects, tap on objects, navigate through the alleys of the shop, and pass by other virtual people within the scene. Both young and older adults were able to perform the task optimally and were able to finish it in an average time of 15 minutes, which normally is the case for several such tests in the clinical or laboratory set-up. This further confirmed the feasibility of carrying out the test with older adults. In addition, Corriveau Lecavalier, Ouellet, Boller, and Belleville (2020) validated this VR task against traditional word recall memory tests for both age groups.

In another study, Kourtesis et al. (2020) validated their VR based cognitive battery of tests for attention, executive functioning, memory processes, viz., episodic and prospective memories. Furthermore, the VR environment in their study had a high ecological validity as it mimics events that would normally be part of someone's life. For instance, the scenes involved planning the errands (home, grocery store, library), completing morning kitchen chores of preparing breakfast, personal chores such as taking medications after breakfast, calling a friend at a particular time, recognising items to purchase at the grocery store, returning a book to the library, handing over keys to someone.

Spatial memory, or memory for locations in relation to objects in the environment, progressively decreases in older individuals who meet the criteria for dementia, an age-related condition that presents with cognitive decline. Ijaz, Ahmadpour, Naismith, and Calvo (2019), created a google map navigation-based scene with landmarks in a VR set up and administered the test of recall of landmarks and navigation paths to the landmarks. The same paradigm was also created on a 2D layout and administered on the computer. The study has shown good feasibility for older participants for the VR set up. More importantly, in their study, Ijas et al. reported that participants in the VR testing enjoyed the test compared to the group administered the 2D computerised test.

Teel, Gay, Johnson, and Slobounov (2016) created a spatial memory task on the VR for detecting deficits in post-concussion sports players and found the test to be highly sensitive and specific in differentiating between post-concussion adults and healthy controls.

In order to test for spatial memory for objects, Munoz-Montoya et al. (2018) created an AR app, which had two phases, a) The configuration phase, where the environment is scanned by the app, b) the object configuration phase where objects are placed in the augmented environment by the examiner. Their study had participants who were part of the AR group, acquaint themselves with the location of the objects in the environment and recall the locations of each object. For comparison, the noAR group also acquainted themselves with the environment through the app; however, they had to memorise the location of the objects on photographs. In comparison to the noAR group in the study, the AR group performed significantly better, probably because encoding of the information of the object in real-time environment may have facilitated a greater impression for later recall.

In terms of spatial memory testing, the use of immersive technologies provides the *spatial* aspect of this type of memory, which lacks in traditional testing.

To summarise, immersive technologies have demonstrated their merit in their utility for cognitive assessments, particularly in regards to testing for cognition in an almost real setup, and across age groups. In keeping with the needs, VR and AR have been adapted in ways that have allowed to measure different cognitive faculties.

4. COGNITION-BASED INTERVENTIONS USING IMMERSIVE TECHNOLOGIES

Different terms are used for cognition-based interventions and these include cognitive remediation, cognitive rehabilitation, cognitive retraining, and cognitive neurorehabilitation. Cognition-based interventions target cognitive processes of individuals that are compromised. These non-invasive interventions are created to improve the productivity of an individual that could positively impact their quality of life (e.g., Messinis, 2019; Shah, 2017).

Cognitive impairment is an outcome following damage to or degeneration in the brain, whereas cognitive decline is an outcome of ageing. Consequently, both types of deterioration can show compromise or sub-optimal abilities and skills in one's daily life. Such brain damage can have several psychological and cognitive consequences on an individual's life. For instance, after sustaining a stroke, the patient may report severe memory issues, such as forgetting where they kept their keys, forgetting to lock their house before leaving, unable to pay attention for a longer period of time. Cognitive deficits may reduce socialising and interacting with family and friends, travelling, being less engaged in daily chores (e.g., Lara et al., 2019), and may also reduce their involvement in important decision-making processes such as financial decisions (e.g., Darby & Dickerson, 2017). Therefore, individuals who have their physical abilities restored continue to experience cognitive deficits, which are left unaddressed (e.g., Kapoor, Lanctôt, Bayley, Kiss, Herrmann, Murray, & Swartz, 2017). Even among the elderly, cognitive decline can take place and can manifest in terms of forgetfulness (e.g., forgetting to consume medications), and inattentiveness, which although may not be frequent, can have negative consequences and compromise the overall quality of life (Hill et al., 2017).

So far, cognitive interventions similar to assessments have been administered in the paper-pencil and computerised modes. For a number of years and even now, these interventions have been adapted using immersive technologies. The following section covers the use of immersive technologies in cognition-based interventions in neurological conditions of brain injury, dementia, and stroke and in elderly individuals who do not present with any neurological condition.

4.1 Stroke

Stroke is a neurological condition characterised by a lack of blood circulation in the brain following a bleed in the cerebral blood vessels. Cognitive deficits are reported following stroke, and the prevalence rate can range between 28-92% (van Rijsbergen, Mark, de Kort, & Sitskoorn, 2014; Nakling, et al., 2017), with predominant complaints in the areas of memory and attention (Evans, et al., 2019). Activities of daily living (ADLs) include daily routines that are also impacted. These include activities such as brushing teeth, ablutions, eating, getting dressed, et cetera. A point to note, although ADLs come across as non-cognitive, they do depend on cognition. For instance, wearing clothes requires one to find the clothes (involves memory), check if the cloth is clean or needs laundry (decision making/ executive function), and wear it in an upright manner (involves visuo-spatial/ perceptual ability). Following a stroke, ADLs are compromised to the extent that external help is required for some time.

The first few months following a stroke are deemed crucial for implementing the cognitive intervention (Cho & Lee, 2019; Coleman et al., 2017). Several studies have demonstrated the positive effects of VR based cognitive interventions for stroke patients. Cho and Lee (2019) compared VR based cognitive training with computerised training for stroke patients and found the former to have significantly higher scores on memory than the latter. Gamito et al. (2015) found a similar effect, with VR based cognitive intervention showing increased improvement in memory and attention compared to patients who did not receive any intervention (wait-list group). Their VR module included daily life activities such as grocery shopping, navigating to the market, finding a virtual person wearing specific clothing, and calculation, which covered cognitive functions of working memory, visuo-spatial ability, attention, and short term memory, respectively. In terms of ADLs, these activities need to be performed recurrently, a form of practice that is required for the activity to become a regular part of one's life. In this sense, then, VR based training help in achieving this goal; with auditory and visual prompts within the VR environment, studies have demonstrated its usefulness for stroke patients (Cho & Lee, 2019).

4.2 Traumatic Brain Injury

Traumatic brain injury or TBI is any change in brain functioning caused due to pathology from an external force or trauma to the head such as being struck by an object or forces produced during a blast or an explosion, or the head striking an object (e.g., during sporting activities), or an object penetrating through the skull and into the brain (e.g., bullets), (Menon, Schwab, Wright, & Maas, 2010). Cognitive impairments following TBI are well documented. Studies have shown that following TBI; some patients had an overall compromise in-memory processing and global cognition which includes other cognitive faculties of attention, executive function, short and long term memories, and visuo-spatial abilities (e.g., de Freitas Cardoso et al., 2019; Azouvi, Arnould, Dromer, & Vallat- Azouvi, 2017).

VR based interventions have been used for some time now to rehabilitate TBI patients. In a recent study, Ettenhofer et al. (2019) enforced a driving simulator task where TBI patients practised their driving skills which had an inbuilt component for cognitive abilities along with guidance and feedback from the clinician and an in-built automated system. For instance, the participant was expected to steer around unfilled potholes only and brake for forward vehicles; this taps into executive functioning and may be analogous to the Stroop task. Their study showed that TBI patients who underwent this intervention had significant improvements in their working memory capacity and selective attention. Another study that used a different VR paradigm shared similar results with improvements in executive functioning and attention (De Luca et al., 2019).

4.3 Mild Cognitive Impairment and Neurocognitive Disorders

Mild cognitive impairment (MCI) occurs in the elderly group and is characterised by a cognitive decline to a greater extent in comparison to the individual's age and education level. However, this decline does not necessarily interfere with one's daily life (Gauthier et al., 2006). MCI can progress into neurocognitive disorders (NCDs, formerly known as dementia), a clinical condition characterised by global impairment in cognition and functional abilities that could be accompanied by behavioural and psychological problems (Gustafson, 1996; NICE, 2007).

As in other conditions, researchers have attempted using VR based interventions on MCI patients to check for its effects on overall cognition. Torpil, Sahin, Pekçetin and Uyanik (2021) demonstrated that VR based intervention games improved the MCI patients' attention, visuo-spatial perceptual abilities, and orientation. In another set of studies, an improvement in executive functioning (Liao et al., 2020; Wall et al., 2018), ADLs, and global cognition, verbal memory (Liao et al., 2020), and visuo-spatial memory (Park et al., 2019) were observed following VR based intervention for the MCI group.

In terms of NCDs, a recent study by Oliviera et al. (2021) showed a significant change in global cognition among NCD patients who underwent VR based cognitive intervention. Many more studies are required to check for the usability of VR based training for the NCD group. Lecouvey et al. (2019), conducted a VR trial on mild Alzheimer's disease patients, using the concept of a virtual town, and driving through the environment by means of a steering wheel and pedal gears, representing a car. Two scenes were involved, with the first scene used for familiarising patients with the VR environment and navigating through it using the driving gear, and the second scene was of interest to test for prospective memory. In all, seven intentions were to be recalled, and patients showed impairment in their recalls compared to healthy controls. According to the authors, this task was sensitive to pick up such memory deficits and could be used on patients.

Why cognition-based interventions work in the VR setup?

- Enriching and ecologically valid environment
- Generalising effects from the VR set up to real life; positive effects are seen in the real world
- Following damage to the brain, motivation, interest can be at its lowest level; immersive technology-based interventions show promise for its positive effects
- Making games enjoyable is key to motivating patients; additionally, challenging oneself allows for greater growth

4.4 Older Individuals

Given that the older population is vulnerable to cognitive decline, several attempts are being made to enforce cognitive training to them. Several recent studies have already been attempted on the older population using exergames or games which involve a motor/exercise component. For instance, Arleti et al. (2020) created the SocialBike VR exergame for older people, which targets both the motor and cognitive components, a dual task. Herein, the participant is cycling on a stationary bike (motor component). The VR scene involves navigating on a path, and the cognitive task involves specific instructions on pressing the button if they see an animal whose name begins with a specific letter on the side of the pathway (cognitive component). The authors have further added a social component wherein the participant can either compete with other players or play as part of a group, which is competing with another group. This home-based task has been studied for feasibility, and preliminary data suggests that the task has high usability characteristic (Pedroli et al., 2018).

In an exergame setup, Huang (2020) had their participants above the age of 50 years play fruit Ninja based on actions using gestures and arm movements in an immersive or non-immersive environment. Their performances on executive function were measured at baseline, after the first session, and after four weeks of the exergame session. There were significant differences in performances after the intervention on executive functioning for the immersive condition only.

In another study, Gamito et al. (2020) assessed the usefulness of an exergame which involved ADL based activities while also indulging in daily life routines, which have a cognitive component. The game had increasing levels of difficulty based on the type of task, e.g., complete a daily hygiene task to purchasing items from and calculating the amount to be paid at the grocery store. Tasks also had cognitive components embedded within, e.g., remembering a list of items to buy (~ verbal memory), selecting ingredients for a cake at the store (~ selective attention). Interestingly, the study found significant improvements in executive functioning, global cognition, and attention in participants who were part of the VR group, as compared to the controls who were part of traditional retraining methods.

An exhaustive review by Corregidor-Sanchez et al. (2020) showed promising results for the use of VR based cognitive training in non-disabled older people for their ADLs. However, further research and clinical trials are required.

In summary, using VR predominantly for cognition-based interventions are showing promise. Undoubtedly, many more studies are required to establish its absolute utility for cognitive interventions, because the positive effects are seen globally rather than specifically for all cognitive faculties (e.g., Maggio et al., 2019).

5. FEASIBILITY OF USING IMMERSIVE TECHNOLOGY-BASED ASSESSMENTS AND INTERVENTIONS

The need for immersive technologies and its use in the clinical sphere is driven by the *elegant simplicity* criterion, which means that the objectivity of testing needs to be clear at the outset (Rizzo, 1998). If this point were to have been raised in the '90s, probably the need for using immersive technologies would not have arisen as immensely. However, we are in an era of continued technological development. Cognitive assessments and interventions have indeed come a long way. In the initial times, cognitive testing used paper-pencil versions, and eventually, the tests and modules were adapted for computer use, followed by a migration of these testing tools to smart devices such as tablets and smartphones. Indeed, the use of immersive technologies can facilitate scientific rigour for fields of cognitive psychology and neuropsychology (Parsons & Duffield, 2020).

Immersive technologies offer advantages in that they facilitate heightened improvement in psychometric rigour. VR based testing ensures high standards for controlling the testing environment by keeping the virtual environment consistent, allows for the greater ecological validity of the test due to its ability to re-create a real environment, and furthermore, control conditions that could otherwise vary, for instance, navigation-based assessments/retraining (Roberts et al. 2019). The aforementioned sections have addressed the utility of immersive technologies based on studies that were conducted on healthy controls and patients with different neurological conditions. Psychometric properties have been established, and studies demonstrate that immersive technology use is feasible.

Studies take into consideration several factors of such technology use and predominantly follow a stringent protocol in creating cognitive tools. For instance, Oliviera et al. (2016), created the ECO-VR with increased planning for the task that would be feasible for cognitive testing of older adults. They carefully chose items/stimuli and created a virtual environment by taking expert opinions, ran multiple pilot studies to check for acceptability of instructions and task requirements for assessing cognition, administration time and practicality, standardised the instructions, and examine the scoring of responses. After several iterations, ECO-VR showed evidence for validity and was deemed feasible for older adults.

Peleg-Adler, Lanir, and Korman (2018) checked for the feasibility of using an AR application for route planning among older and younger adults. This ecologically valid task required participants to plan their bus trip from source to destination, either by means of a direct route or a combined route that required a change of transportation lines. Participants had to explore which route would be the shortest and quickest by using the information from the AR application or the non-AR application. The AR application simply required the participant to raise the smartphone to the map (the specific station name), and a display with bus times would show up. By comparison, the non-AR application had many more steps that required choosing the route, choosing the station name from the list of stations, and then the bus schedule for that station. This study had some interesting findings and observations which can be of great use to future AR app creators and researchers. Older participants found the app user friendly and useful as all information is presented together. Furthermore, performance between the older and younger adults was more or less the same, although, in terms of speed, older adults took more time; however, this was true for both the AR and non-AR interfaces. Older participants also were more likely to move the device frequently to perhaps get accustomed to the AR interface. Finally, the AR task took on an intuitive mode of performance wherein participants were quick to adapt to it, whereas the non-AR app had a learning curve, and this was true for both groups.

In another study, Chung, Pagnini, and Langer (2016) had two groups of participants in the AR and a screen-based navigation system. During the learning phase, participants had to tour a site using these systems, and learn the paths that led from one landmark to another, with occasional prompts on the availability of shorter paths. During the test phase, participants were asked to get from one point to another in the shortest way possible. It was hypothesised that AR-based learning would have created some form of engagement in the learning of the routes, which would have facilitated those participants to choose the shortest path. And that was indeed the case, in addition to the AR group committing fewer errors and took less time than in the non-AR group. Zhang and Robb (2020) used AR for a working memory retraining task. The N back is considered a type of continuous performance task where a series of stimuli are presented, and the participant is supposed to indicate if the currently presented stimulus was presented *n* steps earlier (where n = 1 or 2 or 3) (Kirchner, 1958). They compared it with the traditional N back training and found the former showing better outcomes on WM than the latter. More importantly, they had participants reporting that the AR was more engaging.

Immersive technologies have brought cognitive psychology and neuropsychology to a highly scientific level because of the amount of control one can exercise in carrying out assessments and treatments for neurological patients (Rizzo, Gambino, Sardo, & Rizzo, 2020). Furthermore, immersive technologies possess the quality of enticing the user. It is believed that immersive technology-based cognitive assessments and interventions have brought about a fun element, which makes the process enjoyable and hence, ensuring greater consent, and hence is better received by individuals (e.g., Abdul et al., 2019). To this end, participants have reported VR/AR-based experiences to be joyous, fun, pleasant (e.g., Salisbury et al., 2016). Indeed, when participants are involved with the technology, chances are the technology is accepted and hence is likely to work positively for participants (Bauer & Andriga, 2020).

6. CRITICAL EVALUATION OF USING IMMERSIVE TECHNOLOGY-BASED ASSESSMENTS AND INTERVENTIONS

Several systematic reviews and meta-analytic studies have demonstrated the psychological and cognitive benefits of VR, with participants reporting greater utility, enjoyability, and benefits of the technology (e.g., Abdul et al., 2019; Moreno et al. 2019) and in differentiating performances between the cognitively impaired and the healthy controls (e.g., Negut, Matu, Sava, & David 2016). While the union between immersive technologies and cognition is assuring in terms of its usability for neurological patients and healthy individuals, there have been accounts of negative effects, resistance, as well as lack of acceptance for such technologies in the realm of behavioural sciences. Some factors are acknowledged in the following points.

1. Negative effects of using immersive technologies: Several past studies have reported incidences of simulator sickness, which is similar to motion sickness that typically occurs during a VR experience (Duzmasnka, Strojny, & Strojny, 2018). Consequently, participants are averse to the idea of continuing with VR based assessments or interventions. Studies on VR use have reported dropouts due to simulator sickness (e.g., Ettenhofer et al., 2019) or have reported complaints of physical problems such as headache, fatigue, eye strain, and blurred vision (e.g., Salisbury et al., 2016). Hence, a greater onus rests on the clinician/researcher to figure how their patients/participants are faring during such tasks. Salisbury et al. (2016) strongly recommend strong communication between participants and the clinician/researchers about the task and provide adequate demonstrations to assure them about the technology. Additionally, the manner in which the test is conducted would also predict participation compliance. Time duration of immersive technology-based assessments and interventions is a crucial aspect. Hence, providing additional breaks between two tests or trials can help reduce the incidence of simulator sickness and increase participation (e.g., Roberts et al., 2019). Several studies have also confirmed that keeping the test/intervention up to a short period of time (up to 15 minutes) is received positively by participants, especially in the elderly group (e.g., Bauer & Andriga, 2019).

Clinicians also need to decide on who can avail of immersive technology-based assessments and interventions. Fragile patients are less likely to receive such technologies positively due to their co-morbidities (Lecouvey et al., 2019). In such cases, reverting to traditional or mobile devices for assessments/interventions would be feasible.

2. Challenging infrastructure: Schiza et al. (2019) address the potential issue of slow acceptance of immersive technologies. While in the past, hardware requirements were tough to fulfil, in current times, software requirements are not necessarily easy to work with. A vital requirement in the software infrastructure is the need for flexibility in it, that would allow clinicians to customise the virtual environment. Unquestionably, the progress in this technology has been vast, and hence today, one can avail of many other integrations such as motion sensors, haptics, and feedback loops.

3. Cost and benefits: Salisbury et al. (2016) raised a pertinent requirement for the acceptance of new technology in the healthcare sector. Is the new technology cost-efficient? Is it affordable? The costs that come with immersive technologies can be quite high. Hardware and software costs can be unaffordable for some emerging economies, making these technologies difficult to implement (e.g., Salisbury et al., 2016). However, in the past decade, attempts have been made to reduce these costs for greater acceptance (Parsons et al., 2015). In recent times, low-cost technologies are available and are showing promise for interventions, as they also have the added advantage of being portable and can be used in one's personal space (Schiza et al., 2019).

Parsons et al. (2015) have also acknowledged that it is likely that virtual environments may become redundant, given the constant change our realities undergo. For instance, at one point, going to the grocery store for purchases used to be a norm, however in the past (recent) years, several countries have adopted e-commerce platforms for making purchases online, which is becoming a norm. Accommodating these changes in a virtual environment is also important, however it can become a costly choice, and hence use of immersive technologies may not become as frequent. Bearing these costs will essentially overtake its benefits. Hence, software developers will have to take into account the requirement of customisation to adapt to the ever-changing nature of reality.

4. Test characteristics: Most research reviewed thus far in this chapter cover tasks that have a real-world application and hence are likely to show greater acceptability among participants. However, it is also important to evaluate the type of intervention that is being imparted to patients. Merriman et al. (2019), in their qualitative study, take cognisance of the relevance of tasks that are designed for patients for it to be a successful intervention. Moreover, if interventions have a strong real-world component, it is likely to be well received by both patients and caregivers. In this regard then, immersive technologies stand a strong chance to continue its role for assessments and interventions.
5. Need for further research: Much research confirm the credibility of immersive technology use in cognitive interventions. Primarily, interventions for executive functions,, visuo-spatial abilities, have shown strong effects, however, mixed reviews for interventions of memory, and attention are present (Riva, Mancuso, Cavedoni, & Stramba-Badiale, 2020). This calls for more research studies to confirm conclusively the role of such technologies for interventions.

7. SUMMARY AND CONCLUSION

Are immersive technologies here to stay? This can be evaluated from three points of view, viz; the immersive technologies' benefits to the society, their roles in assessments, and the users' beliefs about the roles of these technologies in assessments. Krohn et al. (2019) have provided VR-based dimensions to evaluate its use in the field of clinical neuropsychology. These include, ecological relevance, technical and user feasibility, task adaptation, user motivation, quantification of performance, and pitfalls. From the user's perspective, Norcini et al. (2011) provide criteria for sound psychological assessments, which include the tests' psychometric properties, feasibility, acceptability, and modifications based on users' feedback. In keeping with these sets of criteria, the users' openness to accepting such technologies, and based on the evidence on immersive technologies as discussed in this chapter, it is clear that these have successfully demonstrated their worth in improving testing and intervention protocols.

To conclude, clinicians have worked towards studying cognitive deficits in an objective manner. In fact, clinicians (e.g., Goldstein – 1878 - 1965) in the 20th century were already advanced in their outlook for assessments and interventions as they were already envisioning the creation of ecologically valid modules. With immersive technologies, cognitive psychology and neuropsychology are indeed reaching a full circle (figure 3), and the primary goal of creating and using ecologically valid cognitive tools and interventions is happening.

Figure 3.

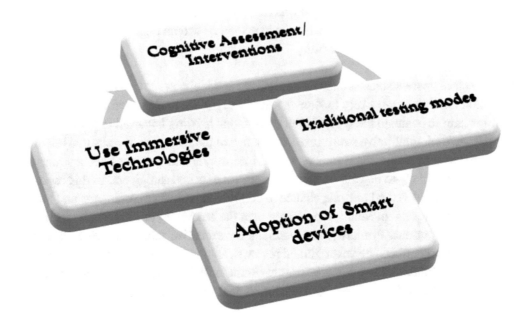

Technology advances are already enforced in areas such as education, shopping, and gaming. In this regard then, people are already getting familiar with these technologies. Hence, implementing these technologies on a larger scale than its current status in the area of cognition is the next likely outcome. Overall, its positives features can take cognition-based tasks to a competitive position and stay at par with the many other advancements in the medical and para-medical fields.

REFERENCES

Abdul, S. S., Malwade, S., Nursetyo, A. A., Sood, M., Bhatia, M., ... Li, J. (2019). Virtual reality among the elderly: A usefulness acceptance study from Taiwan. *BMC Geriatrics*, *19*(1), 223. doi:10.118612877-019-1218-8 PMID:31426766

Anastasi, A. (1976). *Psychological testing* (4th ed.). Macmillan.

Arleti, S., Colombo, V., Spoladore, D., Pedroli, E., Serino, S., ... Sacco, M. (2020). A social virtual reality-based application for the physical and cognitive training of the elderly at home. *Sensors (Basel)*, *19*(2), 261. doi:10.339019020261 PMID:30634719

Azouvi, P., Arnould, A., Dromer, E., & Vallat-Azouvi, C. (2017). Neuropsychology of traumatic brain injury: An expert overview. *Revue Neurologique*, *173*(7-8), 461–472. doi:10.1016/j.neurol.2017.07.006 PMID:28847474

Bauer, A. C. M., & Andringa, G. (2020). The potential of immersive virtual reality for cognitive training in elderly. *Gerontology*, *66*(6), 614–623. doi:10.1159/000509830 PMID:32906122

Bayne, T., Brainard, D., Byrne, R. W., Chittka, L., Clayton, N., Heyes, C., Mather, J., Ölveczky, B., Shadlen, M., Suddendorf, T., & Webb, B. (2019). What is Cognition? *Current Biology*, *29*(13), R608–R616. doi:10.1016/j.cub.2019.05.044 PMID:31287972

Chaytor, N., & Schmitter-Edgecombe, M. (2003). The Ecological Validity of Neuropsychological Tests: A Review of the Literature on Everyday Cognitive Skills. *Neuropsychology Review*, *13*(4), 181–197. doi:10.1023/B:NERV.0000009483.91468.fb PMID:15000225

Cho, D.-R., & Lee, S.-H. (2019). Effects of virtual reality immersive training with computerized cognitive training on cognitive function and activities of daily living performance in patients with acute stage stroke. *Medicine*, *98*(11), e14752. doi:10.1097/MD.0000000000014752 PMID:30882644

Chung, J., Pagnini, F., & Langer, E. (2016). Mindful navigation for pedestrians: Improving engagement with augmented reality. *Technology in Society*, *45*, 29–33. doi:10.1016/j.techsoc.2016.02.006

Cicero, M. T. (2001). Cicero on the ideal orator (de oratore) (J. M. May & J. Wisse, Trans.). Oxford, UK: Oxford University Press. (Original publication 55 BCE)

Climent, G., Rodríguez, C., García, T., Areces, D., Mejías, M., Aierbe, A., Moreno, M., Cueto, E., Castellá, J., & Feli González, M. (2021). New virtual reality tool (Nesplora Aquarium) for assessing attention and working memory in adults: A normative study. *Applied Neuropsychology. Adult*, *28*(4), 403–415. doi:10.1080/23279095.2019.1646745 PMID:31382773

Coleman, E. R., Moudgal, R., Lang, K., Hyacinth, H. I., Awosika, O. O., Kissela, B. M., & Feng, W. (2017). Early Rehabilitation After Stroke: A Narrative Review. *Current Atherosclerosis Reports*, *19*(12), 59. doi:10.100711883-017-0686-6 PMID:29116473

Corregidor-Sánchez, A.-I., Segura-Fragoso, A., Criado-Álvarez, J.-J., Rodríguez-Hernández, M., Mohedano-Moriano, A., & Polonio-López, B. (2020). Effectiveness of Virtual Reality Systems to Improve the Activities of Daily Life in Older People. *International Journal of Environmental Research and Public Health*, *17*(17), 6283. doi:10.3390/ijerph17176283 PMID:32872313

Corriveau Lecavalier, N., Ouellet, E., Boller, B., & Belleville, S. (2020). Use of immersive virtual reality to assess episodic memory: A validation study in older adults. *Neuropsychological Rehabilitation*, *30*(3), 462–480. doi:10.1080/09602011.2018.1477684 PMID:29807474

Crowder, R. G. (1976). *Principles of learning and memory*. Lawrence Erlbaum.

Darby, R. R., & Dickerson, B. C. (2017). Dementia, Decision Making, and Capacity. *Harvard Review of Psychiatry*, *25*(6), 270–278. doi:10.1097/HRP.0000000000000163 PMID:29117022

de Freitas Cardoso, M. G., Faleiro, R. M., de Paula, J. J., Kummer, A., Caramelli, P., Teixeira, A. L., de Souza, L. C., & Miranda, A. S. (2019). Cognitive Impairment Following Acute Mild Traumatic Brain Injury. *Frontiers in Neurology*, *10*, 198. doi:10.3389/fneur.2019.00198 PMID:30906278

De Luca, R., Maggio, M. G., Maresca, G., Latella, D., Cannavò, A., Sciarrone, F., Lo Voi, E., Accorinti, M., Bramanti, P., & Calabrò, R. S. (2019b). Improving cognitive function after traumatic brain injury: A clinical trial on the potential use of the semi-immersive virtual reality. *Behavioural Neurology*, 1–7. Advance online publication. doi:10.1155/2019/9268179 PMID:31481980

Duzmanska, N., Strojny, P., & Strojny, A. (2018). Can simulator sickness be avoided? A review on temporal aspects of simulator sickness. *Frontiers in Psychology*, *9*, 2132. doi:10.3389/fpsyg.2018.02132 PMID:30459688

Eling, P. (2019). History of Neuropsychological Assessment. *Frontiers of Neurology and Neuroscience*, *44*, 164–178. doi:10.1159/000494963 PMID:31220853

Ettenhofer, M. L., Guise, B., Brandler, B., Bittner, K., Gimbel, S. I., Cordero, E., Nelson Schmitt, S., Williams, K., Cox, D., Roy, M. J., & Chan, L. (2019). Neurocognitive driving rehabilitation in virtual environments (NeuroDRIVE): A pilot clinical trial for chronic traumatic brain injury. *NeuroRehabilitation*, *44*(4), 531–544. doi:10.3233/NRE-192718 PMID:31256093

Evans, F. A., Wong, D., Lawson, D. W., Withiel, T. D., & Stolwyk, R. J. (2019). What are the most common memory complaints following stroke? A frequency and exploratory factor analysis of items from the everyday memory questionnaire- revised. *The Clinical Neuropsychologist*, *34*(3), 498–511. doi:10.1080/13854046.2019.1652349 PMID:32189571

Gamito, P., Oliveira, J., Coelho, C., Morais, D., Lopes, P., Pacheco, J., Brito, R., Soares, F., Santos, N., & Barata, A. F. (2017). Cognitive training on stroke patients via virtual reality-based serious games. *Disability and Rehabilitation*, *39*(4), 385–388. doi:10.3109/09638288.2014.934925 PMID:25739412

Gamito, P., Oliviera, J., Alves, C., Santos, N., Coelho, C., & Brito, R. (2020). Virtual reality based cognitive stimulation to improve cognitive functioning in community elderly: A controlled study. *Cyberpsychology, Behavior, and Social Networking*, *23*(3), 150–158. doi:10.1089/cyber.2019.0271 PMID:32031888

Gauthier, S., Reisberg, B., Zaudig, M., Petersen, R. C., Ritchie, K., Broich, K., Belleville, S., Brodaty, H., Bennett, D., Chertkow, H., Cummings, J. L., de Leon, M., Feldman, H., Ganguli, M., Hampel, H., Scheltens, P., Tierney, M. C., Whitehouse, P., & Winblad, B. (2006). International Psychogeriatric Association Expert Conference on mild cognitive impairment. *Lancet*, *367*(9518), 1262–1270. doi:10.1016/S0140-6736(06)68542-5 PMID:16631882

Giglioli, C. I. A., Vidal, B. C., & Raya, A. M. (2019). A Virtual Versus an Augmented Reality Cooking Task Based-Tools: A Behavioral and Physiological Study on the Assessment of Executive Functions. *Frontiers in Psychology*, *10*, 2529. doi:10.3389/fpsyg.2019.02529 PMID:31798497

Graham, J. R., & Naglieri, J. A. (2012). Handbook of psychology: Vol. 10. *Assessment psychology*. John Wiley & Sons Inc.

Gustafson, L. (1996). What is dementia? *Acta Neurologica Scandinavica*, *94*(s168), 22–24. doi:10.1111/j.1600-0404.1996.tb00367.x PMID:8997414

Hill, N. L., McDermott, C., Mogle, J., Munoz, E., DePasquale, N., Wion, R., & Whitaker, E. (2017). Subjective cognitive impairment and quality of life: A systematic review. *International Psychogeriatrics*, *29*(12), 1965–1977. doi:10.1017/S1041610217001636 PMID:28829003

Huang, K.-T. (2020). Exergaming executive functions: An immersive virtual reality-based cognitive training for adults aged 50 and older. *Cyberpsychology, Behavior, and Social Networking*, *23*(3), 143–151. doi:10.1089/cyber.2019.0269 PMID:31794673

Ijaz, K., Ahmadpour, N., Naismith, S. L., & Calvo, R. A. (2019). An Immersive Virtual Reality Platform for Assessing Spatial Navigation Memory in Predementia Screening: Feasibility and Usability Study. *JMIR Mental Health*, *6*(9), e13887. doi:10.2196/13887 PMID:31482851

Jansari, A., Devlin, A., Agnew, R., Akesson, K., Murphy, L., & Leadbetter, T. (2014). Ecological Assessment of Executive Functions: A New Virtual Reality Paradigm. *Brain Impairment*, *15*(2), 71–87. doi:10.1017/BrImp.2014.14

Jin, R., Pilozzi, A., & Huang, X. (2020). Current cognition tests, potential virtual reality applications, and serious games in cognitive assessment and non-pharmacological therapy for neurocognitive disorders. *Journal of Clinical Medicine*, *9*(10), 3287. doi:10.3390/jcm9103287 PMID:33066242

Kapoor, A., Lanctôt, K. L., Bayley, M., Kiss, A., Herrmann, N., Murray, B. J., & Swartz, R. H. (2017). "Good Outcome" Isn't Good Enough: Cognitive Impairment, Depressive Symptoms, and Social Restrictions in Physically Recovered Stroke Patients. *Stroke*, *48*(6), 1688–1690. doi:10.1161/STROKEAHA.117.016728 PMID:28438907

Khosrow-Pour, M. (2014). *Encyclopaedia of Information Science and Technology* (3rd ed.). IGI Global.

Kirchner, W. K. (1958). Age differences in short-term retention of rapidly changing information. *Journal of Experimental Psychology*, *55*(4), 352–358. doi:10.1037/h0043688 PMID:13539317

Kourtesis, P., Korre, D., Collina, S., Doumas, L. A., & MacPherson, S. E. (2020). Guidelines for the development of immersive virtual reality software for cognitive neuroscience and neuropsychology: The development of virtual reality everyday assessment lab (VR-EAL), a neuropsychological test battery in immersive virtual reality. *Frontiers of Computer Science*, *1*, 12. Advance online publication. doi:10.3389/fcomp.2019.00012

Krohn, S., Tromp, J., Quinque, E. M., Belger, J., Klotzsche, F., Gaebler, M., ... Finke, C. (2019, July 21-24). *Multidimensional assessment of virtual reality applications in clinical neuropsychology: The "VR-Check" protocol* [Paper presentation]. International Conference on Virtual Rehabilitation (ICVR) 2019, Tel Aviv, Israel. 10.1109/ICVR46560.2019.8994590

Lara, E., Caballero, F. F., Rico-Uribe, L. A., Olaya, B., Haro, J. M., Ayuso-Mateos, J. L., & Miret, M. (2019). Are loneliness and social isolation associated with cognitive decline? *International Journal of Geriatric Psychiatry*, *34*(11), 1613–1622. doi:10.1002/gps.5174 PMID:31304639

Lecouvey, G., Morand, A., Gonneaud, J., Piolino, P., Orriols, E., Pélerin, A., Ferreira Da Silva, L., de La Sayette, V., Eustache, F., & Desgranges, B. (2019). An Impairment of Prospective Memory in Mild Alzheimer's Disease: A Ride in a Virtual Town. *Frontiers in Psychology*, *10*, 241. doi:10.3389/fpsyg.2019.00241 PMID:30809174

Lezak, M. D., Howieson, D. B., Bigler, E. D., & Tranel, D. (2012). *Neuropsychological Assessment* (5th ed.). Oxford University Press.

Liao, Y. Y., Tseng, H.-Y., Lin, Y.-J., Wang, C.-J., & Hsu, W.-C. (2020). Using virtual reality-based training to improve cognitive function, instrumental activities of daily living and neural efficiency in older adults with mild cognitive impairment. *European Journal of Physical and Rehabilitation Medicine*, *56*(1), 47–57. doi:10.23736/S1973-9087.19.05899-4 PMID:31615196

Maggio, M. G., Maresca, G., De Luca, R., Stagnitti, M. C., Porcari, B., Ferrera, M. C., Galletti, F., Casella, C., Manuli, A., & Calabrò, R. S. (2019). The Growing Use of Virtual Reality in Cognitive Rehabilitation: Fact, Fake or Vision? A Scoping Review. *Journal of the National Medical Association*, *111*(4), 457–463. doi:10.1016/j.jnma.2019.01.003 PMID:30739728

Menon, D. K., Schwab, K., Wright, D. W., & Maas, A. I. (2010). Demographics and Clinical Assessment Working Group of the International and Interagency Initiative toward Common Data Elements for Research on Traumatic Brain Injury and Psychological Health. Position statement: Definition of traumatic brain injury. *Archives of Physical Medicine and Rehabilitation*, *91*(11), 1637–1640. doi:10.1016/j.apmr.2010.05.017 PMID:21044706

Messinis, L., Kosmidis, M. H., Nasios, G., Dardiotis, E., & Tsaousides, T. (2019). Cognitive neurorehabilitation in acquired neurological brain injury. *Behavioural Neurology*, *1-4*, 8241951. doi:10.1155/2019/8241951 PMID:31781294

Moreno, A., Wall, K. J., Thangavelu, K., Craven, L., Ward, E., & Dissanayaka, N. N. (2019). A systematic review of the use of virtual reality and its effects on cognition in individuals with neurocognitive disorders. *Alzheimer's & Dementia: Translational Research & Clinical Interventions*, *5*(1), 834–850. doi:10.1016/j.trci.2019.09.016 PMID:31799368

Munoz-Montoya, F., Juan, M-C., Mendez-Lopez, M., Molla, R., Abad, F., & Fidalgo, C. (2021). SLAM-based augmented reality for the assessment of short-term spatial memory. A comparative study of visual versus tactile stimuli. *PLOS ONE, 16*(2). doi: .pone.0245976 doi:10.1371/journal

Nakling, A. E., Aarsland, D., Næss, H., Wollschlaeger, D., Fladby, T., Hofstad, H., & Wehling, E. (2017). Cognitive Deficits in Chronic Stroke Patients: Neuropsychological Assessment, Depression, and Self-Reports. *Dementia and Geriatric Cognitive Disorders. Extra*, *7*(2), 283–296. doi:10.1159/000478851 PMID:29033974

National Collaborating Centre for Mental Health (UK). (2007). *Dementia: A NICE-SCIE guideline on supporting people with dementia and their carers in health and social care*. British Psychological Society.

Negut, A., Matu, S., Sava, F. A., & David, D. (2016). Virtual reality measures in neuropsychological assessment: A meta-analytic review. *The Clinical Neuropsychologist*, *30*(2), 165–184. doi:10.1080/138 54046.2016.1144793 PMID:26923937

Norcini, J., Anderson, B., Bollela, V., Burch, V., Costa, M. J., Duvivier, R., Galbraith, R., Hays, R., Kent, A., Perrott, V., & Roberts, T. (2011). Criteria for good assessment: Consensus statement and recommendations from the Ottawa 2010 Conference. *Medical Teacher*, *33*(3), 206–214. doi:10.3109/014215 9X.2011.551559 PMID:21345060

Oliviera, C., Lopes Filho, B., Sugarman, M., Esteves, C., Lima, M., Moret-Tatay, C., ... Argimon, I. (2016). Development and Feasibility of a Virtual Reality Task for the Cognitive Assessment of Older Adults: The ECO-VR. *The Spanish Journal of Psychology*, *19*, E95. doi:10.1017jp.2016.96 PMID:27955716

Oliviera, J., Gamito, P., Souto, T., Conde, R., Ferreira, M., Corotnean, T., ... Neto, T. (2021). Virtual Reality-Based Cognitive Stimulation on People with Mild to Moderate Dementia due to Alzheimer's Disease: A Pilot Randomized Controlled Trial. *International Journal of Environmental Research and Public Health, 18*(10), 5290. doi:10.3390/ijerph18105290 PMID:34065698

Ouellet, É., Boller, B., Corriveau-Lecavalier, N., Cloutier, S., & Belleville, S. (2018). The virtual shop: A new immersive virtual reality environment and scenario for the assessment of everyday memory. *Journal of Neuroscience Methods, 303*, 126–135. doi:10.1016/j.jneumeth.2018.03.010 PMID:29581009

Park, E., Yun, B. J., Min, Y. S., Lee, Y.-S., Moon, S.-J., Huh, J.-W., Cha, H., Chang, Y., & Jung, T.-D. (2019). Effects of a mixed reality-based cognitive training system compared to a conventional computer-assisted cognitive training system on mild cognitive impairment: A pilot study. *Cognitive and Behavioral Neurology, 32*(3), 172–178. doi:10.1097/WNN.0000000000000197 PMID:31517700

Parsons, D. T., & Barnett, M. (2018). Virtual apartment -based Stroop for assessing distractor inhibition in healthy aging. *Applied Neuropsychology. Adult, 26*(2), 144–154. doi:10.1080/23279095.2017.1373 281 PMID:28976213

Parsons, D. T., Carlew, A. R., Magtoto, J., & Stonecipher, K. (2015). The potential of function-led virtual environments for ecologically valid measures of executive function in experimental and clinical neuropsychology. *Neuropsychological Rehabilitation*, 1–31. doi:10.1080/09602011.2015.1109524 PMID:26558491

Parsons, T., & Duffield, T. (2020). Paradigm Shift Toward Digital Neuropsychology and High-Dimensional Neuropsychological Assessments [Review]. *Journal of Medical Internet Research, 22*(12), e23777. doi:10.2196/23777 PMID:33325829

Parsons, T. D. (2015). Ecological validity in virtual reality-based neuropsychological assessment. In K.-P. Mehdi (Ed.), *Encyclopaedia of Information Science and Technology* (3rd ed., pp. 214–223). IGI Global. doi:10.4018/978-1-4666-5888-2.ch095

Pedroli, E., Greci, L., Colombo, D., Serino, S., Cipresso, P., Arlati, S., Mondellini, M., Boilini, L., Giussani, V., Goulene, K., Agostoni, M., Sacco, M., Stramba-Badiale, M., Riva, G., & Gaggioli, A. (2018). Characteristics, usability, and users experience of a system combining cognitive and physical therapy in a virtual environment: Positive bike. *Sensors (Basel), 18*(7), 2343. doi:10.3390/s18072343 PMID:30029502

Peleg-Adler, R., Lanir, J., & Korman, M. (2018). The effects of aging on the use of handheld augmented reality in a route planning task. *Computers in Human Behavior, 81*, 52–62. doi:10.1016/j.chb.2017.12.003

Raspelli, S., Pallavicini, F., Carelli, L., Morganti, F., Poletti, B., Corra, B., ... Riva, G. (2011). Validation of a Neuro Virtual Reality-based version of the Multiple Errands Test for the assessment of executive functions. *Studies in Health Technology and Informatics, 167*, 92–97. PMID:21685648

Raz, S., Bar-Haim, Y., Sadeh, A., & Dan, O. (2014). Reliability and validity of the online continuous performance test among young adults. *Assessment, 21*(1), 108–118. doi:10.1177/1073191112443409 PMID:22517923

Riva, G., Mancuso, V., Cavedoni, S., & Stramba-Badiale, C. (2020). Virtual reality in neurorehabilitation: A review of its effects on multiple cognitive domains. *Expert Review of Medical Devices*, *17*(10), 1035–1061. doi:10.1080/17434440.2020.1825939 PMID:32962433

Rizzo, A., Gambino, G., Sardo, P., & Rizzo, V. (2020). Being in the Past and Perform the Future in a Virtual World: VR Applications to Assess and Enhance Episodic and Prospective Memory in Normal and Pathological Aging. *Frontiers in Human Neuroscience*, *14*, 297. doi:10.3389/fnhum.2020.00297 PMID:32848672

Rizzo, A. A., Buckwalter, J. G., Neumann, U., Kesselman, C., & Thiebaux, M. (1998). Basic issues in the application of virtual reality for the assessment and rehabilitation of cognitive impairments and functional disability. *Cyberpsychology & Behavior*, *1*(1), 59–79. doi:10.1089/cpb.1998.1.59

Roberts, A. C., Yeap, Y. W., Seah, H. S., Chan, E., Soh, C. K., & Christopoulos, G. I. (2019). Assessing the suitability of virtual reality for psychological testing. *Psychological Assessment*, *31*(3), 318–328. doi:10.1037/pas0000663 PMID:30802117

Rosvold, H. E., Mirsky, A. F., Sarason, I., Bransome, E. D. Jr, & Beck, L. H. (1956). A continuous performance test of brain damage. *Journal of Consulting Psychology*, *20*(5), 343–350. doi:10.1037/h0043220 PMID:13367264

Salisbury, D. B., Dahdah, M., Driver, S., Parsons, T. D., & Richter, K. M. (2016). Virtual reality and brain computer interface in neurorehabilitation. *Proceedings - Baylor University. Medical Center*, *29*(2), 124–127. doi:10.1080/08998280.2016.11929386 PMID:27034541

Schiza, E., Matsangidou, M., Neolkeous, K., & Pattichis, C. S. (2019). Virtual reality applications for neurological disease: A review. *Frontiers in Robotics and AI*, *6*, 100. doi:10.3389/frobt.2019.00100 PMID:33501115

Shah, U. R. (2017). Cognitive rehabilitation in psychiatry. *Annals of Indian Psychiatry*, *1*(2), 68–75. doi:10.4103/aip.aip_35_17

Shallice, T., & Burgess, P. W. (1991). Deficits in strategy application following frontal lobe damage in man. *Brain*, *114*(Pt 2), 727–741. doi:10.1093/brain/114.2.727 PMID:2043945

Sternberg, S. (1967). Two operations in character recognition: Some evidence from reaction time measurements. *Perception & Psychophysics*, *2*(2), 45–53. doi:10.3758/BF03212460

Sternberg, S. (1969). Memory scanning: Mental processes revealed by reaction-time experiments. *American Scientist*, *57*, 421–457. PMID:5360276

Strauss, E., Sherman, E. M. S., & Spreen, O. (2006). *A compendium of neuropsychological tests: Administration, norms, and commentary* (3rd ed.). Oxford University Press.

Stroop, J. R. (1935). Studies of interference in serial verbal reactions. *Journal of Experimental Psychology*, *18*(6), 643–662. doi:10.1037/h0054651

Teel, E., Gay, M., Johnson, B., & Slobounov, S. (2016). Determining sensitivity/specificity of virtual reality- based neuropsychological tool for detecting residual abnormalities following sport-related concussion. *Neuropsychology*, *30*(4), 474–483. doi:10.1037/neu0000261 PMID:27045961

Torpil, B., Sahin, S., Pekçetin, S., & Uyanik, M. (2021). The effectiveness of a virtual reality-based intervention on cognitive functions in older adults with mild cognitive impairment: A single-blind, randomized controlled trial. *Games for Health Journal*, *10*(2), 109–115. doi:10.1089/g4h.2020.0086 PMID:33058735

Tulving, E., & Craik, F. I. M. (Eds.). (2000). *The Oxford handbook of memory*. Oxford University Press.

Urbina, S. (2014). *Essentials of psychological testing* (2nd ed.). John Wiley & Sons Inc.

van Rijsbergen, M. W., Mark, R. E., de Kort, P. L., & Sitskoorn, M. M. (2014). Subjective cognitive complaints after stroke: A systematic review. *Journal of Stroke and Cerebrovascular Diseases*, *23*(3), 408–420. doi:10.1016/j.jstrokecerebrovasdis.2013.05.003 PMID:23800498

Wall, K., Stark, J., Schillaci, A., Saulnier, E. T., McLaren, E., Striegnitz, K., Cohen, B., Arciero, P., Kramer, A., & Anderson-Hanley, C. (2018). The Enhanced Interactive Physical and Cognitive Exercise System (iPACES™ v2.0): Pilot Clinical Trial of an In-Home iPad-Based Neuro-Exergame for Mild Cognitive Impairment (MCI). *Journal of Clinical Medicine*, *7*(9), 249. doi:10.3390/jcm7090249 PMID:30200183

Wasserman, J. D., & Bracken, B. A. (2003). Psychometric characteristics of assessment procedures. In J. R. Graham & J. A. Naglieri (Eds.), Handbook of psychology: Vol. 10. *Assessment psychology* (pp. 43–66). John Wiley & Sons Inc.

Zhang, B., & Robb, N. (2020). A comparison of the effects of augmented reality N-back training and traditional two-dimensional N-back training for working memory. *SAGE Open*, 1–14.

Section 5
Trends

Chapter 13
Application of Virtual Reality in Cognitive Rehabilitation:
A Road Ahead

Susmita Halder
ⓘ https://orcid.org/0000-0001-6254-3324
St. Xavier's University, Kolkata, India

ABSTRACT

Virtual reality (VR) is defined as a simulation of the real world using computer graphics. The basic components of a VR application or program are interaction and immersion. Human-computer interaction is achieved through multiple sensory channels that allow individuals to explore virtual environments through senses. Immersion is considered the degree to which the individual feels engrossed or enveloped within the virtual environment. Scope of virtual reality is quite wide and varied, including technology, industry, education, and health. In the health sector, it has a significant role in assessment as well as intervention. Specific to human behavior and cognition, virtual reality's (VR) application is for cognitive assessment and rehabilitation. VR offers the potential to develop human testing and training environments that allow for the precise control of complex stimulus presentations in which human cognitive and functional performance can be accurately assessed and rehabilitated.

INTRODUCTION

Scope of VR is quite wide and varied, ranging from technology, industry, education, health, and many more. In health sector, it has significant role in assessment as well as intervention (Duarte et.al.,2020; Koning et.al., 2009). VR consists of an interactive and virtual environment the individual can interact with, created by computer graphics and with different degrees of immersive sensations (Wohlgenannt et.al.,2020). VR can offer almost real experience and ecological demands of the actual world; by creating virtual experience of arranging things, crossing roads, cooking, purchasing things and also classroom situations (Stanton et.al.,1998). These real life-like experiences enhance functionality as well as improve cognitive ability. VR experiences not only enhance brain plasticity, but also engage the client emotionally

DOI: 10.4018/978-1-7998-8371-5.ch013

to the situation. Indeed, VR allows a sense of wellbeing, due to the stimulation of multiple perceptual channels, implemented by the use of auditory and visual feedback, which stimulate the patient's awareness of his performance. The overall VR experiences allow to enhance motivation, compliance to the program, and treatment effect. Finally, it can also be customized according the client's need.

While the use of VR in health sector are vivid, its scope of use in Psychological health and wellbeing is increasing. As psychological assessments as well as interventions primarily depend on active interaction between therapist and the client, VR adds an edge to these interactions making the process more effective. In addition to conventional psychological interventions for which VR has been used, e.g. for phobia or posttraumatic stress, it has wide scope for use in cognitive rehabilitation too (Elbogen et.al.,2019). There is a growing body of literature which suggests application of VR in cognitive assessment and rehabilitation specific to human behavior and cognition is becoming wider (Lim et.al., 2020). VR provides the opportunity to assess the human behavior as accurate as possible by precise testing and controlled training. Further, it allows to improve the cognitive and functional performance, by intervention and rehabilitation (Jin et.al;2020 ; Chua et.al.,2019).

In this background the current chapter will focus and try to address following issues:

- Virtual Reality and its connection with Cognitive rehabilitation
- Its application in improving cognitive impairment in different neurological and mental health problems
- Virtual reality based cognitive training programs and packages
- How the program can be made more realistic and applicable to everyday functioning
- The outcomes and limitations
- Future plans and implications

VIRTUAL REALTY (VR) IN CONNECTION WITH COGNITION

Concept of Cognitive Rehabilitation (CR)

Cognitive Rehabilitation (CR) or neurocognitive rehabilitation refers to non-pharmacological methods of improving cognitive function in people with neurological and severe mental disorders (Cicerone et.al.,2000; Wilson, 2002). CR is a specific term frequently used for cognitive training after Stroke, Traumatic Brain Injury, Multiple Sclerosis, and other neurological and psychiatric disorders (Sohlberg and Mateer; 2001). The primary aim of CR is to repair the cognitive deficits, improve cognitive functions by using compensatory strategies and bring overall positive changes in daily life functioning (Riddoch & Humphreys, 1994). CR program uses certain specially designed techniques and exercises to improve cognitive domains, either by brief repetitive tasks or long-term training exercises that specifically target the impaired component processes (Halder and Mahato, 2018).

In CR, intense repetition of specific exercises is necessary to reorganize the brain in a particular area (Irazok et.al.,2020); however, it places immense demands on both the individual and the trainer. This presents a greater problem when extending the cognitive rehabilitation approach to patients as they are particularly difficult to engage (Wilson and Evans,2020).

While early techniques of CR were paper pencil based, which are still in use; the advent of computerized programs made the task easier and more focused. Now VR appear to further finetune it by aiding in the process. CR can be delivered in different ways; via paper pencil tasks or by computerised programs, of varying length and complexity, or can be undertaken one-on-one by a trained clinician. CR is basically a training-based intervention that aims to improve different domains of cognitive processes; like attention, memory, executive function, social cognition, or metacognition where the primary goal is generalization and sustainability of achieved improvement. However, the training program is not arbitrary, and is based on group of learning principles-based theory of plasticity.

While CR has been extensively applied in neurodegenerative conditions, neurological and brain conditions, major psychiatric conditions and in the recent past in several chronic medical conditions too; there are few limitations too (Cappon et.al.,2016). In terms of applicability, still a question arises as to whether CR is an available option only in case of diagnosed medical or psychiatric conditions or it can be integrated in day to day life with respect to everyday functioning of healthy individuals too. In this regard, maintaining cognitive functioning is a noteworthy concern for adults, and is important in promoting independence, good mood and quality of life (Ord et.al.,2021). Improving performance on cognitive tests is not in itself of benefit; the goals of cognitive remediation are to improve real-world outcomes such as work, socialization, and independent living skills.

VR appears to improve these limitations and the reason why VR adds value or brings new scope in application of CR is that VR based software are thought to be potentially more representative of everyday life situations than paper-and-pencil treatment procedures or limited software. Despite VR based CR interventions in early stage and high costs of VR equipment's, some results point this technology as a new possibility to rehabilitate cognitive and motor functions, stressing its characteristics as a motivator factor. VR is showing immense prospect in therapeutic interventions by creating a virtual environment and including different tasks which are closer to the daily living activities. Another big advantage of this process is its reachability. VR based program by its nature is not restricted to any physical set up like hospital or clinic, it may reach a large population via virtual environment, even to remote places and rural parts of the country. This has potential to cut down cost for clients in terms of follow up visits at clinics or hospitals.

Other than neurological problems, VR has exceptional potential to aid people overcome mental health problems (Valmaggia et.al.,2016). Clinicians use VR to provide a new human-computer interaction paradigm in which users are active participants within a computer generated three-dimensional virtual world. VR based therapeutic program may allow repetition of activities with minimum or no changes and make the client/patient more comfortable with the situation. Also, VR based cognitive rehabilitation program can be customized based on individual's specific strength and weakness to get the maximum benefits (Mancuso et.al.,2020).

Prior to VR, assessment of cognitive functioning and cognitive retraining used to do by using paper-pencil tests and tools, which are still in practise as per requirement. These got updated later to computerized tasks delivered via computer. Using computers made the training program easy to administer, record and training with less error and more precision. In continuation, application of VR has come with a different purpose, it is not exactly replacing the traditional approaches, but it supplements and complement the existing methods and process. The immersive experience which VR gives to client, makes the learning more realistic and potentially the desired change in real life situation is faster.

VR is increasingly being used in the clinical field including mental health and neuroscience. After being applied to evaluate attention, executive function, and memory, VR has begun to be used in the rehabilitation of these cognitive functions. It must be mentioned that the main cause of shifting from paper pencil or computerized training to VR training as in previous paradigms was not ecologically valid or appropriate. Moreover, study findings suggest patients may perform good on tests and showing better performance initially but transfer of training to every day functioning is limited.

VR application also has advantage over standard paper-pencil and computer-based training in terms of precise presentation and control of dynamic multi-sensory 3D stimulus environment, advanced methods of recording behavioural responses, and allow presenting more ecologically relevant stimuli imbedded in a meaningful and familiar context by stimulating naturalistic environment.

VR and Brain connection: VR helps to rewire the brain and increase the neural connections in a stimulated environment. It improves the ability to learn and retain events or incident in more adaptive way at low cost and in less time. VR can be used as the empirical feedback of brain-computer connectivity. Multidimensional approach of VR helps as more realistic way to perceive through neural connectivity. VR has the potential to address and manage brain impairments, disability or disorders (Rose et.al., 2005). VR influences the gross neuroplasticity through synaptic pruning and neural interactions. Synaptic pruning includes programmed reduction in the number of physical synapses between neurons in all sensory–motor systems in the nervous system. This process of pruning is strongly influenced by stimulation from the environment and interactions between neurons during learning—a process termed neural interaction (Eng et.al.,2020).

Attention

In domain of attention, VR training can achieve control over distractions, stimulus load and complexity by alternating responses. Also ecological validity can be systematically increased by introducing virtual environment like classroom, office, home, store, travel places. Components of attention including emotion and attention regulation, selective attention, sustained attention, alternating attention, divided attention, inhibitory, and behavior control are intervened through immersive VR (Climent et.al.,2021). Immersive VR can trigger the emotional, psychological and physiological reactions on the basis of perceived real life situations. The senses of real and maladaptive reactions to the stimulus through immersive VR intervention facilitate the process. VR can hold a patient's attention for a longer period than other methods because it is immersive, interactive, imaginal, and interesting.

Sustained attention training is based on the principles of habituation. In this, VR provides environment to increase attention to include (to practice with more) or to exclude (at initial level) distractors according to need (Benedetti et.al.,2014). Additionally, hand-eye -coordination training is possible which helps to motivate and improve experience of perception. The VRCPAT (Parsons and Rizzo, 2008) is one such battery where difficulty level can be manipulated by changing the presentation of stimulus from simple to complex, or low versus high intensity stimulus. Another VR based tool, The New South Wales Visual Recognition Slide Test (VRST) (George et.al.,2008) is a component to improve the speed of information processing and visual scanning which is associated with attentional abilities. It is found individuals pay more attention in sustained attention tasks in three- dimensional presentations (Smallwood et.al., 2004).

Working Memory (WM)

The concept of WM assumes that a dedicated system maintains and stores information in the short term, and that this system underlies human thought processes. Current views of WM involve a central executive that mediates the flow of information to and from its two slave storage systems: the phonological loop and the visuospatial sketchpad. Virtual Working memory training is known to substantially improve sustained attention in a real-life scenario of classroom learning. Moreover, the use of psychometrically validated VR measurement provides incremental validity beyond that of teacher or parent report of behaviour. The concept underlying VR intervention as a training method for cognitive dysfunctions such as impaired WM is to improve the brain's neuroplasticity by engaging participants in multisensory training. Computerized cognitive interventions to improve working memory also purport to improve ADHD-related inattention and off task behaviour (Coleman et.al.,2019). Such interventions have been shown to improve working memory, executive functioning, and fluid reasoning on standardized neuropsychological measures. One such program, The virtual reality working-memory-training program (VR-WORK-M) is used to improve working memory performance. This program recreates a restaurant environment where participants complete a WM task, which consists in the repetition of a series of items heard through headphones. The WM task in VR-WORK-M is based on both storing and processing information, unlike the free recall paradigm, which deals with storage only and is measured by simple span (Eng et.al.,2020).

Executive Functioning

Executive function is defined as a set of cognitive skills necessary for planning, monitoring and executing a sequence of goal-directed complex actions (Diamond, 2013). It is a set of behavioural competencies that include planning, sequencing, and organizing, controlling, manipulation of simultaneous activities, and cognitive flexibility. Here, VR training targets planning, initiation, multi-tasking, self-awareness in executive functioning which is required for everyday functioning. Developing a comprehensive VR program to target EF could be a tricky task. Virtual environments that replicate real life situations for example, shopping activities usually assesses executive functioning and involves people with cognitive deficits in daily living activities. Whereas, in clinical settings it's difficult to train the client in real life environments and fails to assess and train executive functioning. The use of meaningful context through virtual reality can make easy to evaluate executive functioning limitations and facilitates performance. Some impairments that conciliated the performance manifestations during simulation are omissions, failure in initiation an action and displacement purposelessly.

In one such program, the VR system includes 3 VR games for training 3 core EF: game 1 for inhibitory control (the ability to override a strong internal predisposition or external lure and do what is more appropriate or needed), game 2 for working memory (the ability to hold and process information in mind as needed), and game 3 for cognitive flexibility (the ability to adjust to changing environmental demands and think from different perspectives). Virtual Reality-Based Physical and Cognitive Training (VR) Group package discourages the progressive symptoms of cognitive impairment. It involves physical tasks through cycle-ergometer and two virtual environments for cognitive stimulation (Arlati et. al.,2017). One more assessment tool, named Virtual Reality Cognitive Performance Assessment Test (VRCPAT) (Parsons and Rizzo, 2008) battery has been accepted as useful tool (Ku et.al.,2009) in stroke patients to improve executive functioning through virtual stimulation environment.

Memory

VR promotes content transfer which refers to the cognitive abilities that are already trained. Improvement in content transfer helps to learn or memorize visual stimuli and results in enhancing learning of auditory materials. VR can be suitable for prospective memory as it supports complex, dynamic environments that require coordination of many cognitive functioning. VR related to the information about temporally dated episodes or events, and temporal–spatial relations among these events which improves capacity of episodic memory of the individual. The impact of virtual immersion on memory, possible mnemonic benefits of active or passive cues are engaging with the virtual environment, and the existence and extent of transfer effects from VR to real-life assessments of episodic memory. VR training has been found to promote procedural learning in people with memory impairments, and this learning has been found to transfer to improved real-world performance. The VRCPAT Memory Module (Parsons & Rizzo, 2008) reflects the learning and memory functioning of the patients in accordance to prediction of further functioning. It is a 15 minute measure with 4 phases, Acquisition phase, VR interface and task training phase, Retrieval phase and Debriefing phase.

In virtual environment, information associated with real-like situational cues are used as proxy of measuring capacity. Specific details such as virtual objects, spatial layout and environment would be measured by VR tools and increases the levels of sensory inputs through virtual memory-cues environment (Bailey et.al.,2012). Use of VR is characterised to improve active and passive encoding of episodic memory and includes memory for central and perceptual details, spatiotemporal contextual elements, and binding (Plancher et.al.,2012) (Cushman et al 2008). Acquisition of information in everyday life requires memorization in complex three-dimensional environments. Every day memories are improved with the help of photorealistic virtual environment with verbal and spatial scenary (Windman, 2012).

Visuo-Spatial

VR systems allow visualization of (and interaction with) dynamic virtual 3D environments. Immersive features like a first-person view, stereoscopic displays, and the transfer of real-world movement into virtual space (room scale VR) can provide users of VR with a sense of presence unmatched by screen- or paper-based presentation of spatial information. Additionally, using already available geospatial data and game engines like Unity or Unreal Engine, VR-based 3D spatial representations of real-world space can be created fast and cost-efficiently. The cognition of geographic space is a topic of rising importance in disciplines dealing with spatial visualization, such as spatial cognition and cartography. To shape out an accurate mental representation of the environment, people often use external references. These external sources can be cartographic media, such as "traditional" 2D printed maps or interactive and animated digital spatial representations. The improvement of such cartographic media, with the aim of reducing spatial distortions in cognitive representations of space and to increase the efficiency in map-reading performance, In visuospatial cognitions, utilizing VR technologies for training (and ultimately, also testing) the selected cognitive functions provides an appropriate approach to stimulate the real-life aspect of visuospatial processing, including the processing, representing and storage of complex 3D structural and dynamical relations and contents. Cushman et al (2008) worked on navigational ability in terms of self – orientation, route drawing, and landmark recall and made the scenes like real environment.

It has been found VR is safer and more practical way of understanding and training spatial and navigational deficits. Brooks et al (2004) studied spatial skills by tasks with virtual bungalow with inter connected rooms with objects.

APPLICATION OF VIRTUAL REALITY IN COGNITIVE REHABILITATION

VR for rehabilitation of different cognitive processes, e.g., executive function, memory, spatial capacity, can be effectively planned in VR mode for Acquired Brain Injury (ABI), by developing innovative virtual environments for purpose of rehabilitation. In case of patients with ABI, motor task in a virtual environment demonstrated the ability to improve performance on the task in that environment; the learning did not always transfer to the real-world task (Sharma and Halder, 2021). In ABI patients, their performance and overall satisfaction in a Virtual Environment (VE) training found to be better using either a 3D projection system, compared classical paper-and-pencil, and flat-screen computer rehabilitative tools (Dores et.al.,2009). Immersive VR systems prove capable of evoking a more intense and compelling sense of presence, thanks to the subject-environment interaction allowed, although it is also reported to commonly associated with cyber sickness.

Traumatic Brain Injury

In traumatic brain injury, acute disruption of neural activity and oxidative metabolism with the brain circuit could be observable. Changes in neurotransmitters and neuroendocrine activities are associated with maladaptive behaviours and dysregulation of mood and cognitive functioning. Factor related to cognitive deficits i.e. penetrative brain injury leads to preinjury intelligence and volume of brain tissue lost. Deficits in remembering, planning, organising, encoding and learning lead to difficulties in occupational functioning. Engagement in daily living tasks and providing scope for interaction can help in reducing person's inability to function normally. VR implies to the possibilities to develop specific way in communication patterns with environment; task based as well as by interaction. VR based assessments and training programs aim to measure precise performance and replays of tasks which in turn help in skill development. VR setting for traumatic brain injury includes tasks demanding the improvement of perceptuomotor, visuospatial, orientation, memory and conceptual aspects of tasks and integrating it to daily routine. Impaired incidental memory for objects are improved by four room virtual environment and static display and moving objects in required virtual rooms. Memory recognition functioning is encountered through virtual distraction. Presenting distracting virtual navigation leads to realistic free recall and recognition. Enhancing spatial memory could be focused through motorix memory traces during encoding the navigation by virtual training (De Luca et.al.,2020). Immersive Virtual system equivalent to Wisconsin Card Sorting Test contains a virtual building and ways of exit. The virtual environment comprised of 32 rooms of different shapes and with specific number of rooms include with dead end corridors. Matching strategy have to find out in this system.

Stroke

After having a stroke, difficulty in moving, thinking, and sensing can be seen. This often results in problems with everyday activities such as writing, walking, and driving. VR through interactive video gaming provides rehabilitation therapies to people recovering after stroke. The therapy involves using computer-based programs designed to simulate real life objects and events. Robot training using a virtual environment has recently been shown to enhance stroke rehabilitation. Motor function of the affected arm in stroke affected patients was improved following robot-assisted sensorimotor activity of that arm. VR and interactive video gaming may have some advantages over traditional therapy approaches as they can give people an opportunity to practice everyday activities that are not or cannot be practiced within the hospital environment. Furthermore, there are several features of VR programs that might mean that patients spend more time in therapy: for example, the activity might be more motivating (Jonsdottir et.al.,2021).

Dementia and Mild Cognitive Impairment

In elderly, VR based rehabilitation has been shown significant efficacy in terms of increased attention and motivation to participate. It is encouraging for to do more research in this domain and leading pioneering researchers to explore its use as a neurodiagnostic and cognitive rehabilitation tool. VR computer-based intervention, can used for cognitive stimulation and disease progression evaluation of a wide range of cognitive disorders ranging from mild cognitive impairment (MCI) (Mancuso et.al., 2020) to Alzheimer's disease and various dementias. VR environments have already been successfully used in cognitive rehabilitation and show increased potential for its use in neuropsychological evaluation allowing for greater ecological validity while being more engaging and user friendly. It is always better to try a holistic system, considering the recent research advancements in the domain of health care, and can be intelligently used in cognitive rehabilitation too. Thus looking at research directions, systems, technological frameworks and trends, intervention plan can be made and modified. If clinicians can provide opportunities, persons with cognitive impairments can learn how to navigate and interact within virtual environments.

VR therapy has also been used to engage into activities of daily living in patients with dementia, such as moving in home, kitchen and shopping at a supermarket. VR head-mounted displays (HMDs) have been used to present visual cues overlapping the real visual scene during ambulation of patients with Parkinson's disease. Now research is not only limited to utilize VR for assessment and cognitive rehabilitation of individuals with MCI or with early-stage AD (Diaz Baquero et.al.,2021). By contrast, integrative VR (cognitive and motor rehabilitation) can be used on patients with advance-stage Alzheimer's Disease. VR has been found capable of differentiating older normal controls from those with MCI and from those with early-stage AD by using an entorhinal cortex-based test of virtual reality navigation. (Howett, D et. al. 2019)

VR in Childhood Disorders

The use of VR technologies, can be used both for assessment and intervention in normal children as well as with neurodevelopmental disorders. VR along with recent developments in augmented reality can achieve a high level of relevance and motivation. In the case of children, both VR and AR have been considered positive technologies, since they improve the quality of experience, motivation, and learning. Studies on application of Virtual classroom showing positive results and even found effective for children with 6 years of age (Coleman, B et. al. 2029; Rizzo, 2004; Shahabi, 2007; Parson et. al., 2007; Adama, 2009). A virtual classroom can be used for the assessment and rehabilitation of attention deficits and showed that VR can be used in the assessment of attention as well as cognitive training and can offer better predictive information regarding performance in a real environment. VR & AVC (Rizzo et al 1999) allowed multiple manipulations, including focused or selective attention, sustained, alternative or divided attention tasks on ADHD children.

OUTCOME AND LIMITATIONS

Cognitive Rehabilitation (CR) is already practiced therapeutic process of increasing or improving an individual capacity to process and use incoming information so as to allow increased functioning in everyday life (Sohlberg & Mateer, 1989) along with improving specific cognitive components. CR focuses particularly on self awareness, occupational and social interaction leading to better quality of life. Main approaches in CR are restorative and functional, but there are some weaknesses in both the approaches. In traditional approach the main weakness lies in relying upon test materials or tasks that have less relevance to real world functional cognitive challenges which lacks generalization in real life settings. In contrast, VR program can overcome the major weakness of standard approach by creating an environment more like real like situation by making it functionally relevant, ecologically valid, and optimizing the degree of transfer of training or generalizing or learning to real life situation.

The benefits of VR training over traditional CR can be summarized in terms of a systematically delivered, dynamic but controlled stimulation, provision of interactive stimuli within a complex environment; provision of more ecologically valid rehabilitation scenarios; provision of delivering immediate performance feedback to client, and availability for a more natural and intuitive performance record. It also provide the opportunity to pause treatment and training for discussion and integration of other methods, providing a safe training environment that minimizes risks due to errors; enhancing motivation through the integration of technical mechanisms and real tasks.

VR is a computer-generated technology that enables interactions between the user and virtual environments. The advantages of using VR interventions include enhancing accessibility and cost-effectiveness, creating an immersive experience, and providing immediate feedback based on an individual's performance. However, there are some limitations need to be pointed out. One major drawback of VR system is its high cost and demand of higher technology skills (Park, M. J. et.al 2019). Virtual reality training can be difficult to implement due to lack of competence in technical skills. Therapists' training is required to manage the software and the hardware and to adjust it to each case's needs. VR system also sometimes criticised indicating patients privacy and safety concerns (Burdea, D.C., 2003)

VR may have the potential to provide enhanced scenarios and can solve problems and acquire new skills. Virtual tasks have been described as more interesting and enjoyable by both children and adults, thus obtaining a higher number of repetitions, with positive results on therapist compliance and patient functional outcomes. The basis of VR related functional recovery was sensory feedback during VR training affected neuroplasticity and promoted brain reorganization.

FUTURE DIRECTIONS

Availability of VR in the field of psychological research has increased and it encourages the control over the environment through stimulus representation and response protocols in more ecologically valid way. In therapeutic intervention, VR can create complex scenarios as stimulating exposure with absolute precision with limited time. VR is an advanced technology which includes multimodal sensory input and increases sense of immersion in virtual presented environment in less compound way. VR system describes the virtual environment in presence of details of technical capabilities. It elicits intense emotional responses associated with real life stressful situation quickly. VR improves the relationship between client and therapist within less than expected time limit (Jensen and Konradsen, 2018).

VR technology has become more accessible and available to the population in this decade. The cost of technological assignments has been decreased with the availability of hardware and the demand of dependency of virtual environment emerged massively. Positive research findings and acceptability of this mode among normal an patient population has been surged the need of usage of virtual environment and practice of psychotherapy skills. The excitement around the VR environment is suggesting high requirement of VR and in turn lesser cost value of the technology. It provides opportunity to reproduce real-life scenarios in more adaptive and controlled way depending on the individual needs of the client. VR is a tool that facilitates the application of psychological evaluation in more affordable and available way (Coburn et.al.,2017).

The prime focus of VR is to introduce it as more real-life and personal experience through cinematic outcome. VR therapy is inclined to manualized computer programmes, visual immersion devices and artificially created stimulated environments used widely in spatial cognition and motor control along with social interaction. It includes a set of fancy devices i.e. helmet, trackers, 3D virtual visualizing devices. VR model tries to represent brain model in more realistic way where the individual feels present in real world and emphasizing making perfect device for experiential learning. Low-cost VR devices are presented to cure emotional or cognitive deficits by exposure to immersive virtual environment (Lee, et.al.,2019).

In recent years, with easy availability of computerized devices and internet connection, the application of VR has become more accessible for urban population but in rural or remote areas, its reach need to be widened. Gradual proliferation of technology is required to help increase the usage of VR devices in psychotherapy and assessments of mental health conditions in diverse populations and in different setups. Previously, it was hard to have equipments or facilities of VR due to its high cost and lesser availability in rural areas. But in recent times the decrease in cost of hardware and increased production level has implemented the idea of application of VR technology in educational or therapeutic purpose in more affordable ways (Kenwrigh,2019).

Immersive VR is similar to experience real world circumstances. It stimulates the way of experiences in more convincing way. Using more realistic graphics and visual fluency of situation could improve the virtual experiences of subjects and in case of psychological disorders the subjective reality should be represented through experience of clinical settings. The aim of application of VR technology in clinical settings is to present the individuals' own expectations or experience in exact way.

To reach towards the mass population, standardized procedure should be encouraged but the manipulation of stimulus related to different cultural background is necessary to create more realistic and better outcomes. VR technology has been used as a medium of communication to improve skills or adaptive behaviours. Culture-free VR situation can also be generated, and this would have more generalization. To implicate realistic stimulus, culture-based VR would help to improve capabilities. In the field of VR, the interviewers' bias should be eliminated, and it would be mainly based on human-computer interaction by standardizing the communication. In teaching language and culture, the use of VR technology is also emerging, and it might decrease the cultural biases among different cultures.

Convincing a person's expectations in therapeutic sessions depends on the nature or mode of stimulating virtual environment (Lin et.al., 2020). Each user perceives same virtual environment differently due to presence of individual traits, context specific vocational skills, cultural norms and expectations. Preparing a VR system where every perspective will fit in is difficult and it will increase the expenditure. Development of VR in clinical conditions could be focused on users' subjective and affective state along with mental demand to adapt with virtual environment.

Immersive VR has been identified as a revolutionary tool to intervene psychological disorders and VR technology has the potential to make the psychotherapeutic measures better and cost effective in clinical settings. Use of novel techniques and efficacious ways are identified through the measure of VR. In early generation of VR, the techniques are mostly used as VR exposure therapy for anxiety disorder but with the emerging times, from assessing level of distress to therapeutic measures of different clinical conditions are used without any barrier. VR technology is used to understand the persistence mechanism involved in mental disorders. From heightened social stress reactivity to psychosis liability or the role of cognitive distortion in manifestation of clinical symptomatology are identified and modified by VR technology (North and North 2017).

In preparation of a particular symptom-based treatment planning in regard to psychological conditions, the elements should have emotional or social clues to present it in more realistic and relatable way. It can be used in improving daily living skills by emphasizing on societal skills. VR based cognitive behavioral therapy (VR-CBT) focuses on emotional skills training and integrating emotional regulation skills through elaborating empathy and interpersonal relationships. VR social cognition skills training includes emotional and social stimulus which helps in improving societal functioning of children with autism spectrum disorder (Ke et.al.,2020).

One of the most discussed limitation of VR technology in recent times is that, the use of VR is restricted to laboratory based set-up and its availability is also constraint among mental health professionals. The efficiency to use VR technology is needed to be explored before giving the access to the professionals. It requires more proficiency and practice to demonstrate and apply the functions related to devices. Another factor which is restricting the use of VR technology is the hesitancy towards the provinces of technology in therapists and client. Lack of competency and trust on technology has also limited its use. In future, development of technology in relation to therapeutic measure looks promising, and use of mixed reality would be the preferred way to reach out people. The VR augmented intervention process would be less complicated with huge scope of implications in different clinical population.

SUMMARY

- Availability of VR in the field of psychological research has increased and it encourages the control over the environment through stimulus representation and response protocols in more ecologically valid way.
- In therapeutic intervention, VR can create complex scenarios as stimulating exposure with absolute precision with limited time. VR is an advanced technology which includes multimodal sensory input and increases sense of immersion in virtual presented environment in less compound way.
- VR system describes the virtual environment in presence of details of technical capabilities. It elicits intense emotional responses associated with real life stressful situation quickly. VR improves the relationship between client and therapist within less than expected time limit (Jensen and Konradsen, 2018).
- VR technology has become more accessible and available to the population in this decade. The cost of technological assignments has been decreased with the availability of hardware and the demand of dependency of virtual environment emerged massively.
- Positive research findings and acceptability of this mode among normal an patient population has been surged the need of usage of virtual environment and practice of psychotherapy skills.

- The excitement around the VR environment is suggesting high requirement of VR and in turn lesser cost value of the technology. It provides opportunity to reproduce real-life scenarios in more adaptive and controlled way depending on the individual needs of the client.
- VR is a tool that facilitates the application of psychological evaluation in more affordable and available way (Coburn et.al.,2017).

CONCLUSION

VR has huge potential to aid people overcome mental health problems. Clinicians use VR to provide a new human-computer interaction paradigm in which users are active participants within a computer generated three-dimensional virtual world. VR based therapeutic program may allow repetition of activities with minimum or no changes and make the client/patient more comfortable with the situation. Also, VR based cognitive rehabilitation program can be customized based on individual's specific strength and weakness to get the maximum benefits.

However, basic feasibility issues need to be addressed for this technology to be reasonably and efficiently applied to the cognitive rehabilitation (CR) of persons with mental illness or neurological disorders. Despite important scientific and engineering activity in VR based systems for cognitive and motor rehabilitation, most studies to date have evaluated interventions that were designed to address motor impairments. There are only few randomized controlled studies that include cognitive rehabilitation and/or cognition assessment. Research findings are encouraging but further research is needed, especially to clarify if VR, and more concretely training through the simulation of activities of daily living, is equivalent or more effective than conventional cognitive training.

REFERENCES

Adama, V. S., Schindler, B., & Schmid, T. (2019, September). Using time domain and pearson's correlation to predict attention focus in autistic spectrum disorder from EEG P300 components. In *Mediterranean Conference on Medical and Biological Engineering and Computing* (pp. 1890-1893). Springer.

Arlati, S., Greci, L., Mondellini, M., Zangiacomi, A., Di Santo, S. G., Franchini, F., & Vezzoli, A. (2017, November). A virtual reality-based physical and cognitive training system aimed at preventing symptoms of dementia. In *International Conference on Wireless Mobile Communication and Healthcare* (pp. 117-125). Springer.

Bailey, J., Bailenson, J. N., Won, A. S., Flora, J., & Armel, K. C. (2012, October). Presence and memory: immersive virtual reality effects on cued recall. In *Proceedings of the International Society for Presence Research Annual Conference* (pp. 24-26). Academic Press.

Benedetti, F., Volpi, N. C., Parisi, L., & Sartori, G. (2014, June). Attention training with an easy–to–use brain computer interface. In *International Conference on Virtual, Augmented and Mixed Reality* (pp. 236-247). Springer. 10.1007/978-3-319-07464-1_22

Burdea, G. C. (2003). Virtual rehabilitation—Benefits and challenges. *Methods of Information in Medicine*, *42*(5), 519–523. doi:10.1055-0038-1634378 PMID:14654886

Cappon, D., Jahanshahi, M., & Bisiacchi, P. (2016). Value and efficacy of transcranial direct current stimulation in the cognitive rehabilitation: A critical review since 2000. *Frontiers in Neuroscience, 10*, 157. doi:10.3389/fnins.2016.00157 PMID:27147949

Chua, S. I. L., Tan, N. C., Wong, W. T., Allen, J. C. Jr, Quah, J. H. M., Malhotra, R., & Østbye, T. (2019). Virtual reality for screening of cognitive function in older persons: Comparative study. *Journal of Medical Internet Research, 21*(8), e14821. doi:10.2196/14821 PMID:31373274

Cicerone, K. D., Dahlberg, C., Kalmar, K., Langenbahn, D. M., Malec, J. F., Bergquist, T. F., & Morse, P. A. (2000). Evidence-based cognitive rehabilitation: Recommendations for clinical practice. *Archives of Physical Medicine and Rehabilitation, 81*(12), 1596–1615. doi:10.1053/apmr.2000.19240 PMID:11128897

Climent, G., Rodríguez, C., García, T., Areces, D., Mejías, M., Aierbe, A., Moreno, M., Cueto, E., Castellá, J., & Feli González, M. (2021). New virtual reality tool (Nesplora Aquarium) for assessing attention and working memory in adults: A normative study. *Applied Neuropsychology. Adult, 28*(4), 403–415. doi:10.1080/23279095.2019.1646745 PMID:31382773

Coburn, J. Q., Freeman, I., & Salmon, J. L. (2017). A review of the capabilities of current low-cost virtual reality technology and its potential to enhance the design process. *Journal of Computing and Information Science in Engineering, 17*(3), 031013. doi:10.1115/1.4036921

Coleman, B., Marion, S., Rizzo, A., Turnbull, J., & Nolty, A. (2019). Virtual reality assessment of classroom–related attention: An ecologically relevant approach to evaluating the effectiveness of working memory training. *Frontiers in Psychology, 10*, 1851. doi:10.3389/fpsyg.2019.01851 PMID:31481911

Cushman, L. A., Stein, K., & Duffy, C. J. (2008). Detecting navigational deficits in cognitive aging and Alzheimer disease using virtual reality. *Neurology, 71*(12), 888–895. doi:10.1212/01.wnl.0000326262.67613. fe PMID:18794491

De Luca, R., Portaro, S., Le Cause, M., De Domenico, C., Maggio, M. G., Cristina Ferrera, M., & Calabrò, R. S. (2020). Cognitive rehabilitation using immersive virtual reality at young age: A case report on traumatic brain injury. *Applied Neuropsychology. Child, 9*(3), 282–287. doi:10.1080/21622965.201 9.1576525 PMID:30838889

Diamond, A. (2013). Executive functions. *Annual Review of Psychology, 64*(1), 135–168. doi:10.1146/annurev-psych-113011-143750 PMID:23020641

Diaz Baquero, A. A., Dröes, R. M., Perea Bartolomé, M. V., Irazoki, E., Toribio-Guzmán, J. M., Franco-Martín, M. A., & van der Roest, H. (2021). Methodological Designs Applied in the Development of Computer-Based Training Programs for the Cognitive Rehabilitation in People with Mild Cognitive Impairment (MCI) and Mild Dementia. Systematic Review. *Journal of Clinical Medicine, 10*(6), 1222. doi:10.3390/jcm10061222 PMID:33809445

Dores, R. A., Carvalho, I., Abreu, C., Nunes, J., Leitão, M., & Castro-Caldas, A. (2009). *Virtual Reality: Application to cognitive rehabilitation acquired brain injury.* Academic Press.

Duarte, M. L., Santos, L. R., Júnior, J. G., & Peccin, M. S. (2020). Learning anatomy by virtual reality and augmented reality. A scope review. *Morphologie, 104*(347), 254–266. doi:10.1016/j.morpho.2020.08.004 PMID:32972816

Elbogen, E. B., Dennis, P. A., Van Voorhees, E. E., Blakey, S. M., Johnson, J. L., Johnson, S. C., & Belger, A. (2019). Cognitive rehabilitation with mobile technology and social support for veterans with TBI and PTSD: A randomized clinical trial. *The Journal of Head Trauma Rehabilitation*, *34*(1), 1–10. doi:10.1097/HTR.0000000000000435 PMID:30169439

Eng, C. M., Calkosz, D. M., Yang, S. Y., Williams, N. C., Thiessen, E. D., & Fisher, A. V. (2020, June). Doctoral colloquium—enhancing brain plasticity and cognition utilizing immersive technology and virtual reality contexts for gameplay. In *2020 6th International Conference of the Immersive Learning Research Network (iLRN)* (pp. 395-398). IEEE.

George, S., Clark, M., & Crotty, M. (2008). Validation of the Visual Recognition Slide Test with stroke: A component of the New South Wales occupational therapy off-road driver rehabilitation program. *Australian Occupational Therapy Journal*, *55*(3), 172–179. doi:10.1111/j.1440-1630.2007.00699.x PMID:20887459

Halder, S., & Mahato, A. K. (2018). Cognition in ageing: implications for assessment and intervention. In Handbook of Research on Geriatric Health, Treatment, and Care (pp. 118-133). IGI Global. doi:10.4018/978-1-5225-3480-8.ch007

Howett, D., Castegnaro, A., Krzywicka, K., Hagman, J., Marchment, D., Henson, R., Rio, M., King, J.A., Burgess, N., & Chan, D. (2019) Differentiation of mild cognitive impairment using an entorhinal cortex-based test of virtual reality navigation. *Brain, 142*(6), 1751-1766. doi:10.1093/brain/awz116

Irazoki, E., Contreras-Somoza, L. M., Toribio-Guzmán, J. M., Jenaro-Río, C., van der Roest, H., & Franco-Martín, M. A. (2020). Technologies for cognitive training and cognitive rehabilitation for people with mild cognitive impairment and dementia. A systematic review. *Frontiers in Psychology*, *11*, 648. doi:10.3389/fpsyg.2020.00648 PMID:32373018

Jensen, L., & Konradsen, F. (2018). A review of the use of virtual reality head-mounted displays in education and training. *Education and Information Technologies*, *23*(4), 1515–1529. doi:10.100710639-017-9676-0

Jin, R., Pilozzi, A., & Huang, X. (2020). Current Cognition Tests, Potential Virtual Reality Applications, and Serious Games in Cognitive Assessment and Non-Pharmacological Therapy for Neurocognitive Disorders. *Journal of Clinical Medicine*, *9*(10), 3287. doi:10.3390/jcm9103287 PMID:33066242

Jonsdottir, J., Baglio, F., Gindri, P., Isernia, S., Castiglioni, C., Gramigna, C., Palumbo, G., Pagliari, C., Di Tella, S., Perini, G., Bowman, T., Salza, M., & Molteni, F. (2021). Virtual Reality for Motor and Cognitive Rehabilitation From Clinic to Home: A Pilot Feasibility and Efficacy Study for Persons With Chronic Stroke. *Frontiers in Neurology*, *12*, 440. doi:10.3389/fneur.2021.601131 PMID:33897579

Ke, F., Moon, J., & Sokolikj, Z. (2020). Virtual reality–based social skills training for children with autism spectrum disorder. *Journal of Special Education Technology*, 0162643420945603.

Kenwright, B. (2019). *Virtual Reality: Where Have We Been? Where Are We Now? and Where Are We Going?* Academic Press.

Koning, A. H., Rousian, M., Verwoerd-Dikkeboom, C. M., Goedknegt, L., Steegers, E. A., & van der Spek, P. J. (2009, January). V-scope: design and implementation of an immersive and desktop virtual reality volume visualization system. In MMVR (pp. 136-138). Academic Press.

Ku, K. Y. (2009). Assessing students' critical thinking performance: Urging for measurements using multi-response format. *Thinking Skills and Creativity, 4*(1), 70–76. doi:10.1016/j.tsc.2009.02.001

Lee, J. H., Ku, J., Cho, W., Hahn, W. Y., Kim, I. Y., Lee, S. M., Kang, Y., Kim, D. Y., Yu, T., Wiederhold, B. K., Wiederhold, M. D., & Kim, S. I. (2003). A virtual reality system for the assessment and rehabilitation of the activities of daily living. *Cyberpsychology & Behavior, 6*(4), 383–388. doi:10.1089/109493103322278763 PMID:14511450

Lim, J. E., Wong, W. T., Teh, T. A., Lim, S. H., Allen, J. C. Jr, Quah, J. H. M., ... Tan, N. C. (2020). A Fully-Immersive and Automated Virtual Reality System to Assess the Six Domains of Cognition: Protocol for a Feasibility Study. *Frontiers in Aging Neuroscience, 12*. PMID:33488382

Lin, L. P. L., Huang, S. C. L., & Ho, Y. C. (2020). Could virtual reality effectively market slow travel in a heritage destination? *Tourism Management, 78*, 104027. doi:10.1016/j.tourman.2019.104027

Mancuso, V., Stramba-Badiale, C., Cavedoni, S., Pedroli, E., Cipresso, P., & Riva, G. (2020). Virtual reality meets non-invasive brain stimulation: Integrating two methods for cognitive rehabilitation of mild cognitive impairment. *Frontiers in Neurology, 11*, 1117. doi:10.3389/fneur.2020.566731 PMID:33117261

Mancuso, V., Stramba-Badiale, C., Cavedoni, S., Pedroli, E., Cipresso, P., & Riva, G. (2020). Virtual reality meets non-invasive brain stimulation: Integrating two methods for cognitive rehabilitation of mild cognitive impairment. *Frontiers in Neurology, 11*, 1117. doi:10.3389/fneur.2020.566731 PMID:33117261

North, M. M., & North, S. M. (2017). Virtual reality therapy for treatment of psychological disorders. In *Career Paths in Telemental Health* (pp. 263–268). Springer. doi:10.1007/978-3-319-23736-7_27

Ord, A. S., Shura, R. D., Curtiss, G., Armistead-Jehle, P., Vanderploeg, R. D., Bowles, A. O., & Cooper, D. B. (2021). Number of concussions does not affect treatment response to cognitive rehabilitation interventions following mild TBI in military service members. *Archives of Clinical Neuropsychology, 36*(5), 850–856. doi:10.1093/arclin/acaa119 PMID:33264387

Park, M. J., Kim, D. J., Lee, U., Na, E. J., & Jeon, H. J. (2019). A Literature Overview of Virtual Reality (VR) in Treatment of Psychiatric Disorders: Recent Advances and Limitations. *Frontiers in Psychiatry, 10*, 505. doi:10.3389/fpsyt.2019.00505 PMID:31379623

Parsons, T. D., Bowerly, T., Buckwalter, J. G., & Rizzo, A. A. (2007). A controlled clinical comparison of attention performance in children with ADHD in a virtual reality classroom compared to standard neuropsychological methods. *Child Neuropsychology, 13*(4), 363–381. doi:10.1080/13825580600943473 PMID:17564852

Parsons, T. D., & Rizzo, A. A. (2008). Initial validation of a virtual environment for assessment of memory functioning: Virtual reality cognitive performance assessment test. *Cyberpsychology & Behavior, 11*(1), 17–25. doi:10.1089/cpb.2007.9934 PMID:18275308

Plancher, G., Tirard, A., Gyselinck, V., Nicolas, S., & Piolino, P. (2012). Using virtual reality to characterize episodic memory profiles in amnestic mild cognitive impairment and Alzheimer's disease: Influence of active and passive encoding. *Neuropsychologia, 50*(5), 592–602. doi:10.1016/j.neuropsychologia.2011.12.013 PMID:22261400

Riddoch, M., & Humphreys, G. W. (1994). *Cognitive neuropsychology and cognitive rehabilitation.* Lawrence Erlbaum Associates, Inc.

Rizzo, A. A., Schultheis, M., Kerns, K. A., & Mateer, C. (2004). Analysis of assets for virtual reality applications in neuropsychology. *Neuropsychological Rehabilitation, 14*(1-2), 207–239. doi:10.1080/09602010343000183

Rose, F. D., Brooks, B. M., & Rizzo, A. A. (2005). Virtual reality in brain damage rehabilitation. *Cyberpsychology & Behavior, 8*(3), 241–262. doi:10.1089/cpb.2005.8.241 PMID:15971974

Shahabi, C., Yang, K., Yoon, H., Rizzo, A. A., McLaughlin, M., Marsh, T., & Mun, M. (2007). Immersidata analysis: Four case studies. *Computer, 40*(7), 45–52. doi:10.1109/MC.2007.245

Sharma, P., & Halder, S. (2021). Cognition, Quality of Life And Mood State In Mild Traumatic Brain Injury: A Case Study. *Indian Journal of Mental Health, 8*(1), 112. doi:10.30877/IJMH.8.1.2021.112-116

Smallwood, J., Davies, J. B., Heim, D., Finnigan, F., Sudberry, M., O'Connor, R., & Obonsawin, M. (2004). Subjective experience and the attentional lapse: Task engagement and disengagement during sustained attention. *Consciousness and Cognition, 13*(4), 657–690. doi:10.1016/j.concog.2004.06.003 PMID:15522626

Sohlberg, M. M., & Mateer, C. A. (1989). *Introduction to cognitive rehabilitation: Theory and practice.* The Guilford Press.

Sohlberg, M. M., & Mateer, C. A. (Eds.). (2001). *Cognitive rehabilitation: An integrative neuropsychological approach.* Guilford Press.

Stanton, D., Foreman, N., & Wilson, P. N. (1998, January 1). Uses of virtual reality in clinical training: Developing the spatial skills of children with mobility impairments. *Studies in Health Technology and Informatics*, 219–232. PMID:10350923

Valmaggia, L. R., Latif, L., Kempton, M. J., & Rus-Calafell, M. (2016). Virtual reality in the psychological treatment for mental health problems: An systematic review of recent evidence. *Psychiatry Research, 236*, 189–195. doi:10.1016/j.psychres.2016.01.015 PMID:26795129

Wilson, B. A. (2002). Towards a comprehensive model of cognitive rehabilitation. *Neuropsychological Rehabilitation, 12*(2), 97–110. doi:10.1080/09602010244000020

Wilson, B. A., & Evans, J. (2020). Does cognitive rehabilitation work? Clinical and economic considerations and outcomes. In *Clinical neuropsychology and cost outcome research* (pp. 329–349). Psychology Press. doi:10.4324/9781315787039-23

Windman, V. (2012). iPad Apps for Students with Autism. *Tech & Learning, 32*(7), 28.

Wohlgenannt, I., Simons, A., & Stieglitz, S. (2020). Virtual reality. *Business & Information Systems Engineering, 62*(5), 455–461. doi:10.100712599-020-00658-9

Chapter 14
The Future of Virtual Reality and Deep Learning in Visual Field Testing

Scott E. Lee
University of California, Berkeley, USA

Angelbert Ramos
University of California, Berkeley, USA

Deborah Chen
University of California, Berkeley, USA

Varun Shravah
University of California, Los Angeles, USA

Nikita Chigullapally
University of California, Berkeley, USA

Trinity Rico
University of California, Berkeley, USA

Suzy Chung
University of California, Santa Cruz, USA

Michael Youn
University of California, Berkeley, USA

Allan Lu Lee
University of California, Berkeley, USA

Diane Nguyen
University of California, Berkeley, USA

ABSTRACT

The visual field (VF) examination is a useful clinical tool for monitoring a variety of ocular diseases. Despite its wide utility in eye clinics, the test as currently conducted is subject to an array of issues that interfere in obtaining accurate results. Visual field exams of patients suffering from additional ocular conditions are often unreliable due to interference between the comorbid diseases. To improve upon these shortcomings, virtual reality (VR) and deep learning are being explored as potential solutions. Virtual reality has been incorporated into novel visual field exams to provide a portable, 3D exam experience. Deep learning, a specialization of machine learning, has been used in conjunction with VR, such as in the iGlaucoma application, to limit subjective bias occurring from patients' eye movements. This chapter seeks to analyze and critique how VR and deep learning can augment the visual field experience by improving accuracy, reducing subjective bias, and ultimately, providing clinicians with a greater capacity to enhance patient outcomes.

DOI: 10.4018/978-1-7998-8371-5.ch014

INTRODUCTION

Virtual reality is one of the most promising recent developments in ocular health. From allowing patients to observe ocular diseases affecting their vision to training aspiring physicians in treating ocular diseases, virtual reality has reimagined many aspects of health, including the visual field test. The visual field is one of the main ocular tests used to measure a patient's central and peripheral field of vision and its progression over time. Many ophthalmologists and optometrists use this type of test to detect and monitor progressive ocular diseases, primarily glaucoma. Moreover, this test can further be used to evaluate other medical conditions such as cataracts, macular degeneration, diabetes, stroke, side effects of medications, and more. Despite the versatility and heavy dependence of the test in the medical field, there are a range of issues such as consistent unreliability from the patient's responses and compliance as well as the exclusion of patients with mobility issues and psychological issues. This book chapter will further explain the issues with the current visual field test and how virtual reality and deep learning have the potential to augment the exam to allow for a more accurate portrayal of a patient's visual field to improve patient care.

BACKGROUND

To understand what the visual field is, a comprehensive understanding of vision is necessary. Vision is the ability to process external information taken in via the eyes and transferred to the brain through the optic nerve. When light enters the eye, it travels through the pupil and is refracted by the lens. Eventually the light is projected onto the retina, the functional layer of the eye rich in light-sensitive photoreceptor cells that enable visual perception. The two main photoreceptors are called rods and cones, which are responsible for low light vision and color vision, respectively. When photoreceptors are stimulated by variations in lighting in the ambient environment, the signals are transduced down the optic nerve to communicate this information with the brain. The optic nerve meets with the lateral geniculate nucleus (LGN) in the thalamus to pass on the information to the occipital lobe. The occipital lobe is the associated area of the brain that converts and interprets these signals into robust visual information, allowing us to navigate the world around us (Smith & Czyz, 2020).

The visual field involves the whole area that can be seen by both eyes. Much like the right and left sides of the brain, there are two visual fields: a right visual field and a left visual field. Vision is perceived contralaterally, meaning that the perception of the right visual field is taken in by the opposite side, namely the left side of photoreceptors within the back of the eye and vice versa for the left visual field as shown in Figure 1 (Nieto, M., n.d). While the two fields may seem separate from each other, they superimposed upon one another in the central field to allow depth perception and overall improved visual acuity. When the information from each field comes into the brain through the optic nerve, the fields are interpreted at an area of the brain called the optic chiasm, in which the information coming from the right visual field is transferred to the left occipital lobe and the information from the left visual field goes to the right occipital lobe. In the end, this complex sensory process allows us to see with an in-depth visual field and to interact with the world around us. This comprehensive understanding of vision allows us to create tests to measure how an average individual can see on a day-to-day basis.

Figure 1. A diagram of the human visual pathway and how it is perceived contralaterally (Nieto, M., n.d).

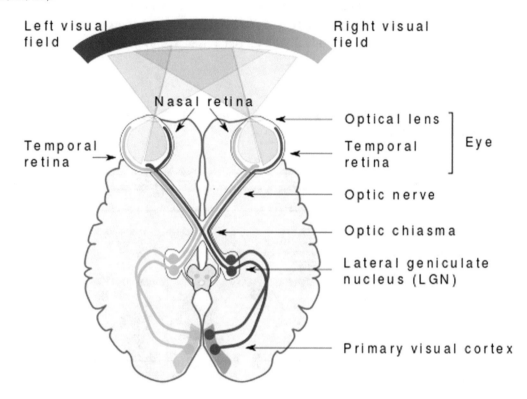

To quantitatively measure the visual field, a test called automated perimetry was developed in the 1970s. This test can be conducted in two distinct ways: kinetically or statically. Kinetic perimetry requires a trained technician to move a physical stimulus in and out of a user's visual field. A user's visual field is then able to be outlined based on the location at which a stimulus is first seen. On the other hand, most modern automated perimeters, such as the Humphrey Visual Field Analyzer, perform static perimetry: the stimulus remains stationary and is instead presented at specific locations with varying intensities and sizes. Both kinetic and static perimetry are reliable, important tools in elucidating field defects and identifying glaucomatous visual field defects in patients. As of today, static perimetry is the only method that has been automated as the standard automated perimetry (SAP), making this test the gold standard for visual field testing.

The most common standard automated perimetry test in the United States is the Humphrey Visual Field test. This test involves the patient fixing their vision on a central fixation light in a curved bowl while pressing a handheld button whenever a flashing light is seen within the bowl. This flashing light is projected at multiple locations around the interior of the bowl at various light intensities. Starting from low intensity, the light is made brighter until the patient can perceive the light and the threshold light sensitivity level of that location in the patient's vision can be determined. The procedure is repeated at other locations until the patient's entire visual field can be generalized and tested. In case the patient moves during the exam, the machine includes an eye gaze tracker and a head tracker with a movable and automated chin rest to account for the patient's movement. The machine also accounted for blind spots and false positives to ensure the accuracy of the results. The visual field test is usually conducted with the supervision of a technician, on a perimetry machine in a dark room. After the patient completes the test, the technician shares the test results to the physician for further patient care and potential diagnosis. Figure 2 and Figure 3 ("Humphrey...", 2013) shows two common printouts of the 24-2 Humphrey Visual Field Test between a healthy individual without diagnosed visual field defects and a glaucoma suspect individual.

Figure 2. A Central 24-2 Threshold Test of a healthy patient's left eye that outlines key aspects of the patient's visual field test results
("Humphrey...", 2013).

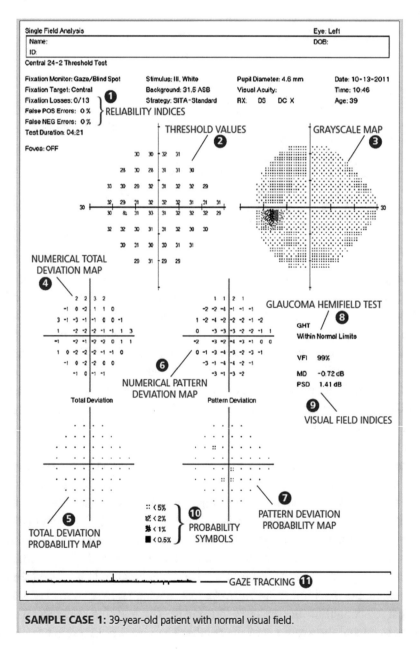

SAMPLE CASE 1: 39-year-old patient with normal visual field.

Figure 3. A Central 24-2 Threshold Test of a glaucoma suspect patient's left eye that outlines key aspects of the patient's visual field test result
("Humphrey...", 2013).

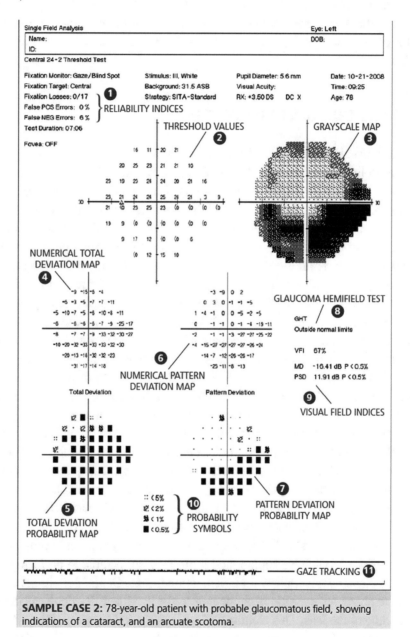

In recent years, different algorithms have been introduced to the Humphrey Visual Field to make it more accurate and efficient. The Swedish Interactive Thresholding Algorithm (SITA), introduced in 2009, has allowed for rapid analysis of results using Bayesian statistical properties (Ng et. al., 2009). SITA Humphrey Visual Field tests are focused on testing stimuli that are likely near a threshold of responses (Carroll & Johnson, 2013). This optimization algorithm also takes into account a user's age to determine perimetry thresholds at specific visual field locations. Results have shown that a user's visual field can be captured in half the time as the standard Humphrey Visual Field, decreasing user fatigue and increasing test reliability (Ng et. al., 2009). Today, SITA is widely used in computer automated Humphrey Visual Fields, although there is still a tremendous amount of potential to improve upon. Though modern technology has been exponentially growing, perimetry tests such as the Humphrey Visual Field have fallen behind.

ISSUES WITH THE CURRENT VISUAL FIELD

While the Humphrey Visual Field provides clinicians with vital information regarding patients' peripheral vision, the test is far from flawless. Indeed, the test as currently performed in ophthalmology and optometry clinics can suffer from a high degree of unreliability. The typical visual field examination currently requires patients to place their heads at the face of the machine and remain as still as possible for five to ten minutes at a time. Meanwhile, the patient focuses intently on various blinking lights inside of the machine and clicks a button for every light the patient can perceive in their peripheral vision. From the evaluation of 1091 visual field exams on the Humphrey visual field, only 54% of the exams were proven reliable. Furthermore, 43% of all testing were found to be unreliable due to a fixation loss of greater than 20%. This data shows that the majority of the unreliability of the test is due to the machine-focused orientation of the exam (Peracha et. al., 2013). This setup already showcases a flaw in the Humphrey Visual Field: the test precludes certain individuals who are unable to withstand the demands of the test. This includes patients with back and spinal issues who may be unable to position their heads in the proper orientation as required by the test. Patients diagnosed with disorders affecting their ability to sit still, such as Parkinson's Disease and cerebral palsy, or those who are claustrophobic will also be at a disadvantage. In terms of stamina, patients who have hypoxia with a limited oxygen tank supply or are lethargic may not complete the test, which can last from five to ten minutes for each eye. Moreover, because visual fields are designed so that an individual must place both their chin and forehead in a specific orientation, the machine cannot accurately fit certain head shapes and accommodate religious headwear such as turbans. Performing the test on such individuals often results in unreliable or invalid test results through no fault of the patient. The Humphrey Visual Field has a clear issue in that it is unable to accommodate every patient, especially those with various ocular conditions.

Patients with ocular conditions including dense cataracts, pterygium, and eyelid conditions such as ptosis, dermatochalasis, ectropion, entropion, and more may not be able to perform well in the visual field due to their vision being impeded by their ocular conditions. Ocular conditions can cause a partial loss of vision due to abnormal conditions happening to the eye itself. Particularly, dense cataracts are caused by the clouding of the lens. This clouding of the lens blurs the vision of the affected eye and can reduce the accuracy with which a patient can perform the visual field test. This decrease in accuracy can cause a misinterpretation of the visual field or even lead to a misdiagnosis. The difference between having dense cataracts compared to no cataracts is significant enough to impact the results of a visual field test. Through studies done on a person's visual field before and after cataract extraction surgery, the juxtaposition of patients' results demonstrates that dense cataracts can cause changes in one's vision (Chen & Budnez, 1998).

Abnormalities of the eyelid can also cause partial vision loss that can negatively affect a patient's visual field performance. Thus these abnormalities can decrease the diagnostic capability and reliability of the test for conditions characterized by visual field defects. Unilateral eyelid drooping as a result of ptosis or dermatochalasis, for instance, can impede detection in the superior portion of the patient's visual field. The patient's poor performance may be attributed to their lid condition and can mask early glaucomatous visual field loss, which by its very nature is subtle and easily missed by visual field analyzers (Brenton et. al., 1986; Broadway, 2012). Again, this data suggests that the accuracy of the Humphrey Visual Field and the diagnostic interpretations of its results can be falsified by comorbid oculoplastic conditions. Ocular conditions are not the only area in which the Humphrey Visual Field falls short as it also depends on the technician that administers the test as well.

The reliance of the Humphrey Visual Field on a technician's ability to correctly administer the test and on a patient's cooperation should not be overlooked, as it is undoubtedly one of the most subjective tests in ophthalmology and optometry clinics. Unlike the Humphrey Visual Field, other routine ocular examinations, such as optical coherence tomography (OCT) or fundus photography, depend nearly entirely on the technician's competence and ability to obtain results, imparting a great degree of objectivity in those tests. The Humphrey Visual Field, on the other hand, burdens the patient with a significant degree of responsibility for obtaining good results, adding a degree of subjectivity to the exam, and reducing its overall reliability. The issue with the Humphrey Visual Field is unreliability because it is a long non-user centered test. The test provides a unique insight into the patient's perception, unlike other ocular examinations. With a heavy dependence on the visual field exam to understand a patient's vision and diagnosis, there is a need to reduce the unreliability resulting from the test as currently performed.

Furthermore, the test is quite costly in terms of resources and time to conduct, as the visual field analyzer machines cost thousands of dollars and the test must be conducted at a medical office under the supervision of a trained technician. The execution of the test also relies in part on the technician's ability to properly convey instructions to the patient. If the technician is unable to effectively communicate the instructions of the exam, as can often be the case if the patient speaks a foreign language or is hearing-impaired, the patient's subsequent lack of understanding may confound the results of the examination, further contributing to its unreliability. An example is a process of ensuring the patient is focused on the fixation point. The machine will flash light into the blindspot of the patient and if the patient's eye is uncentered, then these flashes will be perceived. While technicians are trained to identify and realign the patient, if their instructions are not perceived clearly by the patient, this issue can continue to occur throughout the examination. With the Humphrey Visual Field not being a user-centered test, there can be undetectable errors. In the case of patients who suffer from a mobile disability, the spinal and back strain can add latent variables that hinder test results. It is difficult to objectively deny or verify this claim as it is difficult to test the same patient in their current state versus a seemingly healthy state. With the augmentation of virtual reality and deep learning, these strains can be reduced and the full potential effects of a patient's disability can be studied under the visual field.

VIRTUAL REALITY AND DEEP LEARNING AS SOLUTIONS

Virtual reality addresses the limitations of an in-office visual field machine by accommodating the needs of patients who are normally excluded from the test through the use of a portable virtual reality visual field machine. With the advent of smartphones, tablets, and virtual reality devices, patients can take visual field tests by using mobile applications such as the Moorfields Motion Displacement Test and Melbourne Rapid Fields test (Chang, 2021). These mobile applications are useful for patients who may have difficulty visiting their physicians, as was the case during the COVID-19 pandemic (Ou, 2020). A new issue that arose during the COVID-19 pandemic was the greater number of patients who wore poorly fitted face masks during their standard automated perimetry (SAP) tests, leading to lower test reliability, higher fixation loss, and more false positives, especially since the trial lens of the machine was prone to fog up during the test (Bayram et. al., 2021). Virtual reality devices can be used to overcome these kinds of challenges by augmenting test result accuracy among patients, including those who wear any type of face mask and who can self administer at home.

With the availability of virtual reality goggles and virtual reality programs, patients can take portable visual field exams, allowing patients with mobility issues to take the visual field exam without head and upper body restrictions. Because these novel methods only require goggles and a smartphone with the installed program, administering visual field tests can be more cost-effective as well as more accessible. Unlike other methods of performing the visual field, virtual reality goggles can accommodate the patient's glasses, allowing for patient comfort and a greater capacity for patients to view the various lights within the machine, creating a more accurate response rate.

Because virtual reality can be utilized to simulate a 3D visual field, which is a marked improvement from the current 2D visual field testing, it can help diagnose conditions such as glaucoma and can accurately measure one's visual field. One of the common issues with 2D visual field testing is that patients can often gaze around within the machine rather than fixating on a central point. This leads to false positives and unclear results, as patients end up utilizing their central vision rather than peripheral vision to view the lights. Patients whose peripheral vision has been affected by glaucoma and other diseases tend to unconsciously scan their surroundings more to compensate for this loss. Kasneci, Black, and Wood (2017) studied how glaucoma patients increased their eye movement and had more saccades (rapid eye movements) when reading, driving, walking, and other everyday activities. Eye trackers such as the Pupil Labs eye-tracker, Dikablis Mobile eye-tracker, and Tobii Glasses can be used to improve current virtual reality visual field tests by precisely following the patient's gaze using a more standardized and calibrated reference coordinate system. An electroencephalography device can measure brain activity and electrical signals in the brain, which is especially beneficial for patients who are not able to click a button during the test. Currently, there is an ongoing longitudinal clinical trial using an electroencephalography device called nGoggle to measure the visual fields of patients who are diagnosed with glaucoma, age-related macular degeneration, and other ocular diseases (nGoggle, 2020). Several studies in recent years have sought to test the diagnostic viability of virtual reality devices for glaucomatous testing. Tsapakis and colleagues investigated the effectiveness of using virtual reality glasses in visual field testing and found that the results were highly correlated with that of the 24-2 Humphrey perimeter visual field among patients who were diagnosed with glaucoma (2017).

In another study conducted by Sayed and colleagues (2021), a virtual reality head-mounted display (HMD) showed potential for quantifying monocular and binocular visual field defects comparable to defects identified by a standard automated perimeter. The C3 field analyzer (CFA), which is a virtual reality head-mounted visual field testing machine, has been proven to work relatively well in screening for glaucoma with results comparable to that of the Humphrey Visual Field in identifying glaucoma-suspect patients (Mees, 2020). These studies validate that virtual reality visual fields can be a viable alternative to the standard automated perimetry used in many clinics today.

Similarly, another study conducted by Papageorgiou et.al. (2012) presented a virtual reality driving simulation and eye tracker to explore the connection between real-time eye tracking and visual field defects. By simulating common activities such as driving using virtual reality, researchers may grasp a better understanding of visual field deficits in glaucoma patients and how these deficits affect their peripheral and central vision loss in their daily behavior. This information can be implemented into designing more accurate eye tracking programs in the virtual reality visual field tests, as well as contribute towards new safety measures and customized treatment plans for glaucoma patients.

Virtual reality has also provided new insight into how a patient's visual acuity can affect their peripheral and central vision. In one study, Chow-Wing-Bom and colleagues (2020) created a virtual reality simulation where patients were instructed to perform a visually guided action (i.e. finding a phone) to determine if peripheral vision is largely limited to the "better" eye. Through the use of virtual reality, Chow-Wing-Bom and their colleagues found that as they diminished the vision in the "better eye," there was significantly more head and eye movement to compensate for the loss. Furthermore, when peripheral impairment was only attributed to one eye, there was an increase in response times by only 25% despite greater than 200% vision loss. These findings using virtual reality give physicians new insight into how the worse eye still contributed important visual information towards everyday tasks (Chow-Wing-Bom, 2020). From this study, physicians can have a better understanding of how visual field defects in each eye interact with each other, especially for glaucoma patients whose peripheral vision is greatly affected and sometimes only in one eye.

Even though virtual reality tests have improved the accuracy and quality of visual field tests, it is possible that virtual reality-enhanced visual field tests can still be subjective, similar to SAP tests. To increase the accuracy of the virtual reality visual field test results, researchers are implementing deep learning data collection and analysis to take these advancements a step further to make the visual field exam more objective.

DEEP LEARNING IN VISUAL FIELD TESTING

Deep learning is a rapidly growing field that can assist healthcare workers in potentially diagnosing or predicting future visual field tests from previous visual field tests. As a branch under machine learning that attempts to mimic the human brain in processing large and complex data, deep learning can find patterns in and learn from unstructured data by integrating old knowledge with new knowledge to make new conclusions. Thus, deep learning in conjunction with virtual reality can allow the creation of exams that adapt to each patient's mental and physical capabilities. With a powerful tool like deep learning, clinicians will be able to receive and analyze data, mapping the potential progression of a patient's eye condition. In addition, it will allow us to compare potential interventions, such as eye drop medication versus surgery, to identify which intervention will most improve a patient's vision and to create specialized treatment plans for each patient.

This field of study can play a critical role in addressing some of the previously mentioned issues with the current visual field exam. The largest confounding factor in the visual field exam is a patient's tendency to look away from the fixation light in the center of the machine. However, a virtual reality machine that uses deep learning can adapt to the patient's shifting gaze and move the patient's head or adjust the lights in the bowl so that the patient's gaze is always centered on the fixation light. Researchers are applying the deep learning YOLO (You only look once) model for object detection technology to create a visible-light pupil tracking system. The proposed system first collects data in the form of visual-light images of eyes and creates data sets which are then interpreted by a deep learning network designed for pupil detection. Using a series of neural networks, it is possible that deep learning is trained to detect pupils better and guess their next position. Lastly, the network will be trained with many datasets and calibrated so that it is able to accurately predict pupil locations and gaze points (Ou et al, 2021). This can be applied to the visual field exam, especially for patients who have a hard time looking straight at the fixation dot. The proposed method can be integrated into the exam so that the virtual reality system can predict where the patient's shifting gaze will look next and center the fixation dot so it lands where the patient's gaze will land. This keeps the patient's gaze fixated on the fixation light during the whole exam and helps avoid unreliability due to fixation loss.

Secondly, deep learning can eliminate the communication barrier between the patients and test administrators. Deep learning was used to create virtual assistants such as Siri and Alexa. The companies that created these virtual assistants used a technology called spoken dialogue systems to design and improve the assistants as they interact with and learn from humans. However, there is a new proposed technology called multimodal dialogue systems that can combine speech, image, video, touch, manual gestures, gaze, and head and body movement to design the next generation of virtual assistants (Kepuska & Bohouta, 2018). Having multiple entry routes for information expands the already vast dialogue knowledge base coded within the virtual assistants, which is particularly important for the medical field. The visual field exam, for instance, can be administered without a technician. The virtual assistant would be able to communicate with the patient to give the instructions necessary to administer the test, pause as requested by the patient, monitor and guide the patient throughout the test, and answer any questions the patient has during the visual field exam.

Another advantage of having a virtual test administrator is that there are no limitations on which language the test is administered in. Currently, an office may only be able to accommodate 3 or 4 different languages, however, with a virtual test administrator, the test could be administered in numerous languages with more ease and precision. When technicians administer the visual field exam, language or other communication barriers can lead to an imprecise test, which can necessitate the test to be performed multiple times until a reliable result is reached. This can make the exam very long, tedious, and uncomfortable; however, the virtual assistants can ensure that the exam is administered with more precision so that a proper test result is acquired on the first try. This can make visual field exams quicker and the appointments shorter, leading to more frequent use of the exam and higher patient satisfaction.

One of the key components that make deep learning a successful tool is that it requires an enormous database that spans different ethnic groups, ocular diseases, and ages to accurately predict an output. After gathering the data, researchers use different deep learning models and convolutional neural networks (CNN), a deep learning algorithm that can evaluate an input image and put weight to certain aspects of the photo to filter and differentiate different objects. Current visual fields use a guided progression analysis software (GPA) that quantifies baseline deviations in visual field patterns to monitor the progression of patients' ocular diseases and alert physicians of significant deterioration from these tests (Wang et. al., 2019). Though this form of analysis has become universally accepted, there are still discrepancies and inaccuracies with the GPA. (Giraud, 2010). Deep learning applications can further advance the sophistication of the visual field test by identifying patterns that may not have been detected by current methods of guided progression analysis. For example, a study used a categorization model CascadeNet-5 to analyze over 1.7 million perimetry points of 24-2 Humphrey visual fields from patients in the time range, 1998 to 2018 with a point-wise mean absolute error (PMAE) of 2.47 dB with a 95% CI of 2.45 dB to 2.48 dB. With training, the model was able to predict future Humphrey visual field results within five years of the most recent visual field test with a difference of 0.41 dB (Wen et. al.,

2019). This predictive model can help anticipate glaucoma progression, and thus can be used to assist a clinician's decision-making process and personalize care.

Deep learning is also able to predict successfully a Humphrey visual field from optical coherence tomography (OCT) results (Park, 2020). OCT is an objective test that uses electromagnetic fields to measure the different tissue layers that constitute the retina, cornea, and other parts of the eye. The OCT is a principal tool used to track and detect the progression of glaucoma, ocular hypertension, diabetic retinopathy, and other ocular diseases that are also monitored using the visual field test (American Academy of Ophthalmology, 2021). Because the OCT is considered a reliable, objective test, many ophthalmologists and optometrists rely more on the OCT than visual field results. Park's team used Keras library, TensorFlow, Python, CUDA toolkit 9.0, and Inception V3 to predict visual field results from OCT data of the macular ganglion cell-inner plexiform layer (mGCIPL) and peripapillary retinal nerve fiber layer (pRNFL), which both have lower volumes and thicknesses in patients with glaucoma (Seong et. al., 2010). After using data from 1529 Korean patients who had an OCT and 24-2 Humphrey Visual Field from 2013 to 2018 compared to the visual field data generated from the macular and optic nerve head OCT's results, the researchers calculated a root mean square deviation of 4.70 ± 2.56 dB. Based on the study's predicted visual fields, they are not affected by the patients' age, visual acuity, axial length, and OCT signal strengths of the previous test results, which allows ophthalmologists and optometrists to offer more flexibility to their patients. The study also confirmed that pRNFL is more sensitive to the effects of glaucoma than mGCIPL, which indicated that pRNFL can be a more accurate indicator of glaucoma (Park, 2020). Another study confirmed that deep learning CCN can predict 10-2 Humphrey Visual Field results from the OCT with a mean of 2.84 ± 2.98 dB compared than multiple linear regression's 6.96 ± 5.38 dB and support vector machine's 5.65 ± 5.12 dB with $p<0.001$ using a population of 347 patients (Hashimoto et. al., 2021). Ophthalmologists and optometrists can use visual field test results predicted by deep learning to keep track of the progression of ocular diseases and compare the accuracy of visual field tests for both SAP and virtual reality.

Currently, there is an ongoing trend to incorporate both virtual reality and deep learning in many different fields of medicine including ocular health. There was a recent clinical study that focused on a smartphone virtual reality application called iGlaucoma that combined both virtual reality and deep learning in order to take accurate and precise visual field measurements. The study focused on 5542 patients in China who were separated into two phases. In the first phase, the patients had clinically validated their glaucoma status through three tests of Humphrey visual field maps: pattern deviation probability plots, numerical displays, and numerical pattern deviation plots. The data from the first phase was then used to train the deep learning system from 8424 visual fields and validate 598 visual fields based on the three Humphrey Visual Field maps with high-performance indicators: area under the curve, sensitivity, and specificity. For the six ophthalmologists, their area under the curve is 0.850, sensitivity is 85.8%, and specificity is 84.3%. The study's age-standardized results revealed that iGlaucoma outperformed six ophthalmologists in terms of accurately and quickly detecting glaucoma in patients who have glaucoma after accounting for false positives. This study does have its limitations such as having a small ophthalmologist population primarily focusing on a Chinese population (Li et. al., 2020). Nonetheless, the study showcases the growing possibilities of how virtual reality can bring health equity by bringing these screening diagnostic tools to the smartphones of patients who have low access or lack ocular services as summarized in Table 1.

Table 1. A summary of key studies and their research findings mentioned in this chapter

Study	Research Findings
Tsapakis, 2017; Mees, 2020; and Sayed, 2021	Results of virtual reality devices are similar with results of Humphrey perimeter visual field among glaucoma and glaucoma suspected patients.
Ou et al, 2021	Deep learning can be applied to object detection technology to better detect pupil movement and track gaze, thereby eliminating inaccuracies in visual tests dependent on gaze tracking.
Kepuska & Bohouta, 2018	The integration of multi-modal dialogue systems in virtual assistants can prove extremely useful within several fields, especially ocular health.
Giraud, 2010 and Wang et al, 2019	Artificial intelligence software can monitor the progression of ocular diseases like glaucoma by analyzing discrepancies in visual field patterns to better inform clinical decisions.
Park, 2020 and Seong et. al., 2010	Deep learning can predict potential visual field tests from optical coherence tomography results and vice versa.
Li et al, 2020	iGlaucoma has proven to be a novel mobile application that can accurately and quickly detect glaucomatous visual field tests with the implementation of deep learning and virtual reality.

CONCLUSION

The visual field examination is a vital diagnostic tool in ocular health clinics. For common ailments, such as glaucoma, multiple sclerosis, thyroid eye disease, pituitary gland disorders, or stroke, gradual peripheral vision loss often goes unnoticed by patients until substantial and irreversible damage has occurred. Furthermore, the exam can be utilized to monitor any detrimental side effects of certain medications, such as central vision degradation occurring from the long term usage of hydroxychloroquine. While the visual field is a critical tool, it is far from a perfect test. Patients who suffer from certain other health conditions or those who are simply unable to comprehend the demands of the examination due to communication barriers are much more likely to produce results with a high degree of uncertainty. Unless innovative new avenues for improving the visual field are explored, the exam as currently conducted threatens to preclude a vast number of individuals from receiving the optimal care they deserve. The growing field of virtual reality and deep learning can be the answer to bridging the gap between the utility of the visual field examination and its unreliability.

Using virtual reality technology gives healthcare professionals more flexibility to accommodate those with disabilities. The current visual field machine demands a high range of movement and flexibility of patients' necks and spines. However, many members of the elderly population who have eye problems that warrant the visual field exam, also have back and neck problems which make it hard for them to stretch to properly see the lights in the bowl of the machine. The portability of virtual reality systems and how light they are in weight allow for clinics to more easily administer the test to patients with said neck and back problems, thus surpassing one of the largest hurdles of the current visual field exam.

In addition, the portability of virtual reality technology makes the visual field more accessible for people in rural and underserved areas as smartphones using virtual reality are lighter, smaller, and more cost-effective than the existing Humphrey Visual Field device. Combining virtual reality systems with mobile apps allows patients to monitor their eye health on their own by administering the visual field exam on their own. This can mean fewer in-office visits for patients who are unable to commute to clinics or do not have access to a proper eye clinic nearby. This also allows for a better integration of telehealth in the treatment of eye disease, which is very inconvenient right now as a doctor is not able to examine the health of a patient's eye solely through a computer or phone video chat.

Virtual reality allowed for the creation of virtual assistants who help cross the language barrier between technicians and patients since these assistants can speak infinitely more languages than just one technician. Also, the use of a virtual assistant makes it so a technician is not needed to administer the visual field exam. This makes the test both time and cost-effective as technicians can help other patients in the meantime or prepare other portions of the appointment. This reduces the time and inconvenience of the visual field exam allowing it to be used more frequently and leading to more accurate diagnoses for patients in need.

Virtual reality combined with deep learning not only makes the test more accommodating but also makes it more objective and comprehensive. Using a virtual reality scape allows the exam to test a patient's visual field in a 3-dimensional scope rather than the current 2-dimensional one, allowing for a better and more comprehensive understanding of the patient's field of vision. Deep learning further improves the exam by allowing the OCT to be combined with the visual field exam which makes the visual field more objective and reduces any user error or subjectivity that exists in the current exam. Not only does this potentially provide a more precise measure of a patient's visual field loss, but it also reduces the need for patients to undergo additional, strenuous testing, as clinicians can extract a greater deal of information from the deep learning-enhanced OCT. A common yearly plan for glaucoma patients consists of four doctor's visits spaced three months, during which different exams are performed to monitor the various aspects of glaucoma progression. By extracting more information from the OCT examination, patients can reduce the number of visits they are required to make, disproportionately benefiting lower-income individuals who may be unable to make frequent trips to their ophthalmologist or optometrist due to cost limitations.

Because detecting and treating glaucoma is time-sensitive, there needs to be ongoing research in developing and incorporating smart devices, virtual reality, and deep learning as a screening tool for glaucoma and other ocular diseases to prevent irreversible low vision and blindness. A refined visual field examination will provide clinicians with an enhanced and more accurate view of their patient's disease progression. Although the development of a visual field examination augmented with virtual reality and deep learning is still in its infancy, the potential for this new technology to reduce preventable vision loss and improve patient outcomes is vast.

REFERENCES

American Academy of Ophthalmology. (2021). *What Is Optical Coherence Tomography?* https://www.aao.org/eye-health/treatments/what-is-optical-coherence-tomography

Bayram, N., Gundogan, M., Ozsaygili, C., Vural, E., & Cicek, A. (2021, April 1). The Impacts of Face Mask Use on Standard Automated Perimetry Results in Glaucoma Patients. *Journal of Glaucoma*, *30*(4), 287–292. doi:10.1097/IJG.0000000000001786 PMID:33428353

Brenton, R. S., Phelps, C. D., Rojas, P., & Woolson, R. F. (1986, May 1). Interocular Differences of the Visual Field in Normal Subjects. *Investigative Ophthalmology & Visual Science*, *27*(5), 799–805. PMID:3700029

Broadway, D. C. (2012). Visual Field Testing for Glaucoma – a Practical Guide. *Community Eye Health*, *25*(79–80), 66–70. PMID:23520423

Carroll, J. N., & Johnson, C. A. (2013). *Visual Field Testing: From One Medical Student to Another.* https://eyerounds.org/tutorials/VF-testing/

Chang, R. (n.d.). *The Evolution of Portable Visual Field Testing.* https://www.reviewofophthalmology.com/article/the-evolution-of-portable-visual-field-testing

Chen, P. P., & Budenz, D. L. (1998, March 1). The Effects of Cataract Extraction on the Visual Field of Eyes with Chronic Open-Angle Glaucoma. *American Journal of Ophthalmology*, *125*(3), 325–333. doi:10.1016/S0002-9394(99)80142-1 PMID:9512149

Chow-Wing-Bom, H., Dekker, T. M., & Jones, P. R. (2020, April). The Worse Eye Revisited: Evaluating the Impact of Asymmetric Peripheral Vision Loss on Everyday Function. *Vision Research*, *169*, 49–57. doi:10.1016/j.visres.2019.10.012 PMID:32179339

Galarza, P., Parnasa, E., Guttmann, N., & Joshua, M. (2021, April 14). Artifactual Visual Field Defects Identified on Technically 'Reliable' Visual Field Studies in a Neuro-Ophthalmology Practice. *Eye and Brain*, *13*, 79–88. doi:10.2147/EB.S274523 PMID:33889041

Giraud, J.-M., May, F., Manet, G., Fenolland, J.-R., Meynard, J.-B., Sadat, A.-M., Mouinga, A., Seck, S., & Renard, J.-P. (2010, April 17). Analysis of Progression With GPA (Guided Progression Analysis) and Mean Deviation (MD) Indexes of Automated Perimetry in Ocular Hypertension and Glaucoma. *Investigative Ophthalmology & Visual Science*, *51*(13), 3997.

Hashimoto, Y., Asaoka, R., Kiwaki, T., Sugiura, H., Asano, S., Murata, H., Fujino, Y., Matsuura, M., Miki, A., Mori, K., Ikeda, Y., Kanamoto, T., Yamagami, J., Inoue, K., Tanito, M., & Yamanishi, K. (2021, April 1). Deep Learning Model to Predict Visual Field in Central 10° from Optical Coherence Tomography Measurement in Glaucoma. *The British Journal of Ophthalmology*, *105*(4), 507–513. doi:10.1136/bjophthalmol-2019-315600 PMID:32593978

Humphrey Field Analyzer II-i Single Field Analysis: A Guide to Interpretation. (2013). https://www.zeiss.com/content/dam/Meditec/us/download/Glaucoma%20Landing%20Page/hfasinglefieldguidehfa5268.pdf

Kasneci, E., Black, A. A., & Wood, J. M. (2017). Eye-Tracking as a Tool to Evaluate Functional Ability in Everyday Tasks in Glaucoma. *Journal of Ophthalmology*. doi:10.1155/2017/6425913

Këpuska, V., & Bohouta, G. (2018). Next-Generation of Virtual Personal Assistants (Microsoft Cortana, Apple Siri, Amazon Alexa, and Google Home). *2018 IEEE 8th Annual Computing and Communication Workshop and Conference (CCWC)*, 99–103. doi:10.1109/CCWC.2018.8301638

Li, F., Song, D., Chen, H., Xiong, J., Li, X., Zhong, H., & Tang, G. (2020, September 22). Development and Clinical Deployment of a Smartphone-Based Visual Field Deep Learning System for Glaucoma Detection. *NPJ Digital Medicine*, *3*(1), 1–8. https://doi.org/10.1038/s41746-020-00329-9

Mees, L., Upadhyaya, S., Kumar, P., Kotawala, S., Haran, S., Rajasekar, S., Friedman, D. S., & Venkatesh, R. (2020, February). Validation of a Head-Mounted Virtual Reality Visual Field Screening Device. *Journal of Glaucoma*, *29*(2), 86–91. https://doi.org/10.1097/IJG.0000000000001415

Ng, M., Racette, L., Pascual, J. P., Liebmann, J. M., Girkin, C. A., Lovell, S. L., Zangwill, L. M., Weinreb, R. N., & Sample, P. A. (2009, April 1). Comparing the Full-Threshold and Swedish Interactive Thresholding Algorithms for Short-Wavelength Automated Perimetry. *Investigative Ophthalmology & Visual Science, 50*(4), 1726–1733. https://doi.org/10.1167/iovs.08-2718

NGoggle. (n.d.). *Assessment of Visual Function With a Portable Brain-Computer Interface. Clinical trial registration.* https://clinicaltrials.gov/ct2/show/NCT03760055

Nieto, M. P. (2015). *English: A Simplified Schema of the Human Visual Pathway.* https://commons.wikimedia.org/w/index.php?curid=37868501

Ou, W.-L., Kuo, T.-L., Chang, C.-C., & Fan, C.-P. (2021, January). Deep-Learning-Based Pupil Center Detection and Tracking Technology for Visible-Light Wearable Gaze Tracking Devices. *Applied Sciences (Basel, Switzerland), 11*(2), 851. https://doi.org/10.3390/app11020851

Ou, Y. (n.d.). *The Future of Virtual Reality Visual Field Testing.* Glaucoma Research Foundation. https://www.glaucoma.org/treatment/virtual-reality-visual-field-testing.php

Papageorgiou, E., Hardiess, G., Mallot, H. A., & Schiefer, U. (2012, July 15). Gaze Patterns Predicting Successful Collision Avoidance in Patients with Homonymous Visual Field Defects. *Vision Research, 65*, 25–37. https://doi.org/10.1016/j.visres.2012.06.004

Park, K., Kim, J., & Lee, J. (2020, July 6). A Deep Learning Approach to Predict Visual Field Using Optical Coherence Tomography. *PLoS One, 15*(7), e0234902. https://doi.org/10.1371/journal.pone.0234902

Peracha, M., Hughes, B., Tannir, J., Momi, R., Goyal, A., Juzych, M., Kim, C., McQueen, M., Eby, A., & Fatima, F. (2013, June 16). Assessing the Reliability of Humphrey Visual Field Testing in an Urban Population. *Investigative Ophthalmology & Visual Science, 54*(15), 3920–3920.

Sayed, A., Roongpoovapatr, V., Eleiwa, T., Kashem, R., Abdel-Mottaleb, M., Jumbo, O., Parrish, R., & Abou Shousha, M. (2021, June 21). Measurement of Monocular and Binocular Visual Field Defects with a Virtual Reality Head Mounted Display. *Investigative Ophthalmology & Visual Science, 62*(8), 3512–3512.

Seong, M., Sung, K. R., Choi, E. H., Kang, S. Y., Cho, J. W., Um, T. W., Kim, Y. J., Park, S. B., Hong, H. E., & Kook, M. S. (2010, March 1). Macular and Peripapillary Retinal Nerve Fiber Layer Measurements by Spectral Domain Optical Coherence Tomography in Normal-Tension Glaucoma. *Investigative Ophthalmology & Visual Science, 51*(3), 1446–1452. https://doi.org/10.1167/iovs.09-4258

Skalicky, S. E., & Kong, G. Y. (2019, December). Novel Means of Clinical Visual Function Testing among Glaucoma Patients, Including Virtual Reality. *Journal of Current Glaucoma Practice, 13*(3), 83–87. https://doi.org/10.5005/jp-journals-10078-1265

Smith, A. M., & Czyz, C. N. (2021). Neuroanatomy, Cranial Nerve 2 (Optic). In *StatPearls*. StatPearls Publishing. https://www.ncbi.nlm.nih.gov/books/NBK507907/

Tsapakis, S., Papaconstantinou, D., Diagourtas, A., Droutsas, K., Andreanos, K., Moschos, M. M., & Brouzas, D. (2017). Visual Field Examination Method Using Virtual Reality Glasses Compared with the Humphrey Perimeter. *Clinical Ophthalmology (Auckland, N.Z.)*, *11*, 1431–1443. https://doi.org/10.2147/OPTH.S131160

Wang, M., Shen, L. Q., Pasquale, L. R., Petrakos, P., Formica, S., Boland, M. V., Wellik, S. R., & ... . (2019, January 25). An Artificial Intelligence Approach to Detect Visual Field Progression in Glaucoma Based on Spatial Pattern Analysis. *Investigative Ophthalmology & Visual Science*, *60*(1), 365–375. https://doi.org/10.1167/iovs.18-25568

Wen, J. C., Lee, C. S., Keane, P. A., & Sa Xiao, A. S. (2019, April 5). Forecasting Future Humphrey Visual Fields Using Deep Learning. *PLoS One*, *14*(4), e0214875. https://doi.org/10.1371/journal.pone.0214875

Compilation of References

Aardema, F., O'Connor, K., Côté, S., & Taillon, A. (2010). Virtual Reality Induces Dissociation and Lowers Sense of Presence in Objective Reality. *Cyberpsychology, Behavior, and Social Networking*, *13*(4), 429–435. doi:10.1089/cyber.2009.0164 PMID:20712501

Abbas, J. R., Kenth, J. J., & Bruce, I. A. (2020). The role of virtual reality in the changing landscape of surgical training. *The Journal of Laryngology and Otology*, *134*(10), 863–866. doi:10.1017/S0022215120002078 PMID:33032666

Abdul, S. S., Malwade, S., Nursetyo, A. A., Sood, M., Bhatia, M., ... Li, J. (2019). Virtual reality among the elderly: A usefulness acceptance study from Taiwan. *BMC Geriatrics*, *19*(1), 223. doi:10.118612877-019-1218-8 PMID:31426766

Acharya, S., Bhatt, A. N., Chakrabarti, A., Delhi, V. S., Diehl, J. C., van Andel, E., & Subra, R. (2021). Problem-Based Learning (PBL) in Undergraduate Education: Design Thinking to Redesign Courses. In *Design for Tomorrow—Volume 2* (pp. 349–360). Springer. doi:10.1007/978-981-16-0119-4_28

Adama, V. S., Schindler, B., & Schmid, T. (2019, September). Using time domain and pearson's correlation to predict attention focus in autistic spectrum disorder from EEG P300 components. In *Mediterranean Conference on Medical and Biological Engineering and Computing* (pp. 1890-1893). Springer.

Adefila, A., Opie, J., Ball, S., & Bluteau, P. (2020). Students' engagement and learning experiences using virtual patient simulation in a computer supported collaborative learning environment. *Innovations in Education and Teaching International*, *57*(1), 50–61.

Aebersold, M., & Dunbar, D. M. (2021). Virtual and Augmented Realities in Nursing Education: State of the Science. *Annual Review of Nursing Research*, *39*(1), 225–242. doi:10.1891/0739-6686.39.225 PMID:33431644

Agha, S. (2021). Aligning continuing professional development (CPD) with quality assurance (QA): A perspective of healthcare leadership. *Quality & Quantity*, 1–15.

Al Janabi, H., Aydin, A., Palaneer, S., Macchione, N., Al-Jabir, A., Khan, M., Dasgupta, P., & Ahmed, K. (2019). Effectiveness of the HoloLens mixed-reality headset in minimally invasive surgery: A simulation-based feasibility study. *Surgical Endoscopy*, *34*(3), 1143–1149. doi:10.100700464-019-06862-3 PMID:31214807

Alexander, C., Loeb, A. E., Fotouhi, J., Navab, N., Armand, M., & Khanuja, H. S. (2020). Augmented Reality for Acetabular Component Placement in Direct Anterior Total Hip Arthroplasty. *The Journal of Arthroplasty*, *35*(6), 1636–1641. e3. doi:10.1016/j.arth.2020.01.025 PMID:32063415

Alfalah, S., Falah, J., Alfalah, T., Elfalah, M., Muhaidat, N., & Falah, O. (2018). A Comparative Study Between a Virtual Reality Heart Anatomy System and Traditional Medical Teaching Modalities. *Virtual Reality (Waltham Cross)*.

Ali, M., Al Machot, F., Haj Mosa, A., Jdeed, M., Al Machot, E., & Kyamakya, K. (2018). A globally generalized emotion recognition system involving different physiological signals. *Sensors (Basel)*, *18*(6), 1905. doi:10.339018061905 PMID:29891829

Ali, S., Qandeel, M., Ramakrishna, R., & Yang, C. W. (2018). Virtual Simulation in Enhancing Procedural Training for Fluoroscopy-guided Lumbar Puncture: A Pilot Study. *Academic Radiology*, *25*(2), 235–239. doi:10.1016/j.acra.2017.08.002 PMID:29032887

Alkire, B., Raykar, N., Shrime, M., Weiser, T., Bickler, S., Rose, J., Nutt, C., Greenberg, S., Kotagal, M., Riesel, J., Esquivel, M., Uribe-Letiz, T., Molina, G., Roy, N., Mearat, J., & Farmer, P. (2015). Global access to surgical care: A modelling study. *The Lancet. Global Health*, *3*(6), e316–e323. doi:10.1016/S2214-109X(15)70115-4 PMID:25926087

Alnagrat, A. J. A., Ismail, R. C., & Idrus, S. Z. S. (2021, May). Extended Reality (XR) in Virtual Laboratories: A Review of Challenges and Future Training Directions. *Journal of Physics: Conference Series*, *1874*(1), 012031. doi:10.1088/1742-6596/1874/1/012031

American Academy of Ophthalmology. (2021). *What Is Optical Coherence Tomography?* https://www.aao.org/eye-health/treatments/what-is-optical-coherence-tomography

American Psychiatry Association. (2014). *Manual diagnóstico y estadístico de los trastornos mentales* (5th ed.). Editorial Médica Panamericana.

American Psychological Association. (2002). Criteria for Evaluating Treatment Guidelines. *The American Psychologist*, *57*(12), 1052–1059. doi:10.1037/0003-066X.57.12.1052 PMID:12617064

American Psychological Association. (2013, July 31). *Guidelines for the Practice of Telepsychology*. Retrieved from https://www.apa.org/practice/guidelines/telepsychology

American Psychological Association. (2017). *Clinical Practical Guideline for the Treatment of PTSD*. Retrieved from American Psychological Association: https://www.apa.org/ptsd-guideline

American Psychological Association. (2017). *Ethical principles of psychologists and code of conduct (2002, amended effective June 1, 2010, and January 1, 2017)*. Retrieved from http://www.apa.org/ethics/code/index.html

Anastasi, A. (1976). *Psychological testing* (4th ed.). Macmillan.

Andersen, S. A. W., Mikkelsen, P. T., Konge, L., Cayé-Thomasen, P., & Sørensen, M. S. (2016). Cognitive Load in Mastoidectomy Skills Training: Virtual Reality Simulation and Traditional Dissection Compared. *Journal of Surgical Education*, *73*(1), 45–50. doi:10.1016/j.jsurg.2015.09.010 PMID:26481267

Anderson, A. P., Mayer, M. D., Fellows, A. M., Cowan, D. R., Hegel, M. T., & Buckey, J. C. (2017, June). Relaxation with Immersive Natural Scenes Presented Using Virtual Reality. *Aerospace Medicine and Human Performance*, *88*(6), 520–526. doi:10.3357/AMHP.4747.2017 PMID:28539139

Anderson, P. L., Price, M., Edwards, S. M., Obasaju, M. A., Schmertz, S. K., Zimand, E., & Calamaras, M. R. (2013). Virtual reality exposure therapy for social anxiety disorder: A randomized controlled trial. *Journal of Consulting and Clinical Psychology*, *81*(5), 751–760. doi:10.1037/a0033559 PMID:23796315

Anderson, P. L., Rothbaum, B. O., & Hidges, L. (2005). Virtual reality: Using the virtual world to improve quality of life in the real world. *Bulletin of the Menninger Clinic*, *65*(1), 78–91. Advance online publication. doi:10.1521/bumc.65.1.78.18713 PMID:11280960

Andrade, F. R. H., Mizoguchi, R., & Isotani, S. (2016). The Bright and Dark Sides of Gamification. In A. Micarelli, J. Stamper, & K. Panourgia (Eds.), *Intelligent Tutoring Systems* (pp. 176–186). Lecture Notes in Computer Science. Springer International Publishing. doi:10.1007/978-3-319-39583-8_17

Annala, J., Lindén, J., Mäkinen, M., & Henriksson, J. (2021). Understanding academic agency in curriculum change in higher education. *Teaching in Higher Education*, 1–18. doi:10.1080/13562517.2021.1881772

Antoniou, P., Arfaras, G., Pandria, N., Ntakakis, G., Bambatsikos, E., & Athanasiou, A. (2020). Real-time affective measurements in medical education, using virtual and mixed reality. In *International Conference on Brain Function Assessment in Learning* (pp. 87-95). Springer. 10.1007/978-3-030-60735-7_9

Argyris, C. (1991). Teaching smart people how to learn. *Harvard Business Review, 69*(3).

Arjadi, R., Nauta, M. H., Scholte, W. F., Hollon, S. D., Chowdhary, N., Suryani, A. O., Uiterwaal, C. S. P. M., & Bockting, C. L. (2018). Internet-based behavioural activation with lay counsellor support versus online minimal psychoeducation without support for treatment of depression: A randomised controlled trial in Indonesia. *The Lancet. Psychiatry, 5*(9), 707–716. doi:10.1016/S2215-0366(18)30223-2 PMID:30006262

Arlati, S., Greci, L., Mondellini, M., Zangiacomi, A., Di Santo, S. G., Franchini, F., & Vezzoli, A. (2017, November). A virtual reality-based physical and cognitive training system aimed at preventing symptoms of dementia. In *International Conference on Wireless Mobile Communication and Healthcare* (pp. 117-125). Springer.

Arleti, S., Colombo, V., Spoladore, D., Pedroli, E., Serino, S., ... Sacco, M. (2020). A social virtual reality-based application for the physical and cognitive training of the elderly at home. *Sensors (Basel), 19*(2), 261. doi:10.339019020261 PMID:30634719

Artigas-Pallarés, J. (2009). Dislexia: enfermedad, trastorno o algo distinto. *Rev Neurol, 48*(2), 63-69.

Axelrod, D. (2017). *The Stanford Virtual Heart: Revolutionizing Education on Congenital Heart Defects.* Stanford Children's Health. https://www.stanfordchildrens.org/en/innovation/virtual-reality/stanford-virtual-heart

Aydin, A., Raison, N., Khan, M. S., Dasgupta, P., & Ahmed, K. (2016). Simulation-based training and assessment in urological surgery. *Nature Reviews. Urology, 13*(9), 503–519. doi:10.1038/nrurol.2016.147 PMID:27549358

Ayoub, A., & Pulijala, Y. (2019). The application of virtual reality and augmented reality in Oral & Maxillofacial Surgery. *BMC Oral Health, 19*(1), 1–8. doi:10.118612903-019-0937-8 PMID:31703708

Ayres, P., & Paas, F. (2007a). Can the cognitive load approach make instructional animations more effective? *Applied Cognitive Psychology, 21*(6), 811–820. doi:10.1002/acp.1351

Ayres, P., & Paas, F. (2007b). Making instructional animations more effective: A cognitive load approach. *Applied Cognitive Psychology, 21*(6), 695–700. doi:10.1002/acp.1343

Azizian, M., Liu, M., Khalaji, I., & DiMaio, S. (2019). The da Vinci Surgical System. In The Encyclopedia of medical robotics: Volume 1 Minimally Invasive Surgical Robotics (pp. 3-28). World Scientific. doi:10.1142/9789813232266_0001

Aznar Díaz, I., Romero-Rodríguez, J. M., & Rodríguez-García, A. M. (2018). La tecnología móvil de Realidad Virtual en educación: Una revisión del estado de la literatura científica en España. *EDMETIC. Revista de Educación Mediática y TIC, 7*(1), 256–274. doi:10.21071/edmetic.v7i1.10139

Azouvi, P., Arnould, A., Dromer, E., & Vallat-Azouvi, C. (2017). Neuropsychology of traumatic brain injury: An expert overview. *Revue Neurologique, 173*(7-8), 461–472. doi:10.1016/j.neurol.2017.07.006 PMID:28847474

Bailenson, J. (2018). Protecting Nonverbal Data Tracked in Virtual Reality. *JAMA Pediatrics*, *172*(10), 905–906. doi:10.1001/jamapediatrics.2018.1909 PMID:30083770

Bailey, J., Bailenson, J. N., Won, A. S., Flora, J., & Armel, K. C. (2012, October). Presence and memory: immersive virtual reality effects on cued recall. In *Proceedings of the International Society for Presence Research Annual Conference* (pp. 24-26). Academic Press.

Banakou, D., Hanumanthu, P. D., & Slater, M. (2016). Virtual Embodiment of White People in a Black Virtual Body Leads to a Sustained Reduction in Their Implicit Racial Bias. *Frontiers in Human Neuroscience*, *10*, 601. doi:10.3389/fnhum.2016.00601 PMID:27965555

Bandura, A. (2006). Guide for constructing self-efficacy scales. *Self-Efficacy Beliefs of Adolescents, 5*(1), 307-337.

Bauer, A. C. M., & Andringa, G. (2020). The potential of immersive virtual reality for cognitive training in elderly. *Gerontology*, *66*(6), 614–623. doi:10.1159/000509830 PMID:32906122

Bayne, T., Brainard, D., Byrne, R. W., Chittka, L., Clayton, N., Heyes, C., Mather, J., Ölveczky, B., Shadlen, M., Suddendorf, T., & Webb, B. (2019). What is Cognition? *Current Biology*, *29*(13), R608–R616. doi:10.1016/j.cub.2019.05.044 PMID:31287972

Bayram, N., Gundogan, M., Ozsaygili, C., Vural, E., & Cicek, A. (2021, April 1). The Impacts of Face Mask Use on Standard Automated Perimetry Results in Glaucoma Patients. *Journal of Glaucoma*, *30*(4), 287–292. doi:10.1097/IJG.0000000000001786 PMID:33428353

Beck, J. G., Palyo, S. A., Winer, E. H., Schwagler, B. E., & Ang, E. J. (2007). Virtual reality exposure therapy for PTSD symptoms after a road accident: An uncontrolled case series. *Behavior Therapy*, *38*(1), 39–48. doi:10.1016/j.beth.2006.04.001 PMID:17292693

Beidel, D. C., Frueh, B. C., Neer, S. M., Bowers, C. A., Trachik, B., Uhde, T. W., & Grubaugh, A. (2019). Trauma management therapy with virtual-reality augmented exposure therapy for combat-related PTSD: A randomized controlled trial. *Journal of Anxiety Disorders*, *61*, 64–74. doi:10.1016/j.janxdis.2017.08.005 PMID:28865911

Benedetti, F., Volpi, N. C., Parisi, L., & Sartori, G. (2014, June). Attention training with an easy–to–use brain computer interface. In *International Conference on Virtual, Augmented and Mixed Reality* (pp. 236-247). Springer. 10.1007/978-3-319-07464-1_22

Benítez-Burraco, A. (2010). Neurobiología y neurogenética de la dislexia. *Neurologia (Barcelona, Spain)*, *25*(9), 563–581. doi:10.1016/j.nrl.2009.12.010 PMID:21093706

Bernhardt, S., Nicolau, S., Soler, L., & Doignon, C. (2017). The status of augmented reality in laparoscopic surgery as of 2016. *Medical Image Analysis*, *37*, 66–90. doi:10.1016/j.media.2017.01.007 PMID:28160692

Bettati, P., Chalian, M., Huang, J., Dormer, J. D., Shahedi, M., & Fei, B. (2020). Augmented Reality-Assisted Biopsy of Soft Tissue Lesions. *Proceedings of SPIE—the International Society for Optical Engineering, 11315.* 10.1117/12.2549381

Bevins, F., Bryant, J., Krishnan, C., & Law, J. (2020). *Coronavirus: How should US higher education plan for an uncertain future.* McKinsey.

Bhat, S., Shetty, S., & Shenoy, K.K. (2005). Imaging in implantology. *J Indian Prosthodont Soc, 5*, 10-4.

Bihorac, A., Ozrazgat-Baslanti, T., Ebadi, A., Motaei, A., Madkour, M., Pardalos, P., Lipori, G., Hogan, W., Efron, P., Moore, F., Moldawer, L., Wang, D., Hobson, C., Rashidi, P., Li, X., & Momcilovic, P. (2019). MySurgeryRisk: Development and validation of a machine-learning risk algorithm for major complications and death after surgery. *Annals of Surgery*, *269*(4), 652–662. doi:10.1097/SLA.0000000000002706 PMID:29489489

Billig, J., & Sears, E. (2020). The compounding access problem for surgical care: Innovations in the post-COVID era. *Annals of Surgery*, 272(2), e47–e48. doi:10.1097/SLA.0000000000004085 PMID:32675492

Birchley, G., Ives, J., Huxtable, R., & Blazeby, J. (2020). Conceptualising surgical innovation: An eliminativist proposal. *Health Care Analysis*, 28(1), 73–97. doi:10.100710728-019-00380-y PMID:31327091

Birkfellner, W., Watzinger, F., Wanschitz, F., Ewers, R., & Bergmann, H. (1998). Calibration of tracking systems in a surgical environment. *IEEE Trans Med Imag, 17*, 737-42.

Birsh, J. R. (2011). Connecting research and practice. In J. R. Birsh (Ed.), *Multisensory teaching of basic language skills* (3rd ed., pp. 1–24). Paul H. Brookes Publishing.

Birt, J., Stromberga, Z., Cowling, M., & Moro, C. (2018). Mobile mixed reality for experiential learning and simulation in medical and health sciences education. *Information (Basel)*, 9(2), 31. doi:10.3390/info9020031

Bisson, J., & Andrew, M. (2007). Psychological treatment of post-traumatic stress disorder (PTSD). *Cochrane Database of Systematic Reviews*, 3. PMID:17636720

Blanchard, E. B., & Hickling, E. J. (2004). *After the crash: Psychological assessment and treatment of survivors of motor vehicle accidents*. American Psychological Association. doi:10.1037/10676-000

Blanchard, E. B., Hickling, E. J., Taylor, A. E., & Loos, W. (1995). Psychiatric morbidity associated with motor vehicle accidents. *The Journal of Nervous and Mental Disease*, 183(8), 495–504. doi:10.1097/00005053-199508000-00001 PMID:7643060

Blascovich, J., & McCall, C. (2010). Attitudes in virtual reality. In J. Forgas, W. Crano & J. Cooper (Eds.), The Psychology of Attitudes and Attitude Change. Google Books.

Blaubit Co Ltd. (2019). *Stress Disorder Detection System for Use in Panic Attack Treatment Has Display Section to Display Analyzed Behavioral Data So Virtual Reality (VR) Content Information Outputted by Information Management Department Can Be Revealed to Patient. KR2019061826A*. KPO.

Blei, D. M., Ng, A. Y., & Jordan, M. I. (2003). Latent dirichlet allocation. *The Journal of Machine Learning Research, 3*, 993-1022.

Blumstein, G. (2019). Research: How Virtual Reality Can Help Train Surgeons. *Harvard Business Review*. https://hbr.org/2019/10/research-how-virtual-reality-can-help-train-surgeons

Blumstein, G., Zukotynski, B., Cevallos, N., Ishmael, C., Zoller, S., Burke, Z., Clarkson, S., Park, H., Bernthal, N., & SooHoo, N. F. (2020). Randomized Trial of a Virtual Reality Tool to Teach Surgical Technique for Tibial Shaft Fracture Intramedullary Nailing. *Journal of Surgical Education, 77*(4), 969–977. https://doi-org.ezproxy2.umc.edu/10.1016/j.jsurg.2020.01.002

Bohil, C. J., Alicea, B., & Biocca, F. A. (2011). Virtual reality in neuroscience research and therapy. *Nature Reviews. Neuroscience*, 12(12), 752–762. doi:10.1038/nrn3122 PMID:22048061

Bolinski, F., Etzelmüller, A., Witte, N. A., Beurden, C., Debard, G., Bonroy, B., ... Kleiboer, A. (2021). Physiological and self-reported arousal in virtual reality versus face-to-face emotional activation and cognitive restructuring in university students: A crossover experimental study using wearable monitoring. *Behaviour Research and Therapy*, 142, 103877. doi:10.1016/j.brat.2021.103877 PMID:34029860

Bonsignore, E., Kraus, K., Visconti, A., Hansen, D., Fraistat, A., & Druin, A. (2012). Game design for promoting counterfactual thinking. In *Proceedings of the SIGCHI Conference on Human Factors in Computing Systems, CHI '12*. Association for Computing Machinery. 10.1145/2207676.2208357

Bordnick, P. S., Graap, K. M., Copp, H., Brooks, J., Ferrer, M., & Logue, B. (2004). Utilizing virtual reality to standardize nicotine craving research: A pilot study. *Addictive Behaviors*, *29*(9), 1889–1894. doi:10.1016/j.addbeh.2004.06.008 PMID:15530734

Borgmann, H., Rodríguez Socarrás, M., Salem, J., Tsaur, I., Gomez Rivas, J., Barret, E., & Tortolero, L. (2017). Feasibility and safety of augmented reality-assisted urological surgery using smartglass. *World Journal of Urology*, *35*(6), 967–972. doi:10.100700345-016-1956-6 PMID:27761715

Botella, C., Baños, R. M., Villa, H., Perpiñá, C., & García-Palacios, A. (2000). Virtual Reality in the Treatment of Claustrophobic Fear: A Controlled, Multiple-baseline Design. *Behaviour Research and Therapy*, *31*(3), 583–595. doi:10.1016/S0005-7894(00)80032-5

Botella, C., Fernández-Álvarez, J., Guillén, V., García-Palacios, A., & Baños, R. (2017). Recent Progress in Virtual Reality Exposure Therapy for Phobias: A Systematic Review. *Current Psychiatry Reports*, *19*(42), 1–13. doi:10.100711920-017-0788-4 PMID:28540594

Bouchard, S., Dumoulin, S., Robillard, G., Guitard, T., Klinger, É., Forget, H., Loranger, C., & Roucaut, F. X. (2017). Virtual reality compared with in vivo exposure in the treatment of social anxiety disorder: A three-arm randomised controlled trial. *The British Journal of Psychiatry*, *210*(4), 276–283. doi:10.1192/bjp.bp.116.184234 PMID:27979818

Bozgeyikli, E., Alqasemi, R., Raij, A., Katkoori, S., & Dubeyet, R. (2018). Virtual Reality Interaction Techniques for Individuals with Autism Spectrum Disorder. In *International Conference on Universal Access in Human-Computer Interaction*. Springer. 10.1007/978-3-319-92052-8_6

Brachten, F., Brünker, F., Frick, N. R. J., Ross, B., & Stieglitz, S. (2020). On the ability of virtual agents to decrease cognitive load: An experimental study. *Information Systems and e-Business Management*, *18*(2), 187–207. doi:10.100710257-020-00471-7

Bradley, M. M., & Lang, P. J. (1994). Measuring emotion: The self-assessment manikin and the semantic differential. *Journal of Behavior Therapy and Experimental Psychiatry*, *25*(1), 49–59. doi:10.1016/0005-7916(94)90063-9 PMID:7962581

Braga, R., Camello, L., Costa, V., Raposo, A., Rodrigues, H., & Ventura, P. (2017). Virtual Reality as a Support Tool for the Treatment of Flying Phobia: A Pilot Study. *19th Symposium on Virtual and Augmented Reality (SVR)*. 10.1109/SVR.2017.17

Brandon, E., Freiwirth, R., & Hjersman, J. (2021, May). Special Session—Student Engagement with Reduced Bias in a Virtual Classroom Environment. In *2021 7th International Conference of the Immersive Learning Research Network (iLRN)* (pp. 1-3). IEEE.

Breda, A., & Territo, A. (2016). Virtual Reality Simulators for Robot-assisted Surgery. *European Urology*, *69*(6), 1081–1082. doi:10.1016/j.eururo.2015.11.026 PMID:26688370

Breedon, P., Logan, P., Pearce, D., Edmans, J., Childs, B., & O'Brien, R. (2016). Face to Face: An Interactive Facial Exercise System for Stroke Patients with Facial Weakness. *11th International Conference on Disability, Virtual Reality&Associated Technologies*.

Breining, G. (2018). Future or Fad? Virtual Reality in Medical Education. *AAMCNews*. https://www.aamc.org/news-insights/future-or-fad-virtual-reality-medical-education

Bremner, J. (2019). Simulation-Based Education: Bringing Theory and Practice Together. *Dal News*. https://www.dal.ca/news/2019/11/28/simulation_based-education--bringing-theory-and-practice-togethe.html

Brenton, R. S., Phelps, C. D., Rojas, P., & Woolson, R. F. (1986, May 1). Interocular Differences of the Visual Field in Normal Subjects. *Investigative Ophthalmology & Visual Science, 27*(5), 799–805. PMID:3700029

Bric, J., Lumbard, D., Frelich, M., & Gould, J. (2016). Current state of virtual reality simulation in robotic surgery training: A review. *Surgical Endoscopy, 30*(6), 2169–2178. doi:10.100700464-015-4517-y PMID:26304107

Broadhead, M., Zad, D., MacKinnon, L., & Bacon, L. (2018). A multisensory 3D environment as intervention to aid reading in dyslexia: A proposed framework. *2018 10th International Conference on Virtual Worlds and Games for Serious Applications, VS-Games 2018 - Proceedings*, 1–4.

Broadway, D. C. (2012). Visual Field Testing for Glaucoma – a Practical Guide. *Community Eye Health, 25*(79–80), 66–70. PMID:23520423

Bryant, R. A., Sackville, T., Dang, S. T., Moulds, M., & Guthrie, R. (1999). Treating acute stress disorder: An evaluation of cognitive behavior therapy and supportive counseling techniques. *The American Journal of Psychiatry, 156*(11), 1780–1786. PMID:10553743

Budhiraja, P., Miller, M. R., Modi, A. K., & Forsyth, D. (2017). Rotation Blurring: Use of Artificial Blurring to Reduce Cybersickness in Virtual Reality First Person Shooters. *arXiv 2017*, arXiv:1710.02599

Burdea, G. C. (2003). Virtual rehabilitation—Benefits and challenges. *Methods of Information in Medicine, 42*(5), 519–523. doi:10.1055-0038-1634378 PMID:14654886

Burgess, A., van Diggele, C., Roberts, C., & Mellis, C. (2020). Key tips for teaching in the clinical setting. *BMC Medical Education, 20*(2), 1–7. PMID:33272257

Burgstahler, S. (2009). *Universal Design: Process, Principles, and Applications, DO-IT*. DO-IT.

Buttussi, F., Pellis, T., Cabas Vidani, A., Pausler, D., Carchietti, E., & Chittaro, L. (2013). Evaluation of a 3D serious game for advanced life support retraining. *International Journal of Medical Informatics, 82*(9), 798–809. doi:10.1016/j.ijmedinf.2013.05.007 PMID:23763908

Cabero, J. (Ed.). (2000). *Nuevas tecnologías aplicadas a la educación*. Síntesis.

Cabero, J., & Fernández, J. (2007). *Las TIC para la igualdad*. Publidisa.

Cano, S. R., Alonso, P. S., Benito, V. D., & Villaverde, V. A. (2021). Evaluation of Motivational Learning Strategies for Children with Dyslexia: A FORDYSVAR Proposal for Education and Sustainable Innovation. *Sustainability, 13*(5), 2666. doi:10.3390u13052666

Cao, Z., Jerald, J., & Kopper, R. (2018). Visually-Induced Motion Sickness Reduction via Static and Dynamic Rest Frames. In *2018 IEEE Conference on Virtual Reality and 3D User Interfaces (VR)* (pp. 105-112). IEEE. 10.1109/VR.2018.8446210

Cappon, D., Jahanshahi, M., & Bisiacchi, P. (2016). Value and efficacy of transcranial direct current stimulation in the cognitive rehabilitation: A critical review since 2000. *Frontiers in Neuroscience, 10*, 157. doi:10.3389/fnins.2016.00157 PMID:27147949

Car, J., Carlstedt-Duke, J., Tudor Car, L., Posadzki, P., Whiting, P., Zary, N., Atun, R., Majeed, A., & Campbell, J.Digital Health Education Collaboration. (2019). Digital Education in Health Professions: The Need for Overarching Evidence Synthesis. *Journal of Medical Internet Research, 21*(2), e12913. doi:10.2196/12913 PMID:30762583

Carl, E., Stein, A. T., Levihn-Coon, A., Pogue, J. R., Rothbaum, B., Emmelkamp, P., ... Powers, M. B. (2018). Virtual reality exposure therapy for anxiety and related disorders: A meta-analysis of randomized controlled trials. *Journal of Anxiety Disorders*. Advance online publication. doi:10.1016/j.janxdis.2018.08.003 PMID:30287083

Carroll, J. N., & Johnson, C. A. (2013). *Visual Field Testing: From One Medical Student to Another.* https://eyerounds.org/tutorials/VF-testing/

Cartagena, P. D., Naranjo, J. E., Garcia, C. A., Beltran, C., Castro, M., & Garcia, M. V. (2018). *Virtual Reality-Based System for Hand Rehabilitation Using an Orthosis, w: Augmented Reality, Virtual Reality, and Computer Graphics.* AVR. doi:10.1007/978-3-319-95282-6_8

CDC. (2021). *Disability Impacts All of Us (Disability and Health Data System).* Center for Disease Control.

Chang, E., Hwang, I., Jeon, H., Chun, Y., Kim, H., & Park, C. (2013). Effects of rest frames on cybersickness and oscillatory brain activity. In *Proceedings of the 2013 International Winter Workshop on Brain-Computer Interface (BCI)* (pp. 62–64). IEEE. 10.1109/IWW-BCI.2013.6506631

Chang, R. (n.d.). *The Evolution of Portable Visual Field Testing.* https://www.reviewofophthalmology.com/article/the-evolution-of-portable-visual-field-testing

Chang, T. P. (2020, April 30). *Practical & Academic Considerations for Integrating VR and AR into the Simulation Center Repertoire.* Children's Hospital Los Angeles. https://chla.webex.com/recordingservice/sites/chla/recording/playback/d410d5beaeae46bd9e8756024d091905

Chang, T. P., Beshay, Y., Hollinger, T., & Sherman, J. M. (2019). Comparisons of Stress Physiology of Providers in Real-Life Resuscitations and Virtual Reality-Simulated Resuscitations. *Simulation in Healthcare: Journal of the Society for Simulation in Healthcare, 14*(2), 104–112. doi:10.1097/SIH.0000000000000356

Chang, E., Kim, H. T., & Yoo, B. (2020). Virtual Reality Sickness: A Review of Causes and Measurements. *International Journal of Human-Computer Interaction, 36*(17), 1658–1682. doi:10.1080/10447318.2020.1778351

Chang, J., Tsui, L., Yeung, K., Yip, S., & Leung, G. (2016). Surgical vision: Google Glass and surgery. *Surgical Innovation, 23*(4), 422–426. doi:10.1177/1553350616646477 PMID:27146972

Chan, S. (2021). *Digitally Enabling 'Learning by Doing' in Vocational Education: Enhancing 'Learning as Becoming' Processes.* Springer Nature. doi:10.1007/978-981-16-3405-5

Chaytor, N., & Schmitter-Edgecombe, M. (2003). The Ecological Validity of Neuropsychological Tests: A Review of the Literature on Everyday Cognitive Skills. *Neuropsychology Review, 13*(4), 181–197. doi:10.1023/B:NERV.0000009483.91468.fb PMID:15000225

Chebanova, A. (n.d.). Making Use of Virtual Reality in Healthcare. *Steel Kiwi.* https://steelkiwi.com/blog/making-use-of-virtual-reality-in-healthcare/

Chen, A., Jacobsen, K. H., Deshmukh, A. A., & Cantor, S. B. (2015). The evolution of the disability-adjusted life year (DALY). *Socio-Economic Planning Sciences, 49*, 10–15. doi:10.1016/j.seps.2014.12.002

Cheng, T. S., Lu, Y. C., & Yang, C. S. (2015). Using the multi-display teaching system to lower cognitive load. *Journal of Educational Technology & Society, 18*(4), 128–140.

Chen, K., Barnes-Horowitz, N., Treanor, M., Sun, M., Young, K. S., & Craske, M. G. (2021). Virtual Reality Reward Training for Anhedonia: A Pilot Study. *Frontiers in Psychology, 11*, 613617. doi:10.3389/fpsyg.2020.613617 PMID:33488482

Chen, P. P., & Budenz, D. L. (1998, March 1). The Effects of Cataract Extraction on the Visual Field of Eyes with Chronic Open-Angle Glaucoma. *American Journal of Ophthalmology, 125*(3), 325–333. doi:10.1016/S0002-9394(99)80142-1 PMID:9512149

Chesham, R. K., Malouff, J. M., & Schutte, N. S. (2018). Meta-analysis of the efficacy of virtual reality exposure therapy for social anxiety. *Behaviour Change*, *35*(3), 152–166. doi:10.1017/bec.2018.15

Childs, B. S., Manganiello, M. D., & Korets, R. (2019). Novel Education and Simulation Tools in Urologic Training. *Current Urology Reports*, *20*(12), 81. doi:10.100711934-019-0947-8 PMID:31782033

Chinnock, C. (1994). Virtual reality in surgery and medicine. *Hospital Technology Series*, *13*(18), 1–48. PMID:10172193

Cho, D.-R., & Lee, S.-H. (2019). Effects of virtual reality immersive training with computerized cognitive training on cognitive function and activities of daily living performance in patients with acute stage stroke. *Medicine*, *98*(11), e14752. doi:10.1097/MD.0000000000014752 PMID:30882644

Chou, P.-H., Tseng, P.-T., Wu, Y.-C., Chang, J. P.-C., Tu, Y.-K., Stubbs, B., ... Sui, K.-P. (2021). Efficacy and acceptability of different interventions for acrophobia: A network meta-analysis of randomised controlled trials. *Journal of Affective Disorders*, *282*, 786–794. doi:10.1016/j.jad.2020.12.172 PMID:33601719

Chow-Wing-Bom, H., Dekker, T. M., & Jones, P. R. (2020, April). The Worse Eye Revisited: Evaluating the Impact of Asymmetric Peripheral Vision Loss on Everyday Function. *Vision Research*, *169*, 49–57. doi:10.1016/j.visres.2019.10.012 PMID:32179339

Chua, S. I. L., Tan, N. C., Wong, W. T., Allen, J. C. Jr, Quah, J. H. M., Malhotra, R., & Østbye, T. (2019). Virtual reality for screening of cognitive function in older persons: Comparative study. *Journal of Medical Internet Research*, *21*(8), e14821. doi:10.2196/14821 PMID:31373274

Chung, J., Pagnini, F., & Langer, E. (2016). Mindful navigation for pedestrians: Improving engagement with augmented reality. *Technology in Society*, *45*, 29–33. doi:10.1016/j.techsoc.2016.02.006

Cicero, M. T. (2001). Cicero on the ideal orator (de oratore) (J. M. May & J. Wisse, Trans.). Oxford, UK: Oxford University Press. (Original publication 55 BCE)

Cicerone, K. D., Dahlberg, C., Kalmar, K., Langenbahn, D. M., Malec, J. F., Bergquist, T. F., & Morse, P. A. (2000). Evidence-based cognitive rehabilitation: Recommendations for clinical practice. *Archives of Physical Medicine and Rehabilitation*, *81*(12), 1596–1615. doi:10.1053/apmr.2000.19240 PMID:11128897

Cidrim, L., Braga, P., & Madeiro, F. (2018). Desembaralhando: A Mobile Application for Intervention in the Problem of Dyslexic Children Mirror Writing. *Revista CEFAC*, *20*(1), 13–20. doi:10.1590/1982-0216201820111917

Cidrim, L., & Madeiro, F. (2017). Information and Communication Technology (ICT) applied to dyslexia: Literature review. *Revista CEFAC*, 19(1), 99- 108.Correa, M. R. & González, M. J. A. (2014). Las TIC al servicio de la inclusión educativa. *Digital Education Review*, (25), 108–126.

Cieślik, B., Mazurek, J., Rutkowskic, S., Kiper, P., Turolla, A., & Szczepańska-Gierachae, J. (2020). Virtual reality in psychiatric disorders: A systematic review of reviews. *Complementary Therapies in Medicine*, *52*, 102480. doi:10.1016/j.ctim.2020.102480 PMID:32951730

Ciharova, M., Furukawa, T. A., Efthimiou, O., Karyotaki, E., Miguel, C., Noma, H., Cipriani, A., Riper, H., & Cuijpers, P. (2021). Cognitive restructuring, behavioral activation and cognitive-behavioral therapy in the treatment of adult depression: A network meta-analysis. *Journal of Consulting and Clinical Psychology*, *89*(6), 563–574. doi:10.1037/ccp0000654 PMID:34264703

Cipresso, P., Giglioli, I., Raya, M., & Riva, G. (2018). The past, present, and future of virtual and augmented reality research: A network and cluster analysis of the literature. *Frontiers in Psychology*, *9*, 2086. doi:10.3389/fpsyg.2018.02086 PMID:30459681

Clapp, J. D., Olsen, S. A., Beck, J. G., Palyo, S. A., Grant, D. M., Gudmundsdottir, B., & Marques, L. (2011). The driving behavior survey: Scale construction and validation. *Journal of Anxiety Disorders*, *25*(1), 96–105. doi:10.1016/j.janxdis.2010.08.008 PMID:20832988

Clark, B. (2017). Study: VR Twice as Effective as Morphine at Treating Pain. *TNW News*. https://thenextweb.com/news/study-vr-twice-as-effective-as-morphine-at-treating-pain

Climent, G., Rodríguez, C., García, T., Areces, D., Mejías, M., Aierbe, A., Moreno, M., Cueto, E., Castellá, J., & Feli González, M. (2021). New virtual reality tool (Nesplora Aquarium) for assessing attention and working memory in adults: A normative study. *Applied Neuropsychology. Adult*, *28*(4), 403–415. doi:10.1080/23279095.2019.1646745 PMID:31382773

Coburn, J. Q., Freeman, I., & Salmon, J. L. (2017). A review of the capabilities of current low-cost virtual reality technology and its potential to enhance the design process. *Journal of Computing and Information Science in Engineering*, *17*(3), 031013. doi:10.1115/1.4036921

Cockrell, R. K., Fischer, K., Stevens, L., Robison, E. S., Cooney, T. A., Lagunas, M., & Rahman, S. (2021). OADN Virtual Simulation Reviews: Team Collaboration to Develop an Online Resource to Assist Nurse Educators. *Teaching and Learning in Nursing*, *16*(4), 352–356. Advance online publication. doi:10.1016/j.teln.2021.06.004

Coelho, L., Braga, D., Dias, M., & García-Mateo, C. (2011). An Automatic Voice Pleasantness Classification System Based on Prosodic and Acoustic Patterns of Voice Preference. *Proc. of Interspeech*, 2460.

Coelho, L., & Reis, S. (2021). Ethical Issues of Gamification in Healthcare: The Need to be Involved. In *Handbook of Research on Solving Modern Healthcare Challenges With Gamification* (pp. 1–19). IGI Global. doi:10.4018/978-1-7998-7472-0.ch001

Coleman, B., Marion, S., Rizzo, A., Turnbull, J., & Nolty, A. (2019). Virtual reality assessment of classroom–related attention: An ecologically relevant approach to evaluating the effectiveness of working memory training. *Frontiers in Psychology*, *10*, 1851. doi:10.3389/fpsyg.2019.01851 PMID:31481911

Coleman, E. R., Moudgal, R., Lang, K., Hyacinth, H. I., Awosika, O. O., Kissela, B. M., & Feng, W. (2017). Early Rehabilitation After Stroke: A Narrative Review. *Current Atherosclerosis Reports*, *19*(12), 59. doi:10.100711883-017-0686-6 PMID:29116473

Collins, T., Pizarro, D., Gasparini, S., Bourdel, N., Chauvet, P., Canis, M., Calvet, L., & Bartoli, A. (2021). Augmented Reality Guided Laparoscopic Surgery of the Uterus. *IEEE Transactions on Medical Imaging*, *40*(1), 371–380. doi:10.1109/TMI.2020.3027442 PMID:32986548

Concannon, B. J., Esmail, S., & Roduta Roberts, M. (2019). Head-Mounted Display Virtual Reality in Post-secondary Education and Skill Training. *Frontiers in Education*, *4*(August), 1–23. doi:10.3389/feduc.2019.00080

Condino, S., Turini, G., Parchi, P., Viglialoro, R., Piolanti, N., Gesi, M., Ferrari, M., & Ferrari, V. (2018). How to build a patient-specific hybrid simulator for orthopaedic open surgery: Benefits and limits of mixed-reality using the Microsoft HoloLens. *Journal of Healthcare Engineering*, *2018*, 1–12. Advance online publication. doi:10.1155/2018/5435097 PMID:30515284

Corregidor-Sánchez, A.-I., Segura-Fragoso, A., Criado-Álvarez, J.-J., Rodríguez-Hernández, M., Mohedano-Moriano, A., & Polonio-López, B. (2020). Effectiveness of Virtual Reality Systems to Improve the Activities of Daily Life in Older People. *International Journal of Environmental Research and Public Health*, *17*(17), 6283. doi:10.3390/ijerph17176283 PMID:32872313

Corriveau Lecavalier, N., Ouellet, E., Boller, B., & Belleville, S. (2020). Use of immersive virtual reality to assess episodic memory: A validation study in older adults. *Neuropsychological Rehabilitation*, *30*(3), 462–480. doi:10.1080/09602011.2018.1477684 PMID:29807474

Costa, R. T. D., Carvalho, M. R. D., & Nardi, A. E. (2010). Virtual reality exposure therapy in the treatment of driving phobia. *Psicologia: Teoria e Pesquisa (Brasília)*, *26*(1), 131–137. doi:10.1590/S0102-37722010000100015

Côté, S., & Bouchard, S. (2009). Cognitive mechanisms underlying virtual reality exposure. *Cyberpsychology & Behavior*, *12*(2), 121–129. doi:10.1089/cpb.2008.0008 PMID:19250009

Coyne, L., Merritt, T. A., Parmentier, B. L., Sharpton, R. A., & Takemoto, J. K. (2019). The Past, Present, and Future of Virtual Reality in Pharmacy Education. *American Journal of Pharmaceutical Education*, *83*(3), 7456. doi:10.5688/ajpe7456 PMID:31065173

Crouch, L., Rolleston, C., & Gustafsson, M. (2021). Eliminating global learning poverty: The importance of equalities and equity. *International Journal of Educational Development*, *82*, 102250. doi:10.1016/j.ijedudev.2020.102250

Crowder, R. G. (1976). *Principles of learning and memory*. Lawrence Erlbaum.

Cuetos, F., & Domínguez, A. (2012). *Neurología del lenguaje. Bases e implicaciones clínicas*. Editorial Médica Panamericana.

Cuetos, F., Soriano, M., & Rello, L. (2019). *Dislexia. Ni despiste, ni pereza: Todas las claves para entender el trastorno*. La Esfera de los Libros.

Cuijpers, P. (2017). Four Decades of Outcome Research on Psychotherapies for Adult Depression: An Overview of a Series of Meta-Analyses. *Canadian Psychology*, *58*(1), 7–19. doi:10.1037/cap0000096

Cuijpers, P., Cristea, I. A., Karyotaki, E., Reijnders, M., & Huibers, M. J. (2016). How effective are cognitive behavior therapies for major depression and anxiety disorders? A meta-analytic update of the evidence. *World Psychiatry; Official Journal of the World Psychiatric Association (WPA)*, *15*(3), 245–258. doi:10.1002/wps.20346 PMID:27717254

Cuijpers, P., Noma, H., Karyotaki, E., Vinkers, C. H., Cipriani, A., & Furukawa, T. A. (2020, February). A network meta-analysis of the effects of psychotherapies, pharmacotherapies and their combination in the treatment of adult depression. *World Psychiatry; Official Journal of the World Psychiatric Association (WPA)*, *19*(1), 92–107. doi:10.1002/wps.20701 PMID:31922679

Currie, M. E., McLeod, A. J., Moore, J. T., Chu, M. W. A., Patel, R., Kiaii, B., & Peters, T. M. (2016). Augmented reality system for ultrasound guidance of transcatheter aortic valve implantation. *Innovations*, *11*(1), 31–39. doi:10.1097/imi.0000000000000235 PMID:26938173

Cuschieri, A. (2006). Nature of human error. Implications for surgical practice. *Annals of Surgery*, *244*(5), 642–648. doi:10.1097/01.sla.0000243601.36582.18 PMID:17060751

Cushman, L. A., Stein, K., & Duffy, C. J. (2008). Detecting navigational deficits in cognitive aging and Alzheimer disease using virtual reality. *Neurology*, *71*(12), 888–895. doi:10.1212/01.wnl.0000326262.67613.fe PMID:18794491

Cutolo, F. (2018). Augmented Reality in Image-Guided Surgery. Encyclopedia of Computer Graphics and Games, 1-11. doi:10.1007/978-3-319-08234-9_78-1

Dainer-Best, J., Shumake, J. D., & Beevers, C. G. (2018). Positive Imagery Training Increases Positive Self-Referent Cognition in Depression. *Behaviour Research and Therapy*, *111*, 72–83. doi:10.1016/j.brat.2018.09.010 PMID:30321746

Darby, R. R., & Dickerson, B. C. (2017). Dementia, Decision Making, and Capacity. *Harvard Review of Psychiatry*, *25*(6), 270–278. doi:10.1097/HRP.0000000000000163 PMID:29117022

Dare, A., Grimes, E., Gillies, R., Greenberg, S., Hagander, L., Meara, J., & Leather, A. (2014). Global surgery: Defining an emerging global health field. *Lancet*, *384*(9961), 2245–2247. doi:10.1016/S0140-6736(14)60237-3 PMID:24853601

David, D., Cristea, I., & Hofmann, S. G. (2018, January). Why Cognitive Behavioral Therapy is the Current Gold Standard of psychotherapy. *Frontiers in Psychiatry*, *9*, 4. doi:10.3389/fpsyt.2018.00004 PMID:29434552

Dávila, M., Ceh, J., Balseca, S., & Rendón, M. (2021). Cuidado de enfermería durante el postoperatorio inmediato. *Revista Eugenio Espejo, 15*(2), 18-27. https://bit.ly/3iuDEoE

Davila, D., Helm, M., Frelich, M., Gould, J., & Goldblatt, M. (2018). Robotic skills can be aided by laparoscopic training. *Surgical Endoscopy*, *32*(6), 2683–2688. doi:10.100700464-017-5963-5 PMID:29214515

de Freitas Cardoso, M. G., Faleiro, R. M., de Paula, J. J., Kummer, A., Caramelli, P., Teixeira, A. L., de Souza, L. C., & Miranda, A. S. (2019). Cognitive Impairment Following Acute Mild Traumatic Brain Injury. *Frontiers in Neurology*, *10*, 198. doi:10.3389/fneur.2019.00198 PMID:30906278

De Luca, R., Maggio, M. G., Maresca, G., Latella, D., Cannavò, A., Sciarrone, F., Lo Voi, E., Accorinti, M., Bramanti, P., & Calabrò, R. S. (2019b). Improving cognitive function after traumatic brain injury: A clinical trial on the potential use of the semi-immersive virtual reality. *Behavioural Neurology*, 1–7. Advance online publication. doi:10.1155/2019/9268179 PMID:31481980

De Luca, R., Portaro, S., Le Cause, M., De Domenico, C., Maggio, M. G., Cristina Ferrera, M., & Calabrò, R. S. (2020). Cognitive rehabilitation using immersive virtual reality at young age: A case report on traumatic brain injury. *Applied Neuropsychology. Child*, *9*(3), 282–287. doi:10.1080/21622965.2019.1576525 PMID:30838889

De Marco, M. (2010). Programas informáticos para trastornos de lectoescritura, Dislexia y/o TDAH. In *25 Años de Integración Escolar en España: Tecnología e Inclusión en el ámbito educativo, laboral y comunitario*. Consejería de Educación, Formación y Empleo.

De Visser, H., Watson, M., Salvado, O., & Passenger, J. D. (2011). Progress in virtual reality simulators for surgical training and certification. *The Medical Journal of Australia*, *194*(S4), S38–S40. doi:10.5694/j.1326-5377.2011.tb02942.x PMID:21401487

Dehghani, M., Acikgoz, F., Mashatan, A., & Lee, S. H. (2021). A holistic analysis towards understanding consumer perceptions of virtual reality devices in the post-adoption phase. *Behaviour & Information Technology*, 1–19. doi:10.1080/0144929X.2021.1876767

Dehn, L. B., Kate, L. M. P., Botsch, M., Driessen, M., & Beblo, T. (2017). Training in a comprehensive everyday-like virtual reality environment compared to computerized cognitive training for patients with depression. *Computers in Human Behavior*, *79*, 40–52. doi:10.1016/j.chb.2017.10.019

Del Pozo Jiménez, G., Rodríguez Monsalve, M., Carballido Rodríguez, J., & Castillón Vela, I. (2019). Virtual reality and intracorporeal navigation in urology. Realidad virtual y navegación intraquirúrgica en urología. *Archivos Espanoles de Urologia*, *72*(8), 867–881. PMID:31579046

DeMaria, S., & Levine, A. I. (2013). The use of stress to enrich the simulated environment. In *The comprehensive textbook of healthcare simulation* (pp. 65–72). Springer. doi:10.1007/978-1-4614-5993-4_5

Dennick, R. (2016). Constructivism: Reflections on twenty-five years teaching the constructivist approach in medical education. *International Journal of Medical Education*, *7*, 200–205. doi:10.5116/ijme.5763.de11 PMID:27344115

Desselle, M., Brown, R., James, A., Midwinter, M., Powell, S., & Woodruff, M. (2020). Augmented and virtual reality in surgery. *Computing in Science & Engineering*, *22*(3), 18–26. doi:10.1109/MCSE.2020.2972822

Deterding, S., Sicart, M., Nacke, L., O'Hara, K., & Dixon, D. (2011). Gamification. using game-design elements in non-gaming contexts. In *CHI '11 Extended Abstracts on Human Factors in Computing Systems, CHI EA '11* (pp. 2425–2428). Association for Computing Machinery. doi:10.1145/1979742.1979575

Di Nardo, D., Eberspacher, C., & Palazzini, G. (2020). Technology spreading in healthcare: A novel era in medicine and surgery? *Journal of Gastric Surgery*, *2*(2), 45–48. doi:10.36159/jgs.v2i2.26

Diamond, A. (2013). Executive functions. *Annual Review of Psychology*, *64*(1), 135–168. doi:10.1146/annurev-psych-113011-143750 PMID:23020641

Diana, M., & Marescaux, J. (2015). Robotic surgery. *Journal of British Surgery*, *102*(2), e15–e28. doi:10.1002/bjs.9711 PMID:25627128

Diaz Baquero, A. A., Dröes, R. M., Perea Bartolomé, M. V., Irazoki, E., Toribio-Guzmán, J. M., Franco-Martín, M. A., & van der Roest, H. (2021). Methodological Designs Applied in the Development of Computer-Based Training Programs for the Cognitive Rehabilitation in People with Mild Cognitive Impairment (MCI) and Mild Dementia. Systematic Review. *Journal of Clinical Medicine*, *10*(6), 1222. doi:10.3390/jcm10061222 PMID:33809445

Dickey, R. M., Srikishen, N., Lipshultz, L. I., Spiess, P. E., Carrion, R. E., & Hakky, T. S. (2016). Augmented reality assisted surgery: A urologic training tool. *Asian Journal of Andrology*, *18*(5), 732–734. doi:10.4103/1008-682X.166436 PMID:26620455

Dimaio, S., Kapur, T., Cleary, K., Aylward, S., Kazanzides, P., & Vosburgh, K. (2007). Challenges in image-guided therapy system design. *Neuroimage, 37*, S144-51.

Dingli, A., & Bondin, L. (2019, August). Realtime Adaptive Virtual Reality for Pain Reduction. In *2019 IEEE Conference on Games (CoG)* (pp. 1-4). IEEE. 10.1109/CIG.2019.8848119

Disabled World. (2021). *Disability Statistics: Information*. Charts, Graphs and Tables.

Donker, T., Cornelisz, I., Klaveren, C., Straten, A., Carlbring, P., Cuijpers, P., & Gelder, J.-L. (2019). Effectiveness of Self-guided App-Based Virtual Reality Cognitive Behavior Therapy for Acrophobia: A Randomized Clinical Trial. *JAMA Psychiatry*, *76*(7), 682–690. doi:10.1001/jamapsychiatry.2019.0219 PMID:30892564

Dores, R. A., Carvalho, I., Abreu, C., Nunes, J., Leitão, M., & Castro-Caldas, A. (2009). *Virtual Reality: Application to cognitive rehabilitation acquired brain injury*. Academic Press.

Drewniak, T., Rzepecki, M., Juszczak, K., Kwiatek, W., Bielecki, J., Zieliński, K., Ruta, A., Czekierda, Ł., & Moczulskis, Z. (2011). Obrazowanie guza nerki w trakcie zabiegow nerkooszczednych: Model zwierzecy i zastosowanie kliniczne [Augmented reality for image guided therapy (ARIGT) of kidney tumor during nephron sparing surgery (NSS): animal model and clinical approach]. *Folia Medica Cracoviensia*, *51*(1-4), 77–90. PMID:22891540

Duarte, M. L., Santos, L. R., Júnior, J. G., & Peccin, M. S. (2020). Learning anatomy by virtual reality and augmented reality. A scope review. *Morphologie*, *104*(347), 254–266. doi:10.1016/j.morpho.2020.08.004 PMID:32972816

Duke, J., Guest, M., & Boggess, M. (2010). Age-related safety in professional heavy vehicle drivers: A literature review. *Accident; Analysis and Prevention*, *42*(2), 364–371. doi:10.1016/j.aap.2009.09.026 PMID:20159055

Durgahee, T. (1998). Facilitating reflection: From a sage on stage to a guide on the side. *Nurse Education Today*, *18*(2), 158–164. doi:10.1016/S0260-6917(98)80021-X PMID:9592516

Durham, M., Engel, B., Ferrill, T., Halford, J., Singh, T. P., & Gladwell, M. (2019). Digitally augmented learning in implant dentistry. *Oral and Maxillofacial Surgery Clinics of North America*, *31*(3), 387–398. doi:10.1016/j.coms.2019.03.003 PMID:31153725

Durning, S. J., & Artino, A. R. (2011). Situativity theory: a perspective on how participants and the environment can interact: AMEE Guide no. 52. *Medical Teacher*, *33*(3), 188–199. doi:10.3109/0142159X.2011.550965 PMID:21345059

Duzmanska, N., Strojny, P., & Strojny, A. (2018). Can simulator sickness be avoided? A review on temporal aspects of simulator sickness. *Frontiers in Psychology*, *9*, 2132. doi:10.3389/fpsyg.2018.02132 PMID:30459688

Dymora, P., & Niemiec, K. (2019). Gamification as a supportive tool for school children with dyslexia. *Informatics (MDPI)*, *6*(4), 48. doi:10.3390/informatics6040048

Dyson, A., Farrell, P., Polat, F., Hutcheson., G., & Gallanaugh, F. (2004). Inclusion and Pupil Achievement. London: Department for Education and Skills.

Elbogen, E. B., Dennis, P. A., Van Voorhees, E. E., Blakey, S. M., Johnson, J. L., Johnson, S. C., & Belger, A. (2019). Cognitive rehabilitation with mobile technology and social support for veterans with TBI and PTSD: A randomized clinical trial. *The Journal of Head Trauma Rehabilitation*, *34*(1), 1–10. doi:10.1097/HTR.0000000000000435 PMID:30169439

Elhai, J. D., Grubaugh, A. L., Kashdan, T. B., & Frueh, B. C. (2008). Empirical examination of a proposed refinement to DSM-IV post-traumatic stress disorder symptom criteria using the National Comorbidity Survey Replication data. *The Journal of Clinical Psychiatry*, *69*(4), 597–602. doi:10.4088/JCP.v69n0411 PMID:18294026

Eling, P. (2019). History of Neuropsychological Assessment. *Frontiers of Neurology and Neuroscience*, *44*, 164–178. doi:10.1159/000494963 PMID:31220853

Elliman, J., Loizou, M., & Loizides, F. (2016). Virtual Reality Simulation Training for Student Nurse Education. *8th International Conference on Games and Virtual Worlds for Serious Applications*.

Emmelkamp, P. M., Krijn, M., Hulsbosch, A. M., De Vries, S., Schuemie, M. J., & van der Mast, C. A. (2002). Virtual reality treatment versus exposure in vivo: A comparative evaluation in acrophobia. *Behaviour Research and Therapy*, *40*(5), 509–516. doi:10.1016/S0005-7967(01)00023-7 PMID:12038644

Emmelkamp, P. M., Meyerbröker, K., & Morina, N. (2020). Virtual reality therapy in social anxiety disorder. *Current Psychiatry Reports*, *22*(7), 1–9. doi:10.100711920-020-01156-1 PMID:32405657

Eng, C. M., Calkosz, D. M., Yang, S. Y., Williams, N. C., Thiessen, E. D., & Fisher, A. V. (2020, June). Doctoral colloquium—enhancing brain plasticity and cognition utilizing immersive technology and virtual reality contexts for gameplay. In *2020 6th International Conference of the Immersive Learning Research Network (iLRN)* (pp. 395-398). IEEE.

Eshuis, L. V., van Gelderen, M. J., van Zuiden, M., Nijdam, M. J., Vermetten, E., Olff, M., & Bakker, A. (2020). Efficacy of immersive PTSD treatments: A systematic review of virtual and augmented reality exposure therapy and a meta-analysis of virtual reality exposure therapy. *Journal of Psychiatric Research*. Advance online publication. doi:10.1016/j.jpsychires.2020.11.030 PMID:33248674

Ettenhofer, M. L., Guise, B., Brandler, B., Bittner, K., Gimbel, S. I., Cordero, E., Nelson Schmitt, S., Williams, K., Cox, D., Roy, M. J., & Chan, L. (2019). Neurocognitive driving rehabilitation in virtual environments (NeuroDRIVE): A pilot clinical trial for chronic traumatic brain injury. *NeuroRehabilitation*, *44*(4), 531–544. doi:10.3233/NRE-192718 PMID:31256093

Compilation of References

Evans, F. A., Wong, D., Lawson, D. W., Withiel, T. D., & Stolwyk, R. J. (2019). What are the most common memory complaints following stroke? A frequency and exploratory factor analysis of items from the everyday memory questionnaire- revised. *The Clinical Neuropsychologist, 34*(3), 498–511. doi:10.1080/13854046.2019.1652349 PMID:32189571

Ewers, R., & Schicho, K. (2009). Augmented reality telenavigation in cranio maxillofacial oral surgery. *Studies in Health Technology and Informatics, 150*, 24–25. PMID:19745259

Falconer, C. J., Rovira, A., King, J. A., Gilbert, P., Antley, A., Fearon, P., Ralph, N., Slater, M., & Brewin, C. R. (2016). Embodying Self-compassion within Virtual Reality and its Effects on Patients with Depression. *BJPsych Open, 2*, 74–80.

Farronato, M., Maspero, C., Lanteri, V., Fama, A., Ferrati, F., Pettenuzzo, A., & Farronato, D. (2019). Current state of the art in the use of augmented reality in dentistry: A systematic review of the literature. *BMC Oral Health, 19*(1), 135. doi:10.118612903-019-0808-3 PMID:31286904

Ferreira Reis, A., Wirth, G. J., & Iselin, C. E. (2018). Réalité augmentée en urologie: Actualité et avenir [Augmented reality in urology: present and future]. *Revue Medicale Suisse, 14*(629), 2154–2157. PMID:30484972

Fida, B., Cutolo, F., di Franco, G., Ferrari, M., & Ferrari, V. (2018). Augmented reality in open surgery. *Updates in Surgery, 70*(3), 389–400. doi:10.100713304-018-0567-8 PMID:30006832

Fiorella, L., Van Gog, T., Hoogerheide, V., & Mayer, R. E. (2017). It's all a matter of perspective: Viewing first-person video modeling examples promotes learning of an assembly task. *Journal of Educational Psychology, 109*(5), 653–665. doi:10.1037/edu0000161

Fischer, M., Fuerst, B., Lee, S. C., Fotouhi, J., Habert, S., Weidert, S., Euler, E., Osgood, G., & Navab, N. (2016). Pre-clinical usability study of multiple augmented reality concepts for K-wire placement. *International Journal of Computer Assisted Radiology and Surgery, 11*(6), 1007–1014. doi:10.100711548-016-1363-x PMID:26995603

Fleming, T., Dixon, R., Frampton, C., & Merry, S. (2011). A Pragmatic Randomised Controlled Trial of computerised CBT (SPARX) for symptoms of depression among adolescents excluded from mainstream education. *Behavioural and Cognitive Psychotherapy, 40*(5), 529–541. doi:10.1017/S1352465811000695 PMID:22137185

Fodor, L. A., Coteţ, C. D., Cuijpers, P., Szamoskozi, Ş., David, D., & Cristea, I. A. (2018). The effectiveness of virtual reality based interventions for symptoms of anxiety and depression: A meta-analysis. *Scientific Reports, 8*(1), 10323. Advance online publication. doi:10.103841598-018-28113-6 PMID:29985400

Foohey, S. (2020). *Virtual Resus Room.* https://virtualresusroom.com/

Foronda, C. L., Fernandez-Burgos, M., Nadeau, C., Kelley, C. N., & Henry, M. N. (2020). Virtual Simulation in Nursing Education: A Systematic Review Spanning 1996 to 2018. Simulation in Healthcare. *Journal of the Society for Simulation in Healthcare, 15*(1), 46–54. doi:10.1097/SIH.0000000000000411 PMID:32028447

Fowler, C. (2015). Virtual reality and learning: Where is the pedagogy? *British Journal of Educational Technology, 46*(2), 412–422. doi:10.1111/bjet.12135

Freeman, D., Haselton, P., Freeman, J., Spanlang, B., Kishore, S., Albery, E., Denne, M., Brown, P., Slater, M., & Nickless, A. (2018). Automated psychological therapy using immersive virtual reality for treatment of fear of heights: A single-blind, parallel-group, randomised controlled trial. *Psychiatry, 5*(8), 625–632. doi:10.1016/S2215-0366(18)30226-8 PMID:30007519

Freeman, D., Reeve, S., Robinson, A., Ehlers, A., Clark, D., Spanlang, B., & Slater, M. (2017). Virtual reality in the assessment, understanding, and treatment of mental health disorders. *Psychological Medicine, 47*(14), 2393–2400. doi:10.1017/S003329171700040X PMID:28325167

Furht, B. (Ed.). (2011). *Handbook of Augmented Reality*. doi:10.1007/978-1-4614-0064-6

Gaba, D. M. (2007). The future vision of simulation in healthcare. *Simulation in Healthcare, 2*(2), 126–135. https://doi-org.ezproxy2.umc.edu/10.1097/01.SIH.0000258411.38212.32

Gagnon, K., Young, B., Bachman, T., Longbottom, T., Severin, R., & Walker, M. J. (2020). Doctor of physical therapy education in a hybrid learning environment: Reimagining the possibilities and navigating a "new normal". *Physical Therapy, 100*(8), 1268–1277. doi:10.1093/ptj/pzaa096 PMID:32424417

Galarza, P., Parnasa, E., Guttmann, N., & Joshua, M. (2021, April 14). Artifactual Visual Field Defects Identified on Technically 'Reliable' Visual Field Studies in a Neuro-Ophthalmology Practice. *Eye and Brain, 13*, 79–88. doi:10.2147/EB.S274523 PMID:33889041

Gamito, P., Oliveira, J., Coelho, C., Morais, D., Lopes, P., Pacheco, J., Brito, R., Soares, F., Santos, N., & Barata, A. F. (2017). Cognitive training on stroke patients via virtual reality-based serious games. *Disability and Rehabilitation, 39*(4), 385–388. doi:10.3109/09638288.2014.934925 PMID:25739412

Gamito, P., Oliveira, J., Morais, D., Coelho, C., Santos, N., Alves, C., Galamba, A., Soeiro, M., Yerra, M., French, H., Talmers, L., Gomes, T., & Brito, R. (2018). Cognitive Stimulation of Elderly Individuals with Instrumental Virtual Reality-Based Activities of Daily Life: Pre-Post Treatment Study. *Cyberpsychology, Behavior, and Social Networking, 22*(1), 69–75. doi:10.1089/cyber.2017.0679 PMID:30040477

Gamito, P., Oliveira, J., Rosa, P., Morais, D., Duarte, N., Oliveira, S., & Saraiva, T. (2010). PTSD Elderly War Veterans: A Clinical Controlled Pilot Study. *Cyberpsychology, Behavior, and Social Networking, 13*(1), 43–48. doi:10.1089/cyber.2009.0237 PMID:20528292

Gamito, P., Oliviera, J., Alves, C., Santos, N., Coelho, C., & Brito, R. (2020). Virtual reality based cognitive stimulation to improve cognitive functioning in community elderly: A controlled study. *Cyberpsychology, Behavior, and Social Networking, 23*(3), 150–158. doi:10.1089/cyber.2019.0271 PMID:32031888

Gandolfi, E., Kosko, K. W., & Ferdig, R. E. (2021). Situating presence within extended reality for teacher training: Validation of the extended Reality Presence Scale (XRPS) in preservice teacher use of immersive 360 video. *British Journal of Educational Technology, 52*(2), 824–841. doi:10.1111/bjet.13058

Gautam, G., Benway, B. M., Bhayani, S. B., & Zorn, K. C. (2009). Robot-assisted partial nephrectomy: Current perspectives and future prospects. *Urology, 74*(4), 735–740. doi:10.1016/j.urology.2009.03.041 PMID:19616827

Gautam, S., Jain, A., Gautam, M., Vahia, V. N., & Gautam, A. (2017). Clinical practice guidelines for the management of generalised anxiety disorder (GAD) and panic disorder (PD). *Indian Journal of Psychiatry, 59*(5), S67. doi:10.4103/0019-5545.196975 PMID:28216786

Gauthier, S., Reisberg, B., Zaudig, M., Petersen, R. C., Ritchie, K., Broich, K., Belleville, S., Brodaty, H., Bennett, D., Chertkow, H., Cummings, J. L., de Leon, M., Feldman, H., Ganguli, M., Hampel, H., Scheltens, P., Tierney, M. C., Whitehouse, P., & Winblad, B. (2006). International Psychogeriatric Association Expert Conference on mild cognitive impairment. *Lancet, 367*(9518), 1262–1270. doi:10.1016/S0140-6736(06)68542-5 PMID:16631882

George, S., Clark, M., & Crotty, M. (2008). Validation of the Visual Recognition Slide Test with stroke: A component of the New South Wales occupational therapy off-road driver rehabilitation program. *Australian Occupational Therapy Journal, 55*(3), 172–179. doi:10.1111/j.1440-1630.2007.00699.x PMID:20887459

Gerup, J., Soerensen, C. B., & Dieckmann, P. (2020). Augmented reality and mixed reality for healthcare education beyond surgery: An integrative review. *International Journal of Medical Education, 11*, 1–18. doi:10.5116/ijme.5e01.eb1a PMID:31955150

Giaconia, R. M., Reinherz, H. Z., Silverman, A. B., Pakiz, B., Frost, A. K., & Cohen, E. (1995). Traumas and post-traumatic stress disorder in a community population of older adolescents. *Journal of the American Academy of Child and Adolescent Psychiatry*, *34*(10), 1369–1380. doi:10.1097/00004583-199510000-00023 PMID:7592275

Giglioli, C. I. A., Vidal, B. C., & Raya, A. M. (2019). A Virtual Versus an Augmented Reality Cooking Task Based-Tools: A Behavioral and Physiological Study on the Assessment of Executive Functions. *Frontiers in Psychology*, *10*, 2529. doi:10.3389/fpsyg.2019.02529 PMID:31798497

Gillies, M. (2020). Mel Slater: Becoming a Better Person Through VR Embodiment. *Medium.com* https://medium.com/virtual-reality-virtual-people/mel-slater-becoming-a-better-person-through-vr-embodiment-2c055058d8a4

Giraud, J.-M., May, F., Manet, G., Fenolland, J.-R., Meynard, J.-B., Sadat, A.-M., Mouinga, A., Seck, S., & Renard, J.-P. (2010, April 17). Analysis of Progression With GPA (Guided Progression Analysis) and Mean Deviation (MD) Indexes of Automated Perimetry in Ocular Hypertension and Glaucoma. *Investigative Ophthalmology & Visual Science*, *51*(13), 3997.

Glas, H. (2017). *Image guided surgery and the added value of augmented reality* (Master's thesis). University of Twente. https://bit.ly/3xXsgIh

Goh, P. S., & Sandars, J. (2020). A vision of the use of technology in medical education after the COVID-19 pandemic. *MedEdPublish*, *9*(1), 9. doi:10.15694/mep.2020.000049.1

Gold, J. I., Belmont, K. A., & Thomas, D. A. (2007). The neurobiology of virtual reality pain attenuation. *Cyberpsychology & Behavior*, *10*(4), 536–544. doi:10.1089/cpb.2007.9993 PMID:17711362

Golse, N., Petit, A., Lewin, M., Vibert, E., & Cotin, S. (2021). Augmented Reality during Open Liver Surgery Using a Markerless Non-rigid Registration System. *Journal of Gastrointestinal Surgery*, *25*(3), 662–671. doi:10.100711605-020-04519-4 PMID:32040812

Górski, Buń, Wichniarek, Zawadzki, & Hamrol. (n.d.). Effective Design of Educational Virtual Reality Applications for Medicine using Knowledge-Engineering Techniques. Eurasia Journal of Mathematics, Science and Technology Education, 13(2), 395–416.

Graf, A. C., Jacob, E., Twigg, D., & Nattabi, B. (2020). Contemporary nursing graduates' transition to practice: A critical review of transition models. *Journal of Clinical Nursing*, *29*(15-16), 3097–3107. doi:10.1111/jocn.15234 PMID:32129522

Graham, J. R., & Naglieri, J. A. (2012). Handbook of psychology: Vol. 10. *Assessment psychology*. John Wiley & Sons Inc.

Guha, D., Alotaibi, N. M., Nguyen, N., Gupta, S., McFaul, C., & Yang, V. (2017). Augmented Reality in Neurosurgery: A Review of Current Concepts and Emerging Applications. *The Canadian journal of neurological sciences. Le journal canadien des sciences neurologiques, 44*(3), 235–245.

Guha, D., Alotaibi, N., Nguyen, N., Gupta, S., McFaul, C., & Yang, V. (2017). Augmented reality in neurosurgery: A review of current concepts and emerging applications. *The Canadian Journal of Neurological Sciences*, *44*(3), 235–245. doi:10.1017/cjn.2016.443 PMID:28434425

Gujjar, K. R., van Wijk, A., Kumar, R., & de Jongh, A. (2019). Efficacy of virtual reality exposure therapy for the treatment of dental phobia in adults: A randomized controlled trial. *Journal of Anxiety Disorders*, *62*, 100–108. doi:10.1016/j.janxdis.2018.12.001 PMID:30717830

Gulati, M., Anand, V., Salaria, S.K., Jain, N., & Gupta, S. (2015). Computerized implant-dentistry: advances toward automation. *J Indian Soc Periodontol, 1*, 5-10.

Gumbs, A., De Simone, B., & Chouillard, E. (2020). Searching for a better definition of robotic surgery: Is it really different from laparoscopy? *Mini-invasive Surgery*, *4*. Advance online publication. doi:10.20517/2574-1225.2020.110

Gustafson, L. (1996). What is dementia? *Acta Neurologica Scandinavica, 94*(s168), 22–24. doi:10.1111/j.1600-0404.1996.tb00367.x PMID:8997414

Gutiérrez, A. (2020). ¿Un mundo nuevo? Realidad virtual, realidad aumentada, inteligencia artificial, humanidad mejorada, Internet de las cosas. *Arbor, 196*(797), a572–a572. doi:10.3989/arbor.2020.797n3009

Gutiérrez-Baños, J. L., Ballestero-Diego, R., Truan-Cacho, D., Aguilera-Tubet, C., Villanueva-Peña, A., & Manuel-Palazuelos, J. C. (2015). Urology residents training in laparoscopic surgery. Development of a virtual reality model. *Actas Urologicas Espanolas, 39*(9), 564–572. doi:10.1016/j.acuroe.2015.09.003 PMID:26068072

Gutierrez, J. M., Anorbe-Dıaz, C., & Gonzalez-Marrero, A. (2017). Virtual Technologies Trends in Education. *Eurasia Journal of Mathematics, Science and Technology Education, 13*(2), 469–486.

Hagger, M. S., Hankonen, N., Chatzisarantis, N. L. D., & Ryan, R. M. (2020). Changing Behavior Using Self-Determination Theory. In K. Hamilton, L. D. Cameron, M. S. Hagger, N. Hankonen, & T. Lintunen (Eds.), *The Handbook of Behavior Change, Cambridge Handbooks in Psychology* (pp. 104–119). Cambridge University Press. doi:10.1017/9781108677318.008

Halder, S., & Mahato, A. K. (2018). Cognition in ageing: implications for assessment and intervention. In Handbook of Research on Geriatric Health, Treatment, and Care (pp. 118-133). IGI Global. doi:10.4018/978-1-5225-3480-8.ch007

Hallet, J., Soler, L., Diana, M., Mutter, D., Baumert, T. F., Habersetzer, F., Marescaux, J., & Pessaux, P. (2015). Transthoracic minimally invasive liver resection guided by augmented reality. *Journal of the American College of Surgeons, 220*(5), e55–e60. doi:10.1016/j.jamcollsurg.2014.12.053 PMID:25840539

Hamacher, A., Kim, S. J., Cho, S. T., Pardeshi, S., Lee, S. H., Eun, S. J., & Whangbo, T. K. (2016). Application of Virtual, Augmented, and Mixed Reality to Urology. *International Neurourology Journal, 20*(3), 172–181. doi:10.5213/inj.1632714.357 PMID:27706017

Hamacher, A., Whangbo, T. K., Kim, S. J., & Chung, K. J. (2018). Virtual Reality and Simulation for Progressive Treatments in Urology. *International Neurourology Journal, 22*(3), 151–160. doi:10.5213/inj.1836210.105 PMID:30286577

Hamilton-Basich, M. (2021). *Philips Launches ClarifEye Augmented Reality Surgical Navigation.* Axis Imaging News. https://bit.ly/36QGmj1

Hamilton, D., McKechnie, J., Edgerton, E., & Wilson, C. (2021). Immersive virtual reality as a pedagogical tool in education: A systematic literature review of quantitative learning outcomes and experimental design. *Journal of Computers in Education, 8*(1), 1–32. doi:10.100740692-020-00169-2

HAPI. (2015). Mobility, Universal Design, Health, and Place. Health and Place Initiative.

Harrison, B., Oehmen, R., Robertson, A., Robertson, B., De Cruz, P., Khan, R., & Fick, D. (2017). Through the Eye of the Master: The Use of Virtual Reality in the Teaching of Surgical Hand Preparation. *5th International Conference on Serious Games and Applications for Health.*

Hartman, E., Reynolds, N. P., Ferrarini, C., Messmore, N., Evans, S., Al-Ebrahim, B., & Brown, J. M. (2020). Coloniality-decoloniality and critical global citizenship: Identity, belonging, and education abroad. *Frontiers: The Interdisciplinary Journal of Study Abroad, 32*(1), 33–59. doi:10.36366/frontiers.v32i1.433

Hashimoto, Y., Asaoka, R., Kiwaki, T., Sugiura, H., Asano, S., Murata, H., Fujino, Y., Matsuura, M., Miki, A., Mori, K., Ikeda, Y., Kanamoto, T., Yamagami, J., Inoue, K., Tanito, M., & Yamanishi, K. (2021, April 1). Deep Learning Model to Predict Visual Field in Central 10° from Optical Coherence Tomography Measurement in Glaucoma. *The British Journal of Ophthalmology, 105*(4), 507–513. doi:10.1136/bjophthalmol-2019-315600 PMID:32593978

Hasler, B. S., Kersten, B., & Sweller, J. (2007). Learner control, cognitive load and instructional animation. *Applied Cognitive Psychology*, *21*(6), 713–729. doi:10.1002/acp.1345

Hattab, G., Arnold, M., Strenger, L., Allan, M., Arsentjeva, D., Gold, O., Simpfendörfer, T., Maier-Hein, L., & Speidel, S. (2020). Kidney edge detection in laparoscopic image data for computer-assisted surgery: Kidney edge detection. *International Journal of Computer Assisted Radiology and Surgery*, *15*(3), 379–387. doi:10.100711548-019-02102-0 PMID:31828502

Hawkins, F. H. (2017). *Human factors in flight*. Routledge. doi:10.4324/9781351218580

Hawlitschek, A., & Joeckel, S. (2017). Increasing the effectiveness of digital educational games: The effects of a learning instruction on student's learning, motivation and cognitive load. *Computers in Human Behavior*, *72*, 79–86. doi:10.1016/j.chb.2017.01.040

Hayes, C., & Capper, S. (2020). Illustrating the transcendence of disciplinarity. In *Beyond Disciplinarity* (pp. 40–49). Routledge. doi:10.4324/9781315108377-4

Hayes, C., & Graham, Y. (2020). *Designing a Benchmarking Tool for Testing Posttest Confidence Levels in Emergency Obstetrics Training*. SAGE Publications. doi:10.4135/9781529709285

Hayes, C., Hinshaw, K., & Petrie, K. (2019). Reconceptualizing medical curriculum design in strategic clinical leadership training for the 21st century physician. In *Preparing Physicians to Lead in the 21st Century* (pp. 147–163). IGI Global. doi:10.4018/978-1-5225-7576-4.ch009

Headsets Relaxing Patients During VR Surgery at St. George's. (2019, December 26). Retrieved from https://www.stgeorges.nhs.uk/newsitem/vr-headsets-relaxing-patients-during-surgery-at-st-georges/

Health Quality Ontario. (2019). Internet-Delivered Cognitive Behavioural Therapy for Major Depression and Anxiety Disorders: A Health Technology Assessment. *Ontario Health Technology Assessment Series*, *19*(6), 1–199. PMID:30873251

Hennick, C. (2020). How VR in Healthcare Delivers Pandemic Education and Outreach. *Healthtech Magazine*. https://healthtechmagazine.net/article/2020/10/how-vr-healthcare-delivers-pandemic-education-and-outreach

Heong, Y. M., Ping, K. H., Hamdan, N., Ching, K. B., Yunos, J. M., Mohamad, M. M., ... Azid, N. (2020). Integration of Learning Styles and Higher Order Thinking Skills among Technical Students. *Journal of Technical Education and Training*, *12*(3), 171–179.

Hernández-Sánchez, R. (2017). El cirujano. *Revista de Sanidad Militar*, *71*(2), 177–184. https://bit.ly/3xXV8QX

Hertz, A., George, E., Vaccaro, C. & Brand, T. (2018). Head-to-head comparison of three virtual-reality robotic surgery simulators. *Journal of the Society of Laparoendoscopic & Robotic Surgeons, 22*(1). doi:10.4293/JSLS.2017.00081

Herumurti, D., Yuniarti, A., Rimawan, P., & Yunanto, A. A. (2019, July). Overcoming glossophobia based on virtual reality and heart rate sensors. In *2019 IEEE International Conference on Industry 4.0, Artificial Intelligence, and Communications Technology (IAICT)* (pp. 139-144). IEEE. 10.1109/ICIAICT.2019.8784846

Hervás, C. & Toledo, P. (2007). Las tecnologías como apoyo a la diversidad del alumnado. In *Tecnología educativa* (pp. 233-248). Madrid: McGraw-Hill.

Hessler, K. L., & Henderson, A. M. (2013). Interactive learning research: Application of cognitive load theory to nursing education. *International Journal of Nursing Education Scholarship*, *10*(1), 133–141. doi:10.1515/ijnes-2012-0029 PMID:23813334

Hew, K. F., & Lo, C. K. (2018). Flipped classroom improves student learning in health professions education: A meta-analysis. *BMC Medical Education*, *18*(1), 38. doi:10.118612909-018-1144-z PMID:29544495

Hilburg, R., Patel, N., Ambruso, S., Biewald, M. A., & Farouk, S. S. (2020). Medical education during the coronavirus disease-2019 pandemic: Learning from a distance. *Advances in Chronic Kidney Disease*, *27*(5), 412–417. doi:10.1053/j.ackd.2020.05.017 PMID:33308507

Hill, N. L., McDermott, C., Mogle, J., Munoz, E., DePasquale, N., Wion, R., & Whitaker, E. (2017). Subjective cognitive impairment and quality of life: A systematic review. *International Psychogeriatrics*, *29*(12), 1965–1977. doi:10.1017/S1041610217001636 PMID:28829003

Hilty, D. M., Parish, M. B., Chan, S., Torous, J., Xiong, G., & Yellowlees, P. M. (2020). A comparison of in-person, synchronous and asynchronous telepsychiatry: Skills/competencies, teamwork, and administrative workflow. *Journal of Technology in Behavioral Science*, *5*(3), 273–288. doi:10.100741347-020-00137-8

Hinkle, L., Khoshhal, K., & Metsis, V. (2019, June). Physiological Measurement for Emotion Recognition in Virtual Reality. In *2019 2nd International Conference on Data Intelligence and Security (ICDIS)* (pp. 136-143). IEEE. 10.1109/ICDIS.2019.00028

Hoffman, H. G., Chambers, G. T., Meyer, W. J., III, Arceneaux, L. L., Russell, W. J., Seibel, E. J., Richards, T. L., Sharar, S. R., & Patterson, D. R. (2011). Virtual reality as an adjunctive non-pharmacologic analgesic for acute burn pain during medical procedures. *Annals of Behavioral Medicine, 41*(2), 183–191. https://doi-org.ezproxy2.umc.edu/10.1007/s12160-010-9248-7

Hoffman, H. G., Sharar, S. R., Coda, B., Everett, J. J., Ciol, M., Richards, T., & Patterson, D. R. (2004). Manipulating presence influences the magnitude of virtual reality analgesia. *Pain, 111*(1), 162–168. doi:10.1016/j.pain.2004.06.013 PMID:15327820

Hofmann, S. G., Asnaani, A., Vonk, I. J., Sawyer, A. T., & Fang, A. (2012). The efficacy of cognitive behavioral therapy: A review of meta-analyses. *Cognitive Therapy and Research*, *36*(5), 427–440. doi:10.100710608-012-9476-1 PMID:23459093

Hogg, R. V., Tanis, E. A., & Zimmerman, D. L. (2013). *Probability and statistical inference* (9th ed.). Pearson Education.

Horigome, T., Kurokawa, S., Sawada, K., Kudo, S., Shiga, K., Mimura, M., & Kishimoto, T. (2020). Virtual reality exposure therapy for social anxiety disorder: A systematic review and meta-analysis. *Psychological Medicine*, *50*(15), 2487–2497. doi:10.1017/S0033291720003785 PMID:33070784

Horton, S. (2021). Empathy Cannot Sustain Action in Technology Accessibility. *Frontiers of Computer Science*, *3*, 31.

House, P. M., Pelzl, S., Furrer, S., Lanz, M., Simova, O., Voges, B., Stodieck, S., & Brückner, K. E. (2020). Use of the mixed reality tool "VSI Patient Education" for more comprehensible and imaginable patient educations before epilepsy surgery and stereotactic implantation of DBS or stereo-EEG electrodes. *Epilepsy Research*, *159*, 106247. doi:10.1016/j.eplepsyres.2019.106247 PMID:31794952

Howard, M., & Van Zandt, E. (2021). A meta-analysis of the virtual reality problem: Unequal effects of virtual reality sickness across individual differences. *Virtual Reality (Waltham Cross)*, *25*(4), 1221–1246. Advance online publication. doi:10.100710055-021-00524-3

Howell, H., & Mikeska, J. N. (2021). Approximations of practice as a framework for understanding authenticity in simulations of teaching. *Journal of Research on Technology in Education*, *53*(1), 8–20. doi:10.1080/15391523.2020.1809033

Howett, D., Castegnaro, A., Krzywicka, K., Hagman, J., Marchment, D., Henson, R., Rio, M., King, J.A., Burgess, N., & Chan, D. (2019) Differentiation of mild cognitive impairment using an entorhinal cortex-based test of virtual reality navigation. *Brain, 142*(6), 1751-1766. doi:10.1093/brain/awz116

Hruska, B., Irish, L. A., Pacella, M. L., Sledjeski, E. M., & Delahanty, D. L. (2014). PTSD symptom severity and psychiatric comorbidity in recent motor vehicle accident victims: A latent class analysis. *Journal of Anxiety Disorders, 28*(7), 644–649. doi:10.1016/j.janxdis.2014.06.009 PMID:25124501

Hsieh, M. C., & Lee, J. J. (2017). Preliminary Study of VR and AR Applications in Medical and Healthcare Education. *Journal of Nursing and Health Studies, 3*(1), 1.

Huang, K.-T. (2020). Exergaming executive functions: An immersive virtual reality-based cognitive training for adults aged 50 and older. *Cyberpsychology, Behavior, and Social Networking, 23*(3), 143–151. doi:10.1089/cyber.2019.0269 PMID:31794673

Humpherys, S. L., Bakir, N., & Babb, J. (2021). Experiential learning to foster tacit knowledge through a role play, business simulation. *Journal of Education for Business*, 1–7. doi:10.1080/08832323.2021.1896461

Humphrey Field Analyzer II-i Single Field Analysis: A Guide to Interpretation. (2013). https://www.zeiss.com/content/dam/Meditec/us/download/Glaucoma%20Landing%20Page/hfasinglefieldguidehfa5268.pdf

Hyland, J. R., & Hawkins, M. C. (2008). High-fidelity human simulation in nursing education: A review of literature and guide for implementation. *Teaching and Learning in Nursing, 4*(1), 14–21. doi:10.1016/j.teln.2008.07.004

Ibarra, F. F., Kardan, O., Hunter, M. R., Kotabe, H. P., Meyer, F. A. C., & Berman, M. G. (2017). Image Feature Types and Their Predictions of Aesthetic Preference and Naturalness. *Frontiers in Psychology, 8*, 632. doi:10.3389/fpsyg.2017.00632 PMID:28503158

Ijaz, K., Ahmadpour, N., Naismith, S. L., & Calvo, R. A. (2019). An Immersive Virtual Reality Platform for Assessing Spatial Navigation Memory in Predementia Screening: Feasibility and Usability Study. *JMIR Mental Health, 6*(9), e13887. doi:10.2196/13887 PMID:31482851

ILO. (2007). *Disability in the World of Work: Factsheet*. International Labour Organization.

Institute for Health Metrics and Evaluation (IHME). (2020). Retrieved 2021, from Health Data: http://www.healthdata.org/gbd/about

Integrated Benefits Institute. (2017). *Health and Productivity Benchmarking 2016*. Author.

Iqbal, M., Aydin, A., Lowdon, A., Ahmed, H., Muir, G., Khan, M., Dasgupta, P., & Ahmed, K. (2016). The effectiveness of Google GLASS as a vital signs monitor in surgery: A simulation study. *International Journal of Surgery, 36*, 293–297. doi:10.1016/j.ijsu.2016.11.013 PMID:27833004

Irazoki, E., Contreras-Somoza, L. M., Toribio-Guzmán, J. M., Jenaro-Río, C., van der Roest, H., & Franco-Martín, M. A. (2020). Technologies for cognitive training and cognitive rehabilitation for people with mild cognitive impairment and dementia. A systematic review. *Frontiers in Psychology, 11*, 648. doi:10.3389/fpsyg.2020.00648 PMID:32373018

Iwanaga, J., Loukas, M., Dumont, A. S., & Tubbs, R. S. (2021). A review of anatomy education during and after the COVID-19 pandemic: Revisiting traditional and modern methods to achieve future innovation. *Clinical Anatomy (New York, N.Y.), 34*(1), 108–114. doi:10.1002/ca.23655 PMID:32681805

Jansari, A., Devlin, A., Agnew, R., Akesson, K., Murphy, L., & Leadbetter, T. (2014). Ecological Assessment of Executive Functions: A New Virtual Reality Paradigm. *Brain Impairment, 15*(2), 71–87. doi:10.1017/BrImp.2014.14

Jensen, L., & Konradsen, F. (2018). A review of the use of virtual reality head-mounted displays in education and training. *Education and Information Technologies*, *23*(4), 1515–1529. doi:10.100710639-017-9676-0

Jentsch, F., & Curtis, M. (2017). *Simulation in aviation training*. Routledge. doi:10.4324/9781315243092

Jerdan, S. W., Grindle, M., Woerden, H. C., & Boulos, M. N. (2018). Head-Mounted Virtual Reality and Mental Health: Critical Review of Current Research. *JMIR Serious Games*, *6*(3), e14. doi:10.2196/games.9226 PMID:29980500

Jhuang, A. C., Sun, J. J., Trappey, A. J., Trappey, C. V., & Govindarajan, U. H. (2017, April). Computer supported technology function matrix construction for patent data analytics. In *2017 IEEE 21st International Conference on Computer Supported Cooperative Work in Design (CSCWD)* (pp. 457-462). IEEE. 10.1109/CSCWD.2017.8066737

Jiménez, J. E., Guzmán, R., Rodríguez, C., & Artiles, C. (2009). Prevalencia de las dificultades específicas de aprendizaje: La dislexia en español. *Anales de Psicología*, *25*, 78–85.

Jin, R., Pilozzi, A., & Huang, X. (2020). Current cognition tests, potential virtual reality applications, and serious games in cognitive assessment and non-pharmacological therapy for neurocognitive disorders. *Journal of Clinical Medicine*, *9*(10), 3287. doi:10.3390/jcm9103287 PMID:33066242

Joda, T., & Gallucci, G. O. (2015). The virtual patient in dental medicine. *Clinical Oral Implants Research*, *26*(6), 725–726. doi:10.1111/clr.12379 PMID:24665872

Joda, T., Gallucci, G., Wismeijer, D., & Zitzmann, N. (2019). Augmented and virtual reality in dental medicine: A systematic review. *Computers in Biology and Medicine*, *108*, 93–100. doi:10.1016/j.compbiomed.2019.03.012 PMID:31003184

Johnson, C. E., Kimble, L. P., Gunby, S. S., & Davis, A. H. (2020). Using deliberate practice and simulation for psychomotor skill competency acquisition and retention: A mixed-methods study. *Nurse Educator*, *45*(3), 150–154. doi:10.1097/NNE.0000000000000713 PMID:31246693

Johnston, A., Rae, J., Ariotti, N., Bailey, B., Lilja, A., Webb, R., Ferguson, C., Maher, S., Davis, T. P., Webb, R. I., McGhee, J., & Parton, R. G. (2018). Journey to the centre of the cell: Virtual reality immersion into scientific data. *Traffic (Copenhagen, Denmark)*, *19*(2), 105–110. doi:10.1111/tra.12538 PMID:29159991

Jongerius, C., Hessels, R. S., Romijn, J. A., Smets, E. M., & Hillen, M. A. (2020). The measurement of eye contact in human interactions: A scoping review. *Journal of Nonverbal Behavior*, *44*(3), 1–27. doi:10.100710919-020-00333-3

Jonsdottir, J., Baglio, F., Gindri, P., Isernia, S., Castiglioni, C., Gramigna, C., Palumbo, G., Pagliari, C., Di Tella, S., Perini, G., Bowman, T., Salza, M., & Molteni, F. (2021). Virtual Reality for Motor and Cognitive Rehabilitation From Clinic to Home: A Pilot Feasibility and Efficacy Study for Persons With Chronic Stroke. *Frontiers in Neurology*, *12*, 440. doi:10.3389/fneur.2021.601131 PMID:33897579

Josephsen, J. (2015). Cognitive load theory and nursing simulation: An integrative review. *Clinical Simulation in Nursing*, *11*(5), 259–267. doi:10.1016/j.ecns.2015.02.004

Jud, L., Fotouhi, J., Andronic, O., Aichmair, A., Osgood, G., Navab, N., & Farshad, M. (2020). Applicability of augmented reality in orthopedic surgery–A systematic review. *BMC Musculoskeletal Disorders*, *21*(1), 1–13. doi:10.118612891-020-3110-2 PMID:32061248

Juraschek, M., Büth, L., Posselt, G., & Herrmann, C. (2018). Mixed reality in learning factories. *Procedia Manufacturing*, *23*, 153–158. doi:10.1016/j.promfg.2018.04.009

Kalyvioti, K., & Mikropoulos, T. A. (2013). A virtual reality test for the identification of memory strengths of dyslexic students in Higher Education. *Journal of Universal Computer Science*, *19*(18), 2698–2721.

Kalyvioti, K., & Mikropoulos, T. A. (2014). Virtual Environments and Dyslexia: Review of literature. *Procedia Computer Science*, *27*, 138–147. doi:10.1016/j.procs.2014.02.017

Kamińska, D., Sapiński, T., Wiak, S., Tikk, T., Haamer, R. E., Avots, E., Helmi, A., Ozcinar, C., & Anbarjafari, G. (2019). Virtual Reality and Its Applications in Education: Survey. *Information (Basel)*, *10*(10), 318. doi:10.3390/info10100318

Kamińska, D., Smółka, K., Zwoliński, G., Wiak, S., Merecz-Kot, D., & Anbarjafari, G. (2020). Stress reduction using bilateral stimulation in virtual reality. *IEEE Access: Practical Innovations, Open Solutions*, *8*, 200351–200366.

Kampmann, I. L., Emmelkamp, P. M., Hartanto, D., Brinkman, W.-P., Zijlstra, B. J., & Morina, N. (2016). Exposure to Virtual Social Interactions in the Treatment of Social Anxiety Disorder: A Randomized Controlled Trial. *Behaviour Research and Therapy*, *77*, 147–156. doi:10.1016/j.brat.2015.12.016 PMID:26752328

Kandola, A., Ashdown-Franks, G., Hendrikse, J., Sabiston, C. M., & Stubbs, B. (2019). Physical activity and depression: Towards understanding the antidepressant mechanisms of physical activity. *Neuroscience and Biobehavioral Reviews*, *107*, 525–539. doi:10.1016/j.neubiorev.2019.09.040 PMID:31586447

Kang, J., Diederich, M., Lindgren, R., & Junokas, M. (2021). Gesture patterns and learning in an embodied XR science simulation. *Journal of Educational Technology & Society*, *24*(2), 77–92.

Kapoor, A., Lanctôt, K. L., Bayley, M., Kiss, A., Herrmann, N., Murray, B. J., & Swartz, R. H. (2017). "Good Outcome" Isn't Good Enough: Cognitive Impairment, Depressive Symptoms, and Social Restrictions in Physically Recovered Stroke Patients. *Stroke*, *48*(6), 1688–1690. doi:10.1161/STROKEAHA.117.016728 PMID:28438907

Kardong-Edgren, S., Farra, S., Alinier, G., & Young, H. (2019). A call to unify definitions of virtual reality. *Clinical Simulation in Nursing*, *31*, 28–34. doi:10.1016/j.ecns.2019.02.006

Karunathilake, I. M., & Samarasekera, D. D. (2021). Learning In The 21st Century— 'What's All the Fuss about Change?'. In Educate, Train and Transform: Toolkit on Medical and Health Professions Education (pp. 1-14).Routledge.

Kasneci, E., Black, A. A., & Wood, J. M. (2017). Eye-Tracking as a Tool to Evaluate Functional Ability in Everyday Tasks in Glaucoma. *Journal of Ophthalmology*. doi:10.1155/2017/6425913

Kato, H., & Billinghurst, M. (1999). Marker tracking and HMD calibration for a video-based augmented reality conferencing system. In *IWAR '99 Proceedings of 2nd IEEE and ACM International Workshop on Augmented Reality*. IEEE Computer Society. 10.1109/IWAR.1999.803809

Katz, A. C., Norr, A. M., Buck, B., Fantelli, E., Edwards-Stewart, A., Koenen-Woods, P., Zetocha, K., Smolenski, D. J., Holloway, K., Rothbaum, B. O., Difede, J. A., Rizzo, A., Skopp, N., Mishkind, M., Gahm, G., Reger, G. M., & Andrasik, F. (2020). Changes in physiological reactivity in response to the trauma memory during prolonged exposure and virtual reality exposure therapy for posttraumatic stress disorder. *Psychological Trauma: Theory, Research, Practice, and Policy*, *12*(7), 756–764. doi:10.1037/tra0000567 PMID:32338946

Kaussner, Y., Kuraszkiewicz, A. M., Schoch, S., Markel, P., Hoffmann, S., Baur-Streubel, R., Kenntner-Mabiala, R., & Pauli, P. (2020). Treating patients with driving phobia by virtual reality exposure therapy–a pilot study. *PLoS One*, *15*(1), e0226937. doi:10.1371/journal.pone.0226937 PMID:31910205

Keating, T. C., & Jacobs, J. J. (2021). Augmented Reality in Orthopedic Practice and Education. *The Orthopedic Clinics of North America*, *52*(1), 15–26. doi:10.1016/j.ocl.2020.08.002 PMID:33222981

Ke, F., Moon, J., & Sokolikj, Z. (2020). Virtual reality–based social skills training for children with autism spectrum disorder. *Journal of Special Education Technology*, 0162643420945603.

Kennedy, S. H. (2008). Core symptoms of major depressive disorder: Relevance to diagnosis and treatment. *Dialogues in Clinical Neuroscience, 10*(3), 271–277. doi:10.31887/DCNS.2008.10.3hkennedy PMID:18979940

Kenwright, B. (2019). *Virtual Reality: Where Have We Been? Where Are We Now? and Where Are We Going?* Academic Press.

Këpuska, V., & Bohouta, G. (2018). Next-Generation of Virtual Personal Assistants (Microsoft Cortana, Apple Siri, Amazon Alexa, and Google Home). *2018 IEEE 8th Annual Computing and Communication Workshop and Conference (CCWC)*, 99–103. doi:10.1109/CCWC.2018.8301638

Kerr, R. (2020). Surgery in the 2020s: Implications of advancing technology for patients and the workforce. *Future Healthcare Journal, 7*(1), 46–49. doi:10.7861/fhj.2020-0001 PMID:32104765

Kessing, L. V., & Bukh, J. D. (2017). The clinical relevance of qualitatively distinct subtypes of depression. *World Psychiatry; Official Journal of the World Psychiatric Association (WPA), 16*(3), 318–319. doi:10.1002/wps.20461 PMID:28941112

Khosrow-Pour, M. (2014). *Encyclopaedia of Information Science and Technology* (3rd ed.). IGI Global.

Kierkegaard, S. (2013). Kierkegaard's Writings, II, Volume 2: The Concept of Irony, with Continual Reference to Socrates/ Notes of Schelling's Berlin Lectures. Princeton University Press.

Kim, B. H., & Jo, S. (2018). Deep physiological affect network for the recognition of human emotions. *IEEE Transactions on Affective Computing, 11*(2), 230–243. doi:10.1109/TAFFC.2018.2790939

Kim, G., & Biocca, F. (2018). Immersion in Virtual Reality Can Increase Exercise Motivation and Physical Performance. *International Conference on Virtual, Augmented and Mixed Reality*, 94–102.

Kim, M., Choi, S.-W., Moon, S., Park, H.-I., Hwang, H., Kim, M.-K., & Seok, J.-H. (2020). Treatment Effect of Psycho-education and Training Program Using Virtual Reality Technique in the Patients with Depressive Symptoms. *Journal of Korean Neuropsychiatric Association, 59*(1), 51–60. doi:10.4306/jknpa.2020.59.1.51

Kim, Y., Kim, H., & Kim, Y. (2017). Virtual reality and augmented reality in plastic surgery: A review. *Archives of Plastic Surgery, 44*(3), 179–187. doi:10.5999/aps.2017.44.3.179 PMID:28573091

King, A. M., Gottlieb, M., Mitzman, J., Dulani, T., Schulte, S. J., & Way, D. P. (2019). Flipping the Classroom in Graduate Medical Education: A Systematic Review. *Journal of Graduate Medical Education, 11*(1), 18–29. doi:10.4300/JGME-D-18-00350.2 PMID:30805092

King, O., Borthwick, A., Nancarrow, S., & Grace, S. (2018). Sociology of the professions: What it means for podiatry. *Journal of Foot and Ankle Research, 11*(1), 1–8. doi:10.118613047-018-0275-0 PMID:29942353

Kirchner, W. K. (1958). Age differences in short-term retention of rapidly changing information. *Journal of Experimental Psychology, 55*(4), 352–358. doi:10.1037/h0043688 PMID:13539317

Kirschner, P. A. (2002). Cognitive load theory: Implications of cognitive load theory on the design of learning. *Learning and Instruction, 12*(1), 1–10. doi:10.1016/S0959-4752(01)00014-7

Kong, S. H., Haouchine, N., Soares, R., Klymchenko, A., Andreiuk, B., Marques, B., Shabat, G., Piechaud, T., Diana, M., Cotin, S., & Marescaux, J. (2017). Robust augmented reality registration method for localization of solid organs' tumors using CT-derived virtual biomechanical model and fluorescent fiducials. *Surgical Endoscopy, 31*(7), 2863–2871. doi:10.100700464-016-5297-8 PMID:27796600

Koning, A. H., Rousian, M., Verwoerd-Dikkeboom, C. M., Goedknegt, L., Steegers, E. A., & van der Spek, P. J. (2009, January). V-scope: design and implementation of an immersive and desktop virtual reality volume visualization system. In MMVR (pp. 136-138). Academic Press.

Korea University Research and Business Foundation. (2020). *Virtual Reality-Based Exposure Treatment Method for Patients with Post-traumatic Stress Disorder (PTSD) Involves Adjusting Exposure Intensity of Content According to Stress Index. KR2170379B1.* KPO.

Kosieradzki, M., Lisik, W., Gierwiało, R., & Sitnik, R. (2020). Applicability of Augmented Reality in an Organ Transplantation. *Annals of Transplantation*, *25*, e923597. doi:10.12659/AOT.923597 PMID:32732862

Koufidis, C., Manninen, K., Nieminen, J., Wohlin, M., & Silén, C. (2021). Unravelling the polyphony in clinical reasoning research in medical education. *Journal of Evaluation in Clinical Practice*, *27*(2), 438–450. doi:10.1111/jep.13432 PMID:32573080

Kourtesis, P., Korre, D., Collina, S., Doumas, L. A., & MacPherson, S. E. (2020). Guidelines for the development of immersive virtual reality software for cognitive neuroscience and neuropsychology: The development of virtual reality everyday assessment lab (VR-EAL), a neuropsychological test battery in immersive virtual reality. *Frontiers of Computer Science*, *1*, 12. Advance online publication. doi:10.3389/fcomp.2019.00012

Kozan, K. (2016). The incremental predictive validity of teaching, cognitive and social presence on cognitive load. *The Internet and Higher Education*, *31*, 11–19. doi:10.1016/j.iheduc.2016.05.003

Kraut, A. S., Omron, R., Caretta-Weyer, H., Jordan, J., Manthey, D., Wolf, S. J., Yarris, L. M., Johnson, S., & Kornegay, J. (2019). The Flipped Classroom: A Critical Appraisal. *The Western Journal of Emergency Medicine*, *20*(3), 527–536. doi:10.5811/westjem.2019.2.40979 PMID:31123556

Krijn, M., Emmelkamp, P. M., Biemond, R., de Wilde de Ligny, C., Schuemie, M. J., & van der Mast, C. (2004). Treatment of Acrophobia in Virtual Reality: The Role of Immersion and Presence. *Behaviour Research and Therapy*, *42*, 229–239.

Kritikos, J., Tzannetos, G., Zoitaki, C., Poulopoulou, S., & Koutsouris, D. (2019, March). Anxiety detection from Electrodermal Activity Sensor with movement & interaction during Virtual Reality Simulation. In *2019 9th International IEEE/EMBS Conference on Neural Engineering (NER)* (pp. 571-576). IEEE. 10.1109/NER.2019.8717170

Krohn, S., Tromp, J., Quinque, E. M., Belger, J., Klotzsche, F., Gaebler, M., ... Finke, C. (2019, July 21-24). *Multidimensional assessment of virtual reality applications in clinical neuropsychology: The "VR-Check" protocol* [Paper presentation]. International Conference on Virtual Rehabilitation (ICVR) 2019, Tel Aviv, Israel. 10.1109/ICVR46560.2019.8994590

Ku, K. Y. (2009). Assessing students' critical thinking performance: Urging for measurements using multi-response format. *Thinking Skills and Creativity*, *4*(1), 70–76. doi:10.1016/j.tsc.2009.02.001

Kummer, B., Hazan, R., Merkler, A., Kamel, H., Willey, J., Middlesworth, W., Yaghi, S., Marshall, R., Elkind, M., Boehme, A., & Boehme, A. (2020). A multilevel analysis of surgical category and individual patient-level risk factors for postoperative stroke. *The Neurohospitalist*, *10*(1), 22–28. doi:10.1177/1941874419848590 PMID:31839861

Kunze, K., Minamizawa, K., Lukosch, S., Inami, M., & Rekimoto, J. (2017). Superhuman Sports: Applying Human Augmentation to Physical Exercise. *IEEE Pervasive Computing*, (2), 14–17.

Kurillo, G., Han, J., Nicorici, A., & Bajcsy, R. (2014). *Tele-MFAsT: Kinect-Based Tele-Medicine Tool for Remote Motion and Function Assessment.* MMVR.

Kwon, H., Park, Y., & Han, J. (2018). Augmented reality in dentistry: A current perspective. *Acta Odontologica Scandinavica*, *76*(7), 497–503. doi:10.1080/00016357.2018.1441437 PMID:29465283

Kyaw, B. M., Saxena, N., Posadzki, P., Vseteckova, J., Nikolaou, C. K., George, P. P., Divakar, U., Masiello, I., Kononowicz, A. A., Zary, N., & Tudor Car, L. (2019). Virtual Reality for Health Professions Education: Systematic Review and Meta-Analysis by the Digital Health Education Collaboration. *Journal of Medical Internet Research*, *21*(1), e12959. doi:10.2196/12959 PMID:30668519

Lameras, P., Arnab, S., Dunwell, I., Stewart, C., Clarke, S., & Petridis, P. (2017). Essential features of serious games design in higher education: Linking learning attributes to game mechanics. *British Journal of Educational Technology*, *48*(4), 972–994. doi:10.1111/bjet.12467

Lan, L., Xia, Y., Li, R., Liu, K., Mai, J., Medley, J. A., Obeng-Gyasi, S., Han, L. K., Wang, P., & Cheng, J. X. (2018). A fiber optoacoustic guide with augmented reality for precision breast-conserving surgery. *Light, Science & Applications*, *7*(1), 2. doi:10.103841377-018-0006-0 PMID:30839601

Lara, E., Caballero, F. F., Rico-Uribe, L. A., Olaya, B., Haro, J. M., Ayuso-Mateos, J. L., & Miret, M. (2019). Are loneliness and social isolation associated with cognitive decline? *International Journal of Geriatric Psychiatry*, *34*(11), 1613–1622. doi:10.1002/gps.5174 PMID:31304639

Larsson, P., Västfjäll, D., & Kleiner, M. (2001). The actor-observer effect in virtual reality presentations. *Cyberpsychology & Behavior*, *4*(2), 239–246. doi:10.1089/109493101300117929 PMID:11710250

Laverdière, C., Corban, J., Khoury, J., Ge, S. M., Schupbach, J., Harvey, E. J., Reindl, R., & Martineau, P. A. (2019). Augmented reality in orthopaedics: A systematic review and a window on future possibilities. *The Bone & Joint Journal*, *101-B*(12), 1479–1488. doi:10.1302/0301-620X.101B12.BJJ-2019-0315.R1 PMID:31786992

Lawson, G., Salanitri, D., & Waterfield, B. (2015, August). Vr processes in the automotive industry. In *International Conference on Human-Computer Interaction* (pp. 208-217). Springer.

Leahy, W., & Sweller, J. (2011). Cognitive load theory, modality of presentation and the transient information effect. *Applied Cognitive Psychology*, *25*(6), 943–951. doi:10.1002/acp.1787

Lecouvey, G., Morand, A., Gonneaud, J., Piolino, P., Orriols, E., Pélerin, A., Ferreira Da Silva, L., de La Sayette, V., Eustache, F., & Desgranges, B. (2019). An Impairment of Prospective Memory in Mild Alzheimer's Disease: A Ride in a Virtual Town. *Frontiers in Psychology*, *10*, 241. doi:10.3389/fpsyg.2019.00241 PMID:30809174

Lee, G., & Lee, M. (2018). Can a virtual reality surgical simulation training provide a self-driven and mentor-free skills learning? Investigation of the practical influence of the performance metrics from the virtual reality robotic surgery simulator on the skill learning and associated cognitive workloads. *Surgical Endoscopy*, *32*(1), 62–72. doi:10.100700464-017-5634-6 PMID:28634632

Lee, J. H., Ku, J., Cho, W., Hahn, W. Y., Kim, I. Y., Lee, S. M., Kang, Y., Kim, D. Y., Yu, T., Wiederhold, B. K., Wiederhold, M. D., & Kim, S. I. (2003). A virtual reality system for the assessment and rehabilitation of the activities of daily living. *Cyberpsychology & Behavior*, *6*(4), 383–388. doi:10.1089/109493103322278763 PMID:14511450

Lee, J., Mucksavage, P., Sundaram, C., & McDougall, E. (2011). Best practices for robotic surgery training and credentialing. *The Journal of Urology*, *185*(4), 1191–1197. doi:10.1016/j.juro.2010.11.067 PMID:21334030

Lee, L., & Wong, K. W. (2008). *A Review of Using Virtual Reality for Learning, Transactions on Edutainment* (Vol. 5080). Lecture Notes in Computer Science. Springer.

Lee, S. H. (2018). Research and development of haptic simulator for dental education using virtual reality and use motion. *Int. J. Adv. Smart Conv.*, *7*, 114–120.

Leijte, E., de Blaauw, I., Rosman, C., & Botden, S. (2020). Assessment of validity evidence for the RobotiX robot assisted surgery simulator on advanced suturing tasks. *BMC Surgery*, *20*(1), 1–11. doi:10.118612893-020-00839-z PMID:32787831

Leppink, J., van Gog, T., Paas, F. G. W. C., & Sweller, J. (2015b). Cognitive load theory: Researching and planning teaching to maximise learning. Researching Medical Education. doi:10.1002/9781118838983.ch18

Leppink, J., & van den Heuvel, A. (2015a). The evolution of cognitive load theory and its application to medical education. *Perspectives on Medical Education*, *4*(3), 119–127. doi:10.100740037-015-0192-x PMID:26016429

Leutner, D., Leopold, C., & Sumfleth, E. (2009). Cognitive load and science text comprehension: Effects of drawing and mentally imagining text content. *Computers in Human Behavior*, *25*(2), 284–289. doi:10.1016/j.chb.2008.12.010

Levitt, H. M. (2021). Qualitative generalization, not to the population but to the phenomenon: Reconceptualizing variation in qualitative research. *Qualitative Psychology*, *8*(1), 95–110. doi:10.1037/qup0000184

Lezak, M. D., Howieson, D. B., Bigler, E. D., & Tranel, D. (2012). *Neuropsychological Assessment* (5th ed.). Oxford University Press.

LG Display Co Ltd. (2019). *Display Device for a Virtual Reality Device Used in Military, Architecture, Tourism, Movies, Multimedia or Gaming, Comprises a Display Panel Having Multiple Data Lines, Multiple Gate Lines and Multiple Pixels Arranged in a Matrix. DE102017129795A1*. DPMA.

LG Electronics Inc. (2016). *Wearable Mobile Terminal e.g., Handheld Terminal, for User, Has Controller for Controlling Processor to Transmit Signal for Notifying Emotional State of First User to External Devices in Response to Identified State Corresponding to State. US20160381534A1*. USPTO.

Liang, J. T., Doke, T., Onogi, S., Ohashi, S., Ohnishi, I., Sakuma, I., & Nakajima, Y. (2012). A fluorolaser navigation system to guide linear surgical tool insertion. *International Journal of Computer Assisted Radiology and Surgery*, *7*(6), 931–939. doi:10.100711548-012-0743-0 PMID:22627882

Liao, Y. Y., Tseng, H.-Y., Lin, Y.-J., Wang, C.-J., & Hsu, W.-C. (2020). Using virtual reality-based training to improve cognitive function, instrumental activities of daily living and neural efficiency in older adults with mild cognitive impairment. *European Journal of Physical and Rehabilitation Medicine*, *56*(1), 47–57. doi:10.23736/S1973-9087.19.05899-4 PMID:31615196

Li, F., Song, D., Chen, H., Xiong, J., Li, X., Zhong, H., & Tang, G. (2020, September 22). Development and Clinical Deployment of a Smartphone-Based Visual Field Deep Learning System for Glaucoma Detection. *NPJ Digital Medicine*, *3*(1), 1–8. https://doi.org/10.1038/s41746-020-00329-9

Li, L., Yu, F., Shi, D., Shi, J., Tian, Z., Yang, J., Wang, X., & Jiang, Q. (2017). Application of virtual reality technology in clinical medicine. *American Journal of Translational Research*, *9*(9), 3867–3880. https://bit.ly/3rs5plE PMID:28979666

Lima, E., Rodrigues, P. L., Mota, P., Carvalho, N., Dias, E., Correia-Pinto, J., Autorino, R., & Vilaça, J. L. (2017). Ureteroscopy-assisted Percutaneous Kidney Access Made Easy: First Clinical Experience with a Novel Navigation System Using Electromagnetic Guidance (IDEAL Stage 1). *European Urology*, *72*(4), 610–661. doi:10.1016/j.eururo.2017.03.011 PMID:28377202

Lim, J. E., Wong, W. T., Teh, T. A., Lim, S. H., Allen, J. C. Jr, Quah, J. H. M., ... Tan, N. C. (2020). A Fully-Immersive and Automated Virtual Reality System to Assess the Six Domains of Cognition: Protocol for a Feasibility Study. *Frontiers in Aging Neuroscience*, 12. PMID:33488382

Lin, B.-S., Lee, I.-J., Yang, S.-Y., Lo, Y.-C., Lee, J., & Chen, J.-L. (2018). Design of an Inertial-SensorBased Data Glove for Hand Function Evaluation. *Sensors (Basel)*, *18*(5), 15–45.

Lindner, P., Hamilton, W., Miloff, A., & Carlbring, P. (2019). How to Treat Depression With Low-Intensity Virtual Reality Interventions: Perspectives on Translating Cognitive Behavioral Techniques Into the Virtual Reality Modality and How to Make Anti-Depressive Use of Virtual Reality–Unique Experiences. *Frontiers in Psychiatry, 10*, 792. doi:10.3389/fpsyt.2019.00792 PMID:31736809

Lindner, P., Miloff, A., Fagernäs, S., Andersen, J., Sigeman, M., Andersson, G., Furmark, T., & Carlbring, P. (2019). Therapist-led and self-led one-session virtual reality exposure therapy for public speaking anxiety with consumer hardware and software: A randomized controlled trial. *Journal of Anxiety Disorders, 61*, 45–54. doi:10.1016/j.janxdis.2018.07.003 PMID:30054173

Lindner, P., Miloff, A., Zetterlund, E., Reuterskiöld, L., Andersson, G., & Carlbring, P. (2019). Attitudes Toward and Familiarity With Virtual Reality Therapy Among Practicing Cognitive Behavior Therapists: A Cross-Sectional Survey Study in the Era of Consumer VR Platforms. *Frontiers in Psychology, 10*, 176. doi:10.3389/fpsyg.2019.00176 PMID:30800086

Lin, L. P. L., Huang, S. C. L., & Ho, Y. C. (2020). Could virtual reality effectively market slow travel in a heritage destination? *Tourism Management, 78*, 104027. doi:10.1016/j.tourman.2019.104027

Loeng, S. (2018). Various ways of understanding the concept of andragogy. *Cogent Education, 5*(1), 1496643. doi:10.1080/2331186X.2018.1496643

Logeswaran, A., Munsch, C., Chong, Y. J., Ralph, N., & McCrossnan, J. (2021). The role of extended reality technology in healthcare education: Towards a learner-centred approach. *Future Healthcare Journal, 8*(1), e79–e84. doi:10.7861/fhj.2020-0112 PMID:33791482

Loucks, L., Yasinski, C., Norrholm, S. D., Maples-Keller, J., Post, L., Zwiebach, L., ... Rothbauma, B. O. (2019). You can do that?!: Feasibility of virtual reality exposure therapy in the treatment of PTSD due to military sexual trauma. *Journal of Anxiety Disorders, 61*, 55–63. doi:10.1016/j.janxdis.2018.06.004 PMID:30005843

Luctkar-Flude, M., & Tyerman, J. (2021). The Rise of Virtual Simulation: Pandemic Response or Enduring Pedagogy? *Clinical Simulation in Nursing, 57*, 1–2. doi:10.1016/j.ecns.2021.06.008

Lukas, C. A., Eskofier, B., & Berking, M. (2021). A Gamified Smartphone-Based Intervention for Depression: Randomized Controlled Pilot Trial. *JMIR Mental Health, 8*(7), e16643. doi:10.2196/16643 PMID:34283037

Lungu, A. J., Swinkels, W., Claesen, L., Tu, P., Egger, J., & Chen, X. (2021). A review on the applications of virtual reality, augmented reality and mixed reality in surgical simulation: An extension to different kinds of surgery. *Expert Review of Medical Devices, 18*(1), 47–62. doi:10.1080/17434440.2021.1860750 PMID:33283563

Luo, C., Lan, Y., Luo, X. R., & Li, H. (2021). The effect of commitment on knowledge sharing: An empirical study of virtual communities. *Technological Forecasting and Social Change, 163*, 120438. doi:10.1016/j.techfore.2020.120438

Mace, R., Hardie, G., & Plaice, J. (1991). Accessible environments: Toward universal design. In *Design Interventions: Toward a More Humane Architecture*. Van Nostrand Reinhold.

MacQueen, J. (1967, June). Some methods for classification and analysis of multivariate observations. In *Proceedings of the fifth Berkeley symposium on mathematical statistics and probability* (Vol. 1, No. 14, pp. 281-297). Academic Press.

Madary, M. (2017). The Ethics of Virtual Reality: Risks and Recommendations. In Wirklichkeit(en): Gegenwart neu wahrnehmen - Zukunft kreativ gestalten (pp. 49-55). De Gruyter. doi:10.1515/9783110543711-008

Madary, M., & Metzinger, T. (2016). Real virtuality: A code of ethical conduct: Recommendations for good scientific practice and the consumers of VR technology. *Frontiers in Robotics and AI, 3*. Advance online publication. doi:10.3389/frobt.2016.00003

Maggio, M. G., Maresca, G., De Luca, R., Stagnitti, M. C., Porcari, B., Ferrera, M. C., Galletti, F., Casella, C., Manuli, A., & Calabrò, R. S. (2019). The Growing Use of Virtual Reality in Cognitive Rehabilitation: Fact, Fake or Vision? A Scoping Review. *Journal of the National Medical Association*, *111*(4), 457–463. doi:10.1016/j.jnma.2019.01.003 PMID:30739728

Magic Leap Inc. (2017). *Augmented and Virtual Reality Display Systems and Methods for Determining Optical Prescriptions by Imaging Retina. US20170000343A1*. USPTO.

Malbos, E., Rapee, R. M., & Kavakli, M. (2012). A controlled study of agoraphobia and the independent effect of virtual reality exposure therapy. *The Australian and New Zealand Journal of Psychiatry*, *47*(2), 160–168. doi:10.1177/0004867412453626 PMID:22790176

Mancuso, V., Stramba-Badiale, C., Cavedoni, S., Pedroli, E., Cipresso, P., & Riva, G. (2020). Virtual reality meets non-invasive brain stimulation: Integrating two methods for cognitive rehabilitation of mild cognitive impairment. *Frontiers in Neurology*, *11*, 1117. doi:10.3389/fneur.2020.566731 PMID:33117261

Maples-Keller, J. L., Bunnell, B. E., Kim, S. J., & Rothbaum, B. O. (2017). The Use of Virtual Reality Technology in the Treatment of Anxiety and Other Psychiatric Disorders. *Harvard Review of Psychiatry*, *25*(3), 103–113. doi:10.1097/HRP.0000000000000138 PMID:28475502

Maples-Keller, J. L., Bunnell, B. E., Kim, S.-J., & Rothbaum, B. O. (2017). The Use of Virtual Reality Technology in the Treatment of Anxiety and Other Psychiatric Disorders. *Harvard Review of Psychiatry*, *25*(3), 103–113.

Ma, R., Reddy, S., Vanstrum, E. B., & Hung, A. J. (2021). Innovations in Urologic Surgical Training. *Current Urology Reports*, *22*(4), 26. doi:10.100711934-021-01043-z PMID:33712963

Marín, V. I. (2014). Elusodelblogdeaulacomorecursocomplementariodelaenseñanzapresencialparaelintercambiodeinformacióneinteracciónentreelprofesoradoyalumnadodeprimerañodequímica. *Educación en la Química*, *25*, 183–189.

Martinez, E. (2016). *Dislexia en Adolescentes y Jóvenes Adultos: Caracterización Cognitiva y Afectivo-Motivacional.* http://hdl.handle.net/10550/56210

Marzano, E., Piardi, T., Soler, L., Diana, M., Mutter, D., Marescaux, J., & Pessaux, P. (2013). Augmented reality-guided artery-first pancreatico-duodenectomy. *Journal of Gastrointestinal Surgery*, *17*(11), 1980–1983. doi:10.100711605-013-2307-1 PMID:23943389

Mascitelli, J. R., Schlachter, L., Chartrain, A. G., Oemke, H., Gilligan, J., Costa, A. B., Shrivastava, R. K., & Bederson, J. B. (2018). Navigation-Linked Heads-Up Display in Intracranial Surgery: Early Experience. *Operative Neurosurgery (Hagerstown, Md.)*, *15*(2), 184–193. doi:10.1093/ons/opx205 PMID:29040677

Mathew, P. S., & Pillai, A. S. (2020). Role of Immersive (XR) Technologies in Improving Healthcare Competencies: A Review. *Virtual and Augmented Reality in Education, Art, and Museums*, 23-46.

Mazingi, D., Navarro, S., Bobel, M., Dube, A., Mbanje, C., & Lavy, C. (2020). Exploring the impact of COVID-19 on progress towards achieving global surgery goals. *World Journal of Surgery*, *44*(8), 2451–2457. doi:10.100700268-020-05627-7 PMID:32488665

McCulloch, P., Feinberg, J., Philippou, Y., Kolias, A., Kehoe, S., Lancaster, G., Donovan, J., Petrinic, T., Agha, R., & Pennell, C. (2018). Progress in clinical research in surgery and IDEAL. *Lancet*, *392*(10141), 88–94. doi:10.1016/S0140-6736(18)30102-8 PMID:29361334

McGrath, J. L., Taekman, J. M., Dev, P., Danforth, D. R., Mohan, D., Kman, N., ... Won, K. (2018). Using virtual reality simulation environments to assess competence for emergency medicine learners. *Academic Emergency Medicine*, *25*(2), 186–195. doi:10.1111/acem.13308 PMID:28888070

McKnight, R. R., Pean, C. A., Buck, J. S., Hwang, J. S., Hsu, J. R., & Pierrie, S. N. (2020). Virtual Reality and Augmented Reality-Translating Surgical Training into Surgical Technique. *Current Reviews in Musculoskeletal Medicine*, *13*(6), 663–674. doi:10.100712178-020-09667-3 PMID:32779019

McLay, R. N., McBrien, C., Wiederhold, M. D., & Wiederhold, B. K. (2010). Exposure Therapy with and without Virtual Reality to Treat PTSD while in the Combat Theater: A Parallel Case Series. *Cyberpsychology, Behavior, and Social Networking*, *13*(1), 37–42. doi:10.1089/cyber.2009.0346 PMID:20528291

Mees, L., Upadhyaya, S., Kumar, P., Kotawala, S., Haran, S., Rajasekar, S., Friedman, D. S., & Venkatesh, R. (2020, February). Validation of a Head-Mounted Virtual Reality Visual Field Screening Device. *Journal of Glaucoma*, *29*(2), 86–91. https://doi.org/10.1097/IJG.0000000000001415

Meguerdichian, M., Walker, K., & Bajaj, K. (2016). Working memory is limited: Improving knowledge transfer by optimizing simulation through cognitive load theory. *BMJ Simulation & Technology Enhanced Learning*, *2*(4), 131–138. doi:10.1136/bmjstel-2015-000098

Melnyk, B. M., Tan, A., Hsieh, A. P., Gawlik, K., Arslanian-Engoren, C., Braun, L. T., Dunbar, S., Dunbar-Jacob, J., Lewis, L. M., Millan, A., Orsolini, L., Robbins, L. B., Russell, C. L., Tucker, S., & Wilbur, J. (2021). Critical care nurses' physical and mental health, worksite wellness support, and medical errors. *American Journal of Critical Care*, *30*(3), 176–184. doi:10.4037/ajcc2021301 PMID:34161980

Menon, D. K., Schwab, K., Wright, D. W., & Maas, A. I. (2010). Demographics and Clinical Assessment Working Group of the International and Interagency Initiative toward Common Data Elements for Research on Traumatic Brain Injury and Psychological Health. Position statement: Definition of traumatic brain injury. *Archives of Physical Medicine and Rehabilitation*, *91*(11), 1637–1640. doi:10.1016/j.apmr.2010.05.017 PMID:21044706

Meola, A., Cutolo, F., Carbone, M., Cagnazzo, F., Ferrari, M., & Ferrari, V. (2017). Augmented reality in neurosurgery: A systematic review. *Neurosurgical Review*, *40*(4), 537–548. doi:10.100710143-016-0732-9 PMID:27154018

Messinis, L., Kosmidis, M. H., Nasios, G., Dardiotis, E., & Tsaousides, T. (2019). Cognitive neurorehabilitation in acquired neurological brain injury. *Behavioural Neurology*, *1-4*, 8241951. doi:10.1155/2019/8241951 PMID:31781294

Metaverse. (2021). *Youtube Channel: Metaverse AR Platform.* https://www.youtube.com/channel/UCum7uPJBXug0H-fqNi4AfQmQ

Meulstee, J., Nijsink, J., Schreurs, R., Verhamme, L., Xi, T., Delye, H., Borstlap, W., & Maal, T. (2019). Toward holographic-guided surgery. *Surgical Innovation*, *26*(1), 86–94. doi:10.1177/1553350618799552 PMID:30261829

Meyer, A., Rose, D. H., & Gordon, D. (2014). *Universal design for learning: Theory and Practice.* CAST Professional Publishing.

Meyerbroeker, K., Morina, N., Kerkhof, G., & Emmelkamp, P. (2013). Virtual Reality Exposure Therapy Does Not Provide Any Additional Value in Agoraphobic Patients: A Randomized Controlled Trial. *Psychotherapy and Psychosomatics*, *82*(3), 170–176. doi:10.1159/000342715 PMID:23548832

Michaliszyn, D., Marchand, A., Bouchard, S., Martel, M.-O., & Poirier-Bisson, J. (2010). A Randomized, Controlled Clinical Trial of In Virtuo and In Vivo Exposure for Spider Phobia. *Cyberpsychology, Behavior, and Social Networking*, *13*(6), 689–695. doi:10.1089/cyber.2009.0277 PMID:21142994

Migoya-Borja, M., Delgado-Gómez, D., Carmona-Camacho, R., Porras-Segovia, A., López-Moriñigo, J.-D., Sánchez-Alonso, M., Albarracín García, L., Guerra, N., Barrigón, M. L., Alegría, M., & Baca-García, E. (2020). Feasibility of a Virtual Reality-Based Psychoeducational Tool (VRight) for Depressive Patients. *Cyberpsychology, Behavior, and Social Networking, 23*(4), 246–252. doi:10.1089/cyber.2019.0497 PMID:32207997

Miloff, A., Lindner, P., & Carlbring, P. (2020). The future of virtual reality therapy for phobias: Beyond simple exposures. *Clinical Psychology in Europe, 2*(2), e2913. doi:10.32872/cpe.v2i2.2913

Mitchell, R., & Boyle, B. (2021). Understanding the role of profession in multidisciplinary team innovation: Professional identity, minority dissent and team innovation. *British Journal of Management, 32*(2), 512–528. doi:10.1111/1467-8551.12419

Modern Practice. (2018, October 2). *The Future of Dentistry with Augmented and Virtual Reality.* https://blog.net32.com/the-future-of-dentistry-with-augmented-and-virtual-reality/

Moglia, A., Ferrari, V., Melfi, F., Ferrari, M., Mosca, F., Cuschieri, A., & Morelli, L. (2018). Performances on simulator and da Vinci robot on subjects with and without surgical background. *Minimally Invasive Therapy & Allied Technologies, 27*(6), 309–314. doi:10.1080/13645706.2017.1365729 PMID:28817346

Momartin, S., Silove, D., Manicavasagar, V., & Steel, Z. (2004). Comorbidity of PTSD and depression: Associations with trauma exposure, symptom severity and functional impairment in Bosnian refugees resettled in Australia. *Journal of Affective Disorders, 80*(2-3), 231–238. doi:10.1016/S0165-0327(03)00131-9 PMID:15207936

Monteiro-Junior, R. S., Figueiredo, L. F., Maciel-Pinheiro, P., Abud, E. L., Engedal, K., Barca, M. L., Nascimento, O. J. M., Laks, J., & Deslandes, A. C. (2017). Virtual reality–based physical exercise with exergames (PhysEx) improves mental and physical health of institutionalized older adults. *Journal of the American Medical Directors Association, 18*(5), 454–e1. doi:10.1016/j.jamda.2017.01.001 PMID:28238675

Moreira, D. (2020). Virtual networks and asynchronous communities: methodological reflections on the digital. In *Ethnography in Higher Education* (pp. 177–196). Springer VS. doi:10.1007/978-3-658-30381-5_11

Moreno, A., Wall, K. J., Thangavelu, K., Craven, L., Ward, E., & Dissanayaka, N. N. (2019). A systematic review of the use of virtual reality and its effects on cognition in individuals with neurocognitive disorders. *Alzheimer's & Dementia: Translational Research & Clinical Interventions, 5*(1), 834–850. doi:10.1016/j.trci.2019.09.016 PMID:31799368

Moreno, R. (2007). Optimising learning from animations by minimizing cognitive load: Cognitive and affective consequences of signaling and segmentation methods. *Applied Cognitive Psychology, 21*(6), 765–781. doi:10.1002/acp.1348

Moro, C., Štromberga, Z., Raikos, A., & Stirling, A. (2017). The effectiveness of virtual and augmented reality in health sciences and medical anatomy. *Anatomical Sciences Education, 10*(6), 549–559. doi:10.1002/ase.1696 PMID:28419750

Mortimore, G., Reynolds, J., Forman, D., Brannigan, C., & Mitchell, K. (2021). From expert to advanced clinical practitioner and beyond. *British Journal of Nursing (Mark Allen Publishing), 30*(11), 656–659. doi:10.12968/bjon.2021.30.11.656 PMID:34109817

Muguerza, P., & Canelas, A. (2021). Breaking Boundaries. *PharmaTimes Magazine, 8*(6). http://www.pharmatimes.com/magazine/2021/june_2021/breaking_boundaries

Muhanna, M.A. (2015). Virtual reality and the CAVE: Taxonomy, interaction challenges and research directions. *Journal of King Saud University - Computer and Information Sciences, 27*, 344–361. doi:10.1016/j.jksuci.2014.03.023

Mukherji, B.R., Neuwirth, L.S. & Limonic. (2017). *Making the case for real diversity: Redefining underrepresented minority students in public universities.* Sage Open. doi:10.10.177/2158244017707796

Müller, F., Roner, S., Liebmann, F., Spirig, J. M., Fürnstahl, P., & Farshad, M. (2020). Augmented reality navigation for spinal pedicle screw instrumentation using intraoperative 3D imaging. *The Spine Journal*, *20*(4), 621–628. doi:10.1016/j.spinee.2019.10.012 PMID:31669611

Munoz-Montoya, F., Juan, M-C., Mendez-Lopez, M., Molla, R., Abad, F., & Fidalgo, C. (2021). SLAM- based augmented reality for the assessment of short-term spatial memory. A comparative study of visual versus tactile stimuli. *PLOS ONE*, *16*(2). doi: .pone.0245976 doi:10.1371/journal

Muñoz-Saavedra, L., Miró-Amarante, L., & Domínguez-Morales, M. (2020). Augmented and virtual reality evolution and future tendency. *Applied Sciences (Basel, Switzerland)*, *10*(1), 322. doi:10.3390/app10010322

Mura, G., Carta, M. G., Sancassiani, F., Machado, S., & Prosperini, L. (2018). Active exergames to improve cognitive functioning in neurological disabilities: A systematic review and meta-analysis. *European Journal of Physical and Rehabilitation Medicine*, *54*(3), 450–462. doi:10.23736/S1973-9087.17.04680-9 PMID:29072042

Mu, Y., Hocking, D., Wang, Z. T., Garvin, G. J., Eagleson, R., & Peters, T. M. (2020). Augmented reality simulator for ultrasound-guided percutaneous renal access. *International Journal of Computer Assisted Radiology and Surgery*, *15*(5), 749–757. doi:10.100711548-020-02142-x PMID:32314227

Myles, P., & Maswime, S. (2020). Mitigating the risks of surgery during the COVID-19 pandemic. *Lancet*, *396*(10243), 2–3. doi:10.1016/S0140-6736(20)31256-3 PMID:32479826

Nader, M., & Kruszewski, M. (2013). Wykorzystanie zaawansowanych symulatorów jazdy w badaniach zachowania i umiejętności kierowców. *Prace naukowe Politechniki Warszawskiej*, 321-331.

Nakamoto, M., Ukimura, O., Faber, K., & Gill, I. S. (2012). Current progress on augmented reality visualization in endoscopic surgery. *Current Opinion in Urology*, *22*(2), 121–126. doi:10.1097/MOU.0b013e3283501774 PMID:22249372

Nakling, A. E., Aarsland, D., Næss, H., Wollschlaeger, D., Fladby, T., Hofstad, H., & Wehling, E. (2017). Cognitive Deficits in Chronic Stroke Patients: Neuropsychological Assessment, Depression, and Self-Reports. *Dementia and Geriatric Cognitive Disorders. Extra*, *7*(2), 283–296. doi:10.1159/000478851 PMID:29033974

National Collaborating Centre for Mental Health (UK). (2007). *Dementia: A NICE-SCIE guideline on supporting people with dementia and their carers in health and social care*. British Psychological Society.

National Institute of Neurological Disorder and Stroke. (2016). *Dyslexia Information Page*. http://bit.ly/2IoXY8H

Nedas, T., Challacombe, B., & Dasgupta, P. (2004). Virtual reality in urology. *BJU International*, *94*(3), 255–257. doi:10.1111/j.1464-410X.2004.04975.x PMID:15291846

Negev, M., Dahdal, Y., Khreis, H., Hochman, A., Shaheen, M., Jaghbir, M. T., Alpert, P., Levine, H., & Davidovitch, N. (2021). Regional lessons from the COVID-19 outbreak in the Middle East: From infectious diseases to climate change adaptation. *The Science of the Total Environment*, *768*, 144434. doi:10.1016/j.scitotenv.2020.144434 PMID:33444865

Negrillo-Cárdenas, J., Jiménez-Pérez, J., & Feito, F. (2020). The role of virtual and augmented reality in orthopedic trauma surgery: From diagnosis to rehabilitation. *Computer Methods and Programs in Biomedicine*, *191*, 105407. doi:10.1016/j.cmpb.2020.105407 PMID:32120088

Negut, A., Matu, S., Sava, F. A., & David, D. (2016). Virtual reality measures in neuropsychological assessment: A meta-analytic review. *The Clinical Neuropsychologist*, *30*(2), 165–184. doi:10.1080/13854046.2016.1144793 PMID:26923937

Nelson, B. C., & Erlandson, B. E. (2008). Managing cognitive load in educational multi-user virtual environments: Reflection on design practice. *Educational Technology Research and Development*, *56*(5-6), 619–641. doi:10.100711423-007-9082-1

Nepogodiev, D. (2020). Global guidance for surgical care during the COVID-19 pandemic. *British Journal of Surgery*, *107*(9), 1097–1103. doi:10.1002/bjs.11646 PMID:32293715

Nepogodiev, D., Martin, J., Biccard, B., Makupe, A., Bhangu, A., Ademuyiwa, A., ... Morton, D. (2019). Global burden of postoperative death. *Lancet*, *393*(10170), 401. doi:10.1016/S0140-6736(18)33139-8 PMID:30722955

Neuwirth, L. S., Ebrahimi, A., Mukherji, B. R., & Park, L. (2018). Addressing diverse college students and interdisciplinary learning experiences through online virtual laboratory instruction: A theoretical approach to error-based learning in biopsychology. In A. Ursyn (Ed.), *Visual Approaches to Cognitive Eductaion with Technology Integration*. https://www.igi-global.com/chapter/addressing-diverse-college-students-and-interdisciplinary-learning-experiences-through-online-virtual-laboratory-instructions/195070

Neuwirth, L. S., Ebrahimi, A., Mukherji, B. R., & Park, L. (2019). Addressing diverse college students and interdisciplinary learning experiences through online virtual laboratory instruction: A theoretical approach to error-based learning in biopsychology. *Virtual Reality in Education: Breakthroughs in Research and Practice*, 511-531. https://www.igi-global.com/chapter/addressing-diverse-college-students-and-interdisciplinary-learning-experiences-through-online-virtual-laboratory-instructions/195070

Neuwirth, L. S., Dacius, T. F. Jr, & Mukherji, B. R. (2018). Teaching neuroanatomy through a historical context. *Journal of Undergraduate Neuroscience Education*, *16*(2), E26–E31. PMID:30057504

Neuwirth, L. S., & Ros, M. (2021). Comparisons between first person point-of-view 180° video virtual reality head-mounted display and 3D video computer display in teaching undergraduate neuroscience students stereotaxic surgeries. *Front. Virtual Reality*, *2*, 706653. Advance online publication. doi:10.3389/frvir.2021.706653

Ng, M., Racette, L., Pascual, J. P., Liebmann, J. M., Girkin, C. A., Lovell, S. L., Zangwill, L. M., Weinreb, R. N., & Sample, P. A. (2009, April 1). Comparing the Full-Threshold and Swedish Interactive Thresholding Algorithms for Short-Wavelength Automated Perimetry. *Investigative Ophthalmology & Visual Science*, *50*(4), 1726–1733. https://doi.org/10.1167/iovs.08-2718

NGoggle. (n.d.). *Assessment of Visual Function With a Portable Brain-Computer Interface. Clinical trial registration*. https://clinicaltrials.gov/ct2/show/NCT03760055

Nieto, M. P. (2015). *English: A Simplified Schema of the Human Visual Pathway*. https://commons.wikimedia.org/w/index.php?curid=37868501

Nijmeh, A. D., Goodger, N. M., Hawkes, D., Edwards, P. J., & McGurk, M. (2005). Image-guided navigation in oral and maxillofacial surgery. *British Journal of Oral & Maxillofacial Surgery*, *43*(4), 294–302. doi:10.1016/j.bjoms.2004.11.018 PMID:15993282

Nochaiwong, S., Ruengorn, C., Thavorn, K., Hutton, B., Awiphan, R., Phosuya, C., Ruanta, Y., Wongpakaran, N., & Wongpakaran, T. (2021). Global prevalence of mental health issues among the general population during the coronavirus disease-2019 pandemic: A systematic review and meta-analysis. *Scientific Reports*, *11*(1), 10173. doi:10.103841598-021-89700-8 PMID:33986414

Norcini, J., Anderson, B., Bollela, V., Burch, V., Costa, M. J., Duvivier, R., Galbraith, R., Hays, R., Kent, A., Perrott, V., & Roberts, T. (2011). Criteria for good assessment: Consensus statement and recommendations from the Ottawa 2010 Conference. *Medical Teacher*, *33*(3), 206–214. doi:10.3109/0142159X.2011.551559 PMID:21345060

Norman, G., Grierson, L., Sherbino, J., Hamstra, S., Schmidt, H., & Mamede, S. (2018). Expertise in medicine and surgery. In K. Ericsson, R. Hoffman, A. Kozbelt, & A. Williams (Eds.), *The Cambridge handbook of expertise and expert performance* (pp. 331–355). Cambridge University Press. doi:10.1017/9781316480748.019

Norr, A. M., Smolenski, D. J., Katz, A. C., Rizzo, A. A., Rothbaum, B. O., Difede, J., ... Regera, G. M. (2018). Virtual Reality Exposure vs. Prolonged Exposure for PTSD: Which Treatment for Whom? *Depression and Anxiety*, *35*(6), 523–529. doi:10.1002/da.22751 PMID:29734488

North, M. M., & North, S. M. (2017). Virtual reality therapy for treatment of psychological disorders. In *Career Paths in Telemental Health* (pp. 263–268). Springer. doi:10.1007/978-3-319-23736-7_27

North, M. M., & North, S. M. (2018). The sense of presence exploration in virtual reality therapy. *J. UCS*, *24*(2), 72–84.

North, M. M., North, S. M., & Coble, J. R. (1997). Virtual reality therapy: An effective treatment for psychological disorders. *Studies in Health Technology and Informatics*, 59–70. PMID:10175343

Núñez, M. P., & Santamaría, M. (2016). Una propuesta de mejora de la dislexia a través del procesador de textos: "Adapro. *Revista Educativa Hekademos*, (19), 20–25.

Nyachwaya, J. M., & Gillaspie, M. (2016). Features of representations in general chemistry textbooks: A peek through the lens of the cognitive load theory. *Chemistry Education Research and Practice*, *17*, 58–71. doi:10.1039/C5RP00140D

O'Brolcháin, F., Jacquemard, T., Monaghan, D., O'Connor, N., Novitzky, P., & Gordijn, B. (2016). The Convergence of Virtual Reality and Social Networks: Threats to Privacy and Autonomy. *Science and Engineering Ethics*, *22*(1), 1–29. doi:10.100711948-014-9621-1 PMID:25552240

Obrad, C. (2020). Constraints and consequences of online teaching. *Sustainability*, *12*(17), 6982. doi:10.3390u12176982

Ocloo, J., Garfield, S., Franklin, B. D., & Dawson, S. (2021). Exploring the theory, barriers and enablers for patient and public involvement across health, social care and patient safety: A systematic review of reviews. *Health Research Policy and Systems*, *19*(1), 1–21. doi:10.118612961-020-00644-3 PMID:33472647

OECD. (2018). *The future of education and skills 2030*. OECD.

Okoro, C. A., Hollis, N. T. D., Cyrus, A. C., & Griffin-Blake, S. (2018). Prevalence of Disabilities and Health Care Access by Disability Status and Type Among Adults— United States. *MMWR. Morbidity and Mortality Weekly Report*, *67*(32), 882–887. Advance online publication. doi:10.15585/mmwr.mm6732a3 PMID:30114005

Okoye, K., Rodriguez-Tort, J. A., Escamilla, J., & Hosseini, S. (2021). Technology-mediated teaching and learning process: A conceptual study of educators' response amidst the Covid-19 pandemic. *Education and Information Technologies*, 1–33. PMID:34025205

Oliviera, C., Lopes Filho, B., Sugarman, M., Esteves, C., Lima, M., Moret-Tatay, C., ... Argimon, I. (2016). Development and Feasibility of a Virtual Reality Task for the Cognitive Assessment of Older Adults: The ECO-VR. *The Spanish Journal of Psychology*, *19*, E95. doi:10.1017jp.2016.96 PMID:27955716

Oliviera, J., Gamito, P., Souto, T., Conde, R., Ferreira, M., Corotnean, T., ... Neto, T. (2021). Virtual Reality-Based Cognitive Stimulation on People with Mild to Moderate Dementia due to Alzheimer's Disease: A Pilot Randomized Controlled Trial. *International Journal of Environmental Research and Public Health*, *18*(10), 5290. doi:10.3390/ijerph18105290 PMID:34065698

Oman, S. P., Magdi, Y., & Simon, L. V. (2020). *Past Present and Future of Simulation in Internal Medicine*. StatPearls Publishing.

Ord, A. S., Shura, R. D., Curtiss, G., Armistead-Jehle, P., Vanderploeg, R. D., Bowles, A. O., & Cooper, D. B. (2021). Number of concussions does not affect treatment response to cognitive rehabilitation interventions following mild TBI in military service members. *Archives of Clinical Neuropsychology*, *36*(5), 850–856. doi:10.1093/arclin/acaa119 PMID:33264387

Orr, N., Matthews, B., See, Z. S., Burrell, A., Day, J., & Seengal, D. (2021). Transdisciplinarity in extended reality (XR) research design: Technological transformation and social good (co-creation session at XR+ Creativity Symposium, University of Newcastle, 2020). *Virtual Creativity, 11*(1), 163-179.

Oskam, P. (2005). *Virtual reality exposure therapy (VRET) effectiveness and improvement.* In 2nd Twente University Student Conference on IT, Enschede, The Netherlands.

Otero, A., & Flores, J. (2011). Realidad virtual: Un medio de comunicación de contenidos. Aplicación como herramienta educativa y factores de diseño e implantación en museos y espacios públicos. *Icono 14. Revista de Comunicación Audiovisual y Nuevas Tecnologías, 9*(2), 185–211.

Ottosson, S. (2002). Virtual reality in the product development process. *Journal of Engineering Design, 13*(2), 159–172. doi:10.1080/09544820210129823

Ou, Y. (n.d.). *The Future of Virtual Reality Visual Field Testing.* Glaucoma Research Foundation. https://www.glaucoma.org/treatment/virtual-reality-visual-field-testing.php

Ouellet, É., Boller, B., Corriveau-Lecavalier, N., Cloutier, S., & Belleville, S. (2018). The virtual shop: A new immersive virtual reality environment and scenario for the assessment of everyday memory. *Journal of Neuroscience Methods, 303*, 126–135. doi:10.1016/j.jneumeth.2018.03.010 PMID:29581009

Ougrin, D. (2011). Efficacy of exposure versus cognitive therapy in anxiety disorders: Systematic review and meta-analysis. *BMC Psychiatry, 11*(1), 1–13. doi:10.1186/1471-244X-11-200 PMID:22185596

Ou, W.-L., Kuo, T.-L., Chang, C.-C., & Fan, C.-P. (2021, January). Deep-Learning-Based Pupil Center Detection and Tracking Technology for Visible-Light Wearable Gaze Tracking Devices. *Applied Sciences (Basel, Switzerland), 11*(2), 851. https://doi.org/10.3390/app11020851

Owens, K. P. (2021, July). Competency-Based Experiential-Expertise and Future Adaptive Learning Systems. In *International Conference on Human-Computer Interaction* (pp. 93-109). Springer.

Paas, F. G. W. C., Renkl, A., & Sweller, J. (2010a). Cognitive load theory and instructional design: Recent developments. *Educational Psychologist, 38*(1), 1–4. doi:10.1207/S15326985EP3801_1

Paas, F. G. W. C., Tuovinen, J. E., Tabbers, H., & Van Gerven, P. W. M. (2010b). Cognitive load measurement as a means to advance cognitive load theory. *Educational Psychologist, 38*(1), 63–71. doi:10.1207/S15326985EP3801_8

Paas, F. G. W. C., van Gog, T., & Sweller, J. (2010). Cognitive load theory: New conceptualizations, specifications, and integrative research perspectives. *Educational Psychology Review, 22*(2), 115–121. doi:10.100710648-010-9133-8

Paas, F. G. W. C., & Van Merriënboer, J. J. G. (1994). Instructional control of cognitive load in the training of complex cognitive tasks. *Educational Psychology Review, 6*(4), 351–371. doi:10.1007/BF02213420

Palmer, C. (2019). *Real treatments in virtual worlds: Treating patients in virtual environments is now easier and less expensive, and the number of conditions that the technology can treat has grown.* American Psychological Association. https://www.apa.org/monitor/2019/09/cover-virtual-worlds

Papageorgiou, E., Hardiess, G., Mallot, H. A., & Schiefer, U. (2012, July 15). Gaze Patterns Predicting Successful Collision Avoidance in Patients with Homonymous Visual Field Defects. *Vision Research, 65*, 25–37. https://doi.org/10.1016/j.visres.2012.06.004

Parham, G., Bing, E.G., Cuevas, A., Fisher, B., Skinner, J., & Mwanahamuntu, M. (2019). Creating a low-cost virtual reality surgical simulation to increase surgical oncology capacity and capability. *Ecancer Medical Science.*

Park, C., & Kim, D. G. (2020). Exploring the roles of social presence and gender difference in online learning. *Decision Sciences Journal of Innovative Education*, *18*(2), 291–312. doi:10.1111/dsji.12207

Park, E., Yun, B. J., Min, Y. S., Lee, Y.-S., Moon, S.-J., Huh, J.-W., Cha, H., Chang, Y., & Jung, T.-D. (2019). Effects of a mixed reality-based cognitive training system compared to a conventional computer-assisted cognitive training system on mild cognitive impairment: A pilot study. *Cognitive and Behavioral Neurology*, *32*(3), 172–178. doi:10.1097/WNN.0000000000000197 PMID:31517700

Park, K., Kim, J., & Lee, J. (2020, July 6). A Deep Learning Approach to Predict Visual Field Using Optical Coherence Tomography. *PLoS One*, *15*(7), e0234902. https://doi.org/10.1371/journal.pone.0234902

Park, M. J., Kim, D. J., Lee, U., Na, E. J., & Jeon, H. J. (2019). A Literature Overview of Virtual Reality (VR) in Treatment of Psychiatric Disorders: Recent Advances and Limitations. *Frontiers in Psychiatry*, *10*, 505. doi:10.3389/fpsyt.2019.00505 PMID:31379623

Parsons, D. T., & Barnett, M. (2018). Virtual apartment -based Stroop for assessing distractor inhibition in healthy aging. *Applied Neuropsychology. Adult*, *26*(2), 144–154. doi:10.1080/23279095.2017.1373281 PMID:28976213

Parsons, D. T., Carlew, A. R., Magtoto, J., & Stonecipher, K. (2015). The potential of function-led virtual environments for ecologically valid measures of executive function in experimental and clinical neuropsychology. *Neuropsychological Rehabilitation*, 1–31. doi:10.1080/09602011.2015.1109524 PMID:26558491

Parsons, T. D. (2015). Ecological validity in virtual reality-based neuropsychological assessment. In K.-P. Mehdi (Ed.), *Encyclopaedia of Information Science and Technology* (3rd ed., pp. 214–223). IGI Global. doi:10.4018/978-1-4666-5888-2.ch095

Parsons, T. D. (2021). Ethical challenges of using virtual environments in the assessment and treatments of psychopathological disorders. *Journal of Clinical Medicine*, *10*(3), 378. doi:10.3390/jcm10030378 PMID:33498255

Parsons, T. D., Bowerly, T., Buckwalter, J. G., & Rizzo, A. A. (2007). A controlled clinical comparison of attention performance in children with ADHD in a virtual reality classroom compared to standard neuropsychological methods. *Child Neuropsychology*, *13*(4), 363–381. doi:10.1080/13825580600943473 PMID:17564852

Parsons, T. D., & Rizzo, A. A. (2008). Initial validation of a virtual environment for assessment of memory functioning: Virtual reality cognitive performance assessment test. *Cyberpsychology & Behavior*, *11*(1), 17–25. doi:10.1089/cpb.2007.9934 PMID:18275308

Parsons, T., & Duffield, T. (2020). Paradigm Shift Toward Digital Neuropsychology and High-Dimensional Neuropsychological Assessments [Review]. *Journal of Medical Internet Research*, *22*(12), e23777. doi:10.2196/23777 PMID:33325829

Paul, M., Bullock, K., & Bailenson, J. (2020). Virtual Reality Behavioral Activation as an Intervention for Major Depressive Disorder: Case Report. *JMIR Mental Health*, *7*(11), e24331. doi:10.2196/24331 PMID:33031046

Pazmiño, A., Jácome, J., Santillán, C., & Freire, M. (2019). El uso de las TIC para el aprendizaje de la programación. *Dominio de las Ciencias*, *5*(1), 290–298. doi:10.23857/dc.v5i1.861

Pedroli, E., Greci, L., Colombo, D., Serino, S., Cipresso, P., Arlati, S., Mondellini, M., Boilini, L., Giussani, V., Goulene, K., Agostoni, M., Sacco, M., Stramba-Badiale, M., Riva, G., & Gaggioli, A. (2018). Characteristics, usability, and users experience of a system combining cognitive and physical therapy in a virtual environment: Positive bike. *Sensors (Basel)*, *18*(7), 2343. doi:10.339018072343 PMID:30029502

Peinado, F., Fernández, A., Teba, F., Celada, G., & Acosta, M. A. (2018). El urólogo del futuro y las nuevas tecnologías [The urologist of the future and new technologies]. *Archivos Espanoles de Urologia*, *71*(1), 142–149. PMID:29336344

Peleg-Adler, R., Lanir, J., & Korman, M. (2018). The effects of aging on the use of handheld augmented reality in a route planning task. *Computers in Human Behavior*, *81*, 52–62. doi:10.1016/j.chb.2017.12.003

Pelissolo, A., Zaoui, M., Aguayo, G., Yao, S. N., Roche, S., & Ecochard, R. (2012). Virtual reality exposure therapy versus cognitive behavior therapy for panic disorder with agoraphobia: A randomized comparison study. *Journal of Cyber Therapy and Rehabilitation*, *5*(1), 35–43.

Peracha, M., Hughes, B., Tannir, J., Momi, R., Goyal, A., Juzych, M., Kim, C., McQueen, M., Eby, A., & Fatima, F. (2013, June 16). Assessing the Reliability of Humphrey Visual Field Testing in an Urban Population. *Investigative Ophthalmology & Visual Science*, *54*(15), 3920–3920.

Pérez-Guerrero, A., Aragón, M., & Torres, L. (2017). Dolor postoperatorio: ¿hacia dónde vamos? *Revista de la Sociedad Española del Dolor, 24*(1), 1-3. https://bit.ly/3hTSxlc

Perez-Marcos, D., Chevalley, O., Schmidlin, T., Garipelli, G., Serino, A., Vuadens, P., Tadi, T., Blanke, O., & Millán, J. R. (2017). Increasing Upper Limb Training Intensity in Chronic Stroke Using Embodied Virtual Reality: A Pilot Study. *Journal of Neuroengineering and Rehabilitation*, *14*(119).

Perkonigg, A., Kessler, R. C., Storz, S., & Wittchen, H. U. (2000). Traumatic events and post-traumatic stress disorder in the community: Prevalence, risk factors and comorbidity. *Acta Psychiatrica Scandinavica*, *101*(1), 46–59. doi:10.1034/j.1600-0447.2000.101001046.x PMID:10674950

Pessaux, P., Diana, M., Soler, L., Piardi, T., Mutter, D., & Marescaux, J. (2015). Towards cybernetic surgery: Robotic and augmented reality-assisted liver segmentectomy. *Langenbeck's Archives of Surgery*, *400*(3), 381–385. doi:10.100700423-014-1256-9 PMID:25392120

Pfefferle, M., Shahub, S., Shahedi, M., Gahan, J., Johnson, B., Le, P., Vargas, J., Judson, B. O., Alshara, Y., Li, Q., & Fei, B. (2020). Renal biopsy under augmented reality guidance. *Proceedings of SPIE—the International Society for Optical Engineering, 11315*.

Phipps, L., Sutherland, A., & Seale, J. (Eds.). (2002). *Access All Areas: disability, technology and learning*. JISC TechDis Service and ALT.

Plancher, G., Tirard, A., Gyselinck, V., Nicolas, S., & Piolino, P. (2012). Using virtual reality to characterize episodic memory profiles in amnestic mild cognitive impairment and Alzheimer's disease: Influence of active and passive encoding. *Neuropsychologia*, *50*(5), 592–602. doi:10.1016/j.neuropsychologia.2011.12.013 PMID:22261400

Ploder, O., Wagner, A., & Enislidis, G. (1995). Computer-assisted intraoperative visualization of dental implants. Augmented reality in medicine. *Der Radiologe*, *35*, 569–572. PMID:8588037

Pokorny, M., & Yaxley, J. (2019). Three-dimensional Elastic Augmented Reality for Robot-assisted Laparoscopic Prostatectomy: Pushing the Boundaries, but Cutting it Fine. *European Urology*, *76*(4), 515–516. doi:10.1016/j.eururo.2019.04.025 PMID:31053374

Porpiglia, F., Fiori, C., Checcucci, E., Amparore, D., & Bertolo, R. (2018). Augmented Reality Robot-assisted Radical Prostatectomy: Preliminary Experience. *Urology*, *115*, 184. doi:10.1016/j.urology.2018.01.028 PMID:29548868

Porras, D. C., Siemonsma, P., Inzelberg, R., Zeilig, G., & Plotnik, M. (2018). Advantages of Virtual Reality in the Rehabilitation of Balance and Gait: Systematic Review. *Neurology*, *29*(90), 1017–1025.

Pottle, J. (2019). Virtual reality and the transformation of medical education. *Future Healthcare Journal*, *6*(3), 181–185. doi:10.7861/fhj.2019-0036 PMID:31660522

Powell, W., Rizzo, A., Sharkey, P., & Merrick, J. (2017). Innovations and Challenges in the Use of Virtual Reality Technologies for Rehabilitation. *Journal of Alternative Medical Research, 10*.

Pratt, P., & Arora, A. (2018). Transoral Robotic Surgery: Image Guidance and Augmented Reality. *ORL; Journal for Oto-Rhino-Laryngology and Its Related Specialties, 80*(3-4), 204–212. doi:10.1159/000489467 PMID:29936505

Proniewska, K., Pregowska, A., Dolega-Dlegowski, D., & Dudek, D. (2021). Immersive technologies as a solution for general data protection regulation in Europe and impact on the COVID-19 pandemic. *Cardiology Journal, 28*(1), 23–33. doi:10.5603/CJ.a2020.0102 PMID:32789838

Protopapas, A. (2019). Evolving Concepts of Dyslexia and Their Implications for Research and Remediation. *Frontiers in Psychology, 10*, 2873. doi:10.3389/fpsyg.2019.02873 PMID:31920890

Pynoos, J., Nishita, C., & Perelma, L. (2003). Advancements in the Home Modification Field. *Journal of Housing for the Elderly, 17*(1-2), 105–116. doi:10.1300/J081v17n01_08

Qian, J., McDonough, D. J., & Gao, Z. (2020). The Effectiveness of Virtual Reality Exercise on Individual's Physiological, Psychological and Rehabilitative Outcomes: A Systematic Review. *International Journal of Environmental Research and Public Health, 17*(11), 4133. doi:10.3390/ijerph17114133 PMID:32531906

Qingdao Cybercare Information Technology Co Ltd. (2016). *Driving Virtual Reality Post-Traumatic Stress Disorder Treatment System, has Display Displayed Virtual Scene, which is Matched with User Physiological Data, Vibrator Fixed with Controller, and Physiological Data Output Sent to Controller. CN103405239B.* CNIPA.

Quero, G., Lapergola, A., Soler, L., Shahbaz, M., Hostettler, A., Collins, T., Marescaux, J., Mutter, D., Diana, M., & Pessaux, P. (2019). Virtual and Augmented Reality in Oncologic Liver Surgery. *Surgical Oncology Clinics of North America, 28*(1), 31–44. doi:10.1016/j.soc.2018.08.002 PMID:30414680

Radia, M., Arunakirinathan, M., & Sibley, D. (2018). A Guide to Eyes: Ophthalmic Simulators. *The Bulletin of the Royal College of Surgeons of England, 100*(4), 169–171.

Rahman, R., Wood, M. E., Qian, L., Price, C. L., Johnson, A. A., & Osgood, G. M. (2020). Head-Mounted Display Use in Surgery: A Systematic Review. *Surgical Innovation, 27*(1), 88–100. doi:10.1177/1553350619871787 PMID:31514682

Rao, S. K., & Prasad, R. (2018). Impact of 5G technologies on industry 4.0. *Wireless Personal Communications, 100*(1), 145–159.

Raspelli, S., Pallavicini, F., Carelli, L., Morganti, F., Poletti, B., Corra, B., ... Riva, G. (2011). Validation of a Neuro Virtual Reality-based version of the Multiple Errands Test for the assessment of executive functions. *Studies in Health Technology and Informatics, 167*, 92–97. PMID:21685648

Raz, S., Bar-Haim, Y., Sadeh, A., & Dan, O. (2014). Reliability and validity of the online continuous performance test among young adults. *Assessment, 21*(1), 108–118. doi:10.1177/1073191112443409 PMID:22517923

Rebbani, Z., Azougagh, D., Bahatti, L., & Bouattane, O. (2021). Definitions and Applications of Augmented/Virtual Reality: A Survey. *International Journal (Toronto, Ont.), 9*(3), 279–285. doi:10.30534/ijeter/2021/21932021

Reedy, G. B. (2015). Using cognitive load theory to inform simulation design and practice. *Clinical Simulation in Nursing, 11*(8), 355–360. doi:10.1016/j.ecns.2015.05.004

Reger, G. M., Holloway, K. M., Candy, C., Rothbaum, B. O., Difede, J., Rizzo, A. A., & Gahm, G. A. (2011). Effectiveness of Virtual Reality Exposure Therapy for Active Duty Soldiers in a Military Mental Health Clinic. *Journal of Traumatic Stress, 24*(1), 93–96. doi:10.1002/jts.20574 PMID:21294166

Reger, G. M., Koenen-Woods, P., Zetocha, K., Smolenski, D. J., Holloway, K. M., Rothbaum, B. O., Difede, J. A., Rizzo, A. A., Edwards-Stewart, A., Skopp, N. A., Mishkind, M., Reger, M. A., & Gahm, G. A. (2016). Randomized Controlled Trial of Prolonged Exposure Using Imaginal Exposure vs. Virtual Reality Exposure in Active Duty Soldiers With Deployment-Related Posttraumatic Stress Disorder (PTSD). *Journal of Consulting and Clinical Psychology*, *84*(11), 946–959. doi:10.1037/ccp0000134 PMID:27606699

Reger, G. M., Smolenski, D., Norr, A., Katz, A., Buck, B., & Rothbaum, B. O. (2019). Does Virtual Reality Increase Emotional Engagement During Exposure for PTSD? Subjective Distress During Prolonged and Virtual Reality Exposure Therapy. *Journal of Anxiety Disorders*, *61*, 75–81. doi:10.1016/j.janxdis.2018.06.001 PMID:29935999

Rehasoft. (2019a). *Dislexia, TDAH, Discalculia y Baja Visión*. https://www.rehasoft.com/

Rehasoft. (2019b). *DiTres*. https://www.rehasoft.com/dislexia/ditres/

Rehasoft. (2019c). *DiTex*. https://www.rehasoft.com/dislexia/ditex/

Rehasoft. (2019d). *DiDoc*. https://www.rehasoft.com/dislexia/didoc/

Reinhard, R., Rutrecht, H. M., Hengstenberg, P., Tutulmaz, E., Geissler, B., Hecht, H., & Muttray, A. (2017). The best way to assess visually induced motion sickness in a fixed-base driving simulator. *Transportation Research Part F: Traffic Psychology and Behaviour*, *48*, 74–88. doi:10.1016/j.trf.2017.05.005

Reyna, D., Caraza, R., Gonzalez-Knoell, M., Ayala, A., Martinez, P., Loredo, A., Rosas, R., & Reyes, P. (2018). Virtual Reality for Social Phobia Treatment. *Smart Technology*, *213*, 165–177.

Riches, S., Elghany, S., Garety, P., Rus-Calafell, M., & Valmaggia, L. (2019). Factors Affecting Sense of Presence in a Virtual Reality Social Environment: A Qualitative Study. *Cyberpsychology, Behavior, and Social Networking*, *22*(4), 288–292. doi:10.1089/cyber.2018.0128 PMID:30802148

Riddell, J., Jhun, P., Fung, C. C., Comes, J., Sawtelle, S., Tabatabai, R., Joseph, D., Shoenberger, J., Chen, E., Fee, C., & Swadron, S. P. (2017). Does the Flipped Classroom Improve Learning in Graduate Medical Education? *Journal of Graduate Medical Education*, *9*(4), 491–496. doi:10.4300/JGME-D-16-00817.1 PMID:28824764

Riddoch, M., & Humphreys, G. W. (1994). *Cognitive neuropsychology and cognitive rehabilitation*. Lawrence Erlbaum Associates, Inc.

Riva, G. (2017). Applications of Virtual Environments in Medicine. *Methods of Information in Medicine*, *42*(5), 524–534.

Riva, G., Mancuso, V., Cavedoni, S., & Stramba-Badiale, C. (2020). Virtual reality in neurorehabilitation: A review of its effects on multiple cognitive domains. *Expert Review of Medical Devices*, *17*(10), 1035–1061. doi:10.1080/174344 40.2020.1825939 PMID:32962433

Rizzetto, F., Bernareggi, A., Rantas, S., Vanzulli, A., & Vertemati, M. (2020). Immersive Virtual Reality in surgery and medical education: Diving into the future. *American Journal of Surgery*, *220*(4), 856–857. doi:10.1016/j.amjsurg.2020.04.033 PMID:32386709

Rizzo, A., Schultheis, M. T., & Rothbaum, B. O. (2002). Ethical issues for the use of virtual reality in the psychological sciences. In Ethical issues in clinical neuropsychology (pp. 243-280). Swets & Zeitlinge.

Rizzo, A. A., Buckwalter, J. G., Neumann, U., Kesselman, C., & Thiebaux, M. (1998). Basic issues in the application of virtual reality for the assessment and rehabilitation of cognitive impairments and functional disability. *Cyberpsychology & Behavior*, *1*(1), 59–79. doi:10.1089/cpb.1998.1.59

Rizzo, A. A., Schultheis, M., Kerns, K. A., & Mateer, C. (2004). Analysis of assets for virtual reality applications in neuropsychology. *Neuropsychological Rehabilitation*, *14*(1-2), 207–239. doi:10.1080/09602010343000183

Rizzo, A. S., & Shilling, R. (2017). Clinical Virtual Reality tools to advance the prevention, assessment, and treatment of PTSD. *European Journal of Psychotraumatology*, *8*(sup5), 1414560. doi:10.1080/20008198.2017.1414560 PMID:29372007

Rizzo, A., Gambino, G., Sardo, P., & Rizzo, V. (2020). Being in the Past and Perform the Future in a Virtual World: VR Applications to Assess and Enhance Episodic and Prospective Memory in Normal and Pathological Aging. *Frontiers in Human Neuroscience*, *14*, 297. doi:10.3389/fnhum.2020.00297 PMID:32848672

Rizzo, A., & Talbot, T. (2016). *Virtual Reality Standardized Patients for Clinical Training, w: The Digital Patient*. John Wiley&Sons, Inc.

Robert, I. V. (2021). Formation and development of digital transformation of domestic education on the basis of systemic convergence of pedagogical science and technology. In *SHS Web of Conferences* (Vol. 101, p. 03017). EDP Sciences.

Roberts, A. C., Yeap, Y. W., Seah, H. S., Chan, E., Soh, C. K., & Christopoulos, G. I. (2019). Assessing the suitability of virtual reality for psychological testing. *Psychological Assessment*, *31*(3), 318–328. doi:10.1037/pas0000663 PMID:30802117

Rodríguez-Cano, S., Delgado-Benito, V., Ausín-Villaverde, V., & Martín, L. M. (2021). Design of a Virtual Reality software to promote the learning of students with Dyslexia. *Sustainability*, *13*(15), 8425. doi:10.3390u13158425

Román, M., Cardemil, C., & Carrasco, A. (2011). Enfoque y metodología para evaluar la calidad del proceso pedagógico que incorpora TIC en el aula. *Revista Iberoaméricana de Evaluación Educativa*, *4*(2), 9–35.

Romano, D. M. (2005). Virtual reality therapy. *Developmental Medicine and Child Neurology*, *47*(9), 580–580. doi:10.1111/j.1469-8749.2005.tb01206.x PMID:16138662

Ropelato, S., Menozzi, M., Michel, D., & Siegrist, M. (2020). Augmented Reality Microsurgery: A Tool for Training Micromanipulations in Ophthalmic Surgery Using Augmented Reality. *Simulation in Healthcare*, *15*(2), 122–127.

Ros, M., & Trives, J. V. (2020). *Point-of-view recording device*. US Patent App. 16/341,070.

Rose, A. S., Kim, H., Fuchs, H., & Frahm, J. M. (2019). Development of augmented-reality applications in otolaryngology-head and neck surgery. *The Laryngoscope*, *129*(S3, Suppl 3), S1–S11. doi:10.1002/lary.28098 PMID:31260127

Rose, F. D., Brooks, B. M., & Rizzo, A. A. (2005). Virtual reality in brain damage rehabilitation. *Cyberpsychology & Behavior*, *8*(3), 241–262. doi:10.1089/cpb.2005.8.241 PMID:15971974

Ros, M., Debien, B., Cyteval, C., Molinari, N., Gatto, F., & Lonjon, N. (2020). Applying an immersive tutorial in virtual reality to learning a new technique. *Neuro-Chirurgie*, *66*(4), 212–218. doi:10.1016/j.neuchi.2020.05.006 PMID:32623059

Ros, M., & Neuwirth, L. S. (2020). Increasing global awareness of timely COVID-19 healthcare guidelines through FPV training tutorials: Portable public health crises teaching method. *Nurse Education Today*, *91*(104479), 1–6. doi:10.1016/j.nedt.2020.104479 PMID:32473497

Ros, M., Neuwirth, L. S., Ng, S., Debien, B., Molinari, N., Gatto, F., & Lonjon, N. (2021). The Effects of an Immersive Virtual Reality Application in First Person Point-of-View, Video-Based, on The Learning and Generalized Performance of a Lumbar Puncture Medical Procedure. *Educational Technology Research and Development*, *69*(3), 1529–1556. Advance online publication. doi:10.100711423-021-10003-w

Ros, M., Trives, J. V., & Lonjon, N. (2017). From stereoscopic recording to virtual reality headsets: Designing a new way to learn surgery. *Neuro-Chirurgie, 63*(1), 1–5. doi:10.1016/j.neuchi.2016.08.004 PMID:28233530

Ros, M., Weaver, L., & Neuwirth, L. S. (2020). Virtual reality stereoscopic 180-degree video-based immersive environments: Applications for training surgeons and other medical professionals. In J. E. Stefaniak (Ed.), *Cases on Instructional Design and Performance Outcomes in Medical Education*. IGI Global. doi:10.4018/978-1-7998-5092-2.ch005

Rosvold, H. E., Mirsky, A. F., Sarason, I., Bransome, E. D. Jr, & Beck, L. H. (1956). A continuous performance test of brain damage. *Journal of Consulting Psychology, 20*(5), 343–350. doi:10.1037/h0043220 PMID:13367264

Rothbaum, B. O., Anderson, P., Zimand, E., Hodges, L., Lang, D., & Wilson, J. (2006). Virtual reality exposure therapy and standard (in vivo) exposure therapy in the treatment of fear of flying. *Behavior Therapy, 37*(1), 80–90. doi:10.1016/j.beth.2005.04.004 PMID:16942963

Rothbaum, B., Hodges, L., Kooper, R., Opdyke, D., Williford, J., & North, M. (1995b). Effectiveness of computer-generated (virtual reality) graded exposure in the treatment of acrophobia. *The American Journal of Psychiatry, 152*(4), 626–628. doi:10.1176/ajp.152.4.626 PMID:7694917

Roussin, C. J., & Weinstock, P. (2017). SimZones: An organizational innovation for simulation programs and centers. *Academic Medicine, 92*(8), 1114–1120. doi:10.1097/ACM.0000000000001746 PMID:28562455

Roy, E., Bakr, M. M., & George, R. (2017). The need for virtual reality simulators in dental education: A review. *The Saudi Dental Journal, 29*(2), 41–47. doi:10.1016/j.sdentj.2017.02.001 PMID:28490842

Runciman, M., Darzi, A., & Mylonas, G. (2019). Soft robotics in minimally invasive surgery. *Soft Robotics, 6*(4), 423–443. doi:10.1089oro.2018.0136 PMID:30920355

Ryan, R., & Deci, E. (2005). Toward a Social Psychology of Assimilation: Self-Determination Theory in Cognitive Development and Education. doi:10.1017/CBO9781139152198.014

Salari, N., Hosseinian-Far, A., Jalali, R., Vaisi-Raygani, A., Rasoulpoor, S., Mohammadi, M., Rasoulpoor, S., & Khaledi-Paveh, B. (2020). Prevalence of stress, anxiety, depression among the general population during the COVID-19 pandemic: A systematic review and meta-analysis. *Globalization and Health, 16*(57), 57. Advance online publication. doi:10.118612992-020-00589-w PMID:32631403

Salehi, E., Mehrabi, M., Fatehi, F., & Salehi, A. (2020). Virtual Reality Therapy for Social Phobia: A Scoping Review. *Studies in Health Technology and Informatics, 270*(06), 2020. PMID:32570476

Salisbury, D. B., Dahdah, M., Driver, S., Parsons, T. D., & Richter, K. M. (2016). Virtual reality and brain computer interface in neurorehabilitation. *Proceedings - Baylor University. Medical Center, 29*(2), 124–127. doi:10.1080/08998 280.2016.11929386 PMID:27034541

Samadbeik, M., Yaaghobi, D., Bastani, P., Abhari, S., Rezaee, R., & Garavand, A. (2018). The applications of virtual reality technology in medical groups teaching. *Journal of Advances in Medical Education & Professionalism, 6*(3), 123. https://bit.ly/3xXshMB PMID:30013996

Saputra, M. R. U., Alfarozi, S. A. I., & Nugroho, K. A. (2018). LexiPal: Kinect- based application for dyslexia using multisensory approach and natural user interface. *International Journal of Computer Applications in Technology, 57*(4), 334. doi:10.1504/IJCAT.2018.10014728

Sarika, G., Neelkant, P., Jitender, S., Ravinder, S., & Sanjeev, L. (2015). Oral implant imaging: a review. *Malays J Med Sci, 22*, 7-17.

Sathiyanarayanan, M., & Rajan, S. (2016). MYO Armband for Physiotherapy Healthcare: A Case Study Using Gesture Recognition Application. *8th International Conference on Communication Systems and Networks (COMSNETS)*.

Sayadi, L., Naides, A., Eng, M., Fijany, A., Chopan, M., Sayadi, J., Shaterian, A., Banyard, D., Evans, G., Vyas, R., & Widgerow, A. (2019). The new frontier: A review of augmented reality and virtual reality in plastic surgery. *Aesthetic Surgery Journal, 39*(9), 1007–1016. doi:10.1093/asjjz043 PMID:30753313

Sayed, A., Roongpoovapatr, V., Eleiwa, T., Kashem, R., Abdel-Mottaleb, M., Jumbo, O., Parrish, R., & Abou Shousha, M. (2021, June 21). Measurement of Monocular and Binocular Visual Field Defects with a Virtual Reality Head Mounted Display. *Investigative Ophthalmology & Visual Science, 62*(8), 3512–3512.

Schenkman, N. (2008). Virtual reality training in urology. *The Journal of Urology, 180*(6), 2305–2306. doi:10.1016/j.juro.2008.09.069 PMID:18930286

Schijven, M., & Jakimowicz, J. (2003). Construct validity. *Surgical Endoscopy, 17*(5), 803–810. doi:10.100700464-002-9151-9 PMID:12582752

Schiza, E., Matsangidou, M., Neolkeous, K., & Pattichis, C. S. (2019). Virtual reality applications for neurological disease: A review. *Frontiers in Robotics and AI, 6*, 100. doi:10.3389/frobt.2019.00100 PMID:33501115

Schlairet, M. C., Schlairet, T. J., Sauls, D. H., & Bellflowers, L. (2015). Cognitive load, emotion, and performance in high-fidelity simulation among beginning nursing students: A pilot study. *The Journal of Nursing Education, 54*(3). Advance online publication. doi:10.3928/01484834-20150218-10 PMID:25692940

Schmalstieg, D., & Hollerer, T. (2016). Augmented Reality: Principles and Practice. Addison-Wesley Professional.

Schreuder, H., Persson, J., Wolswijk, R., Ihse, I., Schijven, M., & Verheijen, R. (2014). Validation of a novel virtual reality simulator for robotic surgery. *TheScientificWorldJournal, 2014*, 1–10. Advance online publication. doi:10.1155/2014/507076 PMID:24600328

Schulz, C., Waldeck, S., & Mauer, U. M. (2012). Intraoperative image guidance in neurosurgery: Development, current indications, and future trends. *Radiology Research and Practice, 2012*, 197364. doi:10.1155/2012/197364 PMID:22655196

Scozzari, S., & Gamberini, L. (2011). Virtual reality as a tool for cognitive behavioral therapy: a review. *Virtual reality in psychotherapy, rehabilitation, and assessment*, 63-108.

Selwyn, N. (2004). Reconsidering Political and Popular Understandings of the Digital Divide. *New Media & Society, 6*(3), 341–362. doi:10.1177/1461444804042519

Seo, J. H., Smith, B. M., Cook, M., Malone, E., Pine, M., Leal, S., Bai, Z., Suh, J., & Anatomy Builder, V. R. (2017). Applying a Constructive Learning Method in the Virtual Reality Canine Skeletal System. *International Conference on Applied Human Factors and Ergonomics*, 245–252.

Seong, M., Sung, K. R., Choi, E. H., Kang, S. Y., Cho, J. W., Um, T. W., Kim, Y. J., Park, S. B., Hong, H. E., & Kook, M. S. (2010, March 1). Macular and Peripapillary Retinal Nerve Fiber Layer Measurements by Spectral Domain Optical Coherence Tomography in Normal-Tension Glaucoma. *Investigative Ophthalmology & Visual Science, 51*(3), 1446–1452. https://doi.org/10.1167/iovs.09-4258

Servadei, F., Rossini, Z., Nicolosi, F., Morselli, C., & Park, K. (2018). The role of neurosurgery in countries with limited facilities: Facts and challenges. *World Neurosurgery, 112*, 315–321. doi:10.1016/j.wneu.2018.01.047 PMID:29366998

Sevillano, M., & Rodríguez, R. (2013). Integración de tecnologías de la información y comunicación en educación infantil en Navarra. *Píxel-Bit. Revista de Medios y Educación, 42*, 75–87.

Shaffer, F., & Ginsberg, J. P. (2017). An overview of heart rate variability metrics and norms. *Frontiers in Public Health*, *5*, 258. doi:10.3389/fpubh.2017.00258 PMID:29034226

Shahabi, C., Yang, K., Yoon, H., Rizzo, A. A., McLaughlin, M., Marsh, T., & Mun, M. (2007). Immersidata analysis: Four case studies. *Computer*, *40*(7), 45–52. doi:10.1109/MC.2007.245

Shah, J., Mackay, S., Vale, J., & Darzi, A. (2001). Simulation in urology—A role for virtual reality? *BJU International*, *88*(7), 661–665. doi:10.1046/j.1464-410X.2001.02320.x PMID:11890232

Shah, U. R. (2017). Cognitive rehabilitation in psychiatry. *Annals of Indian Psychiatry*, *1*(2), 68–75. doi:10.4103/aip.aip_35_17

Shallice, T., & Burgess, P. W. (1991). Deficits in strategy application following frontal lobe damage in man. *Brain*, *114*(Pt 2), 727–741. doi:10.1093/brain/114.2.727 PMID:2043945

Sharma, Hunt, Maheshwari, Osborn, Levay, Kaliki, Soares, & Thakork. (2018). A Mixed-Reality Training Environment for Upper Limb Prosthesis Control. *Conf. IEEE Biomed. Circuits Syst. (BioCAS)*.

Sharma, P., & Halder, S. (2021). Cognition, Quality of Life And Mood State In Mild Traumatic Brain Injury: A Case Study. *Indian Journal of Mental Health*, *8*(1), 112. doi:10.30877/IJMH.8.1.2021.112-116

Sheetz, K., Claflin, J., & Dimick, J. (2020). Trends in the adoption of robotic surgery for common surgical procedures. *JAMA Network Open*, *3*(1), e1918911–e1918911. doi:10.1001/jamanetworkopen.2019.18911 PMID:31922557

Sheridan, T. B. (2000, October). Interaction, imagination and immersion some research needs. In *Proceedings of the ACM symposium on Virtual reality software and technology* (pp. 1-7). 10.1145/502390.502392

Sherman, W., Craig, A. B., Sherman, W. R., & Craig, A. B. (Eds.). (2003). *Understanding Virtual Reality: Interface, Application, and Design, The Morgan Kaufmann Series in Computer Graphics*. Morgan Kaufmann. doi:10.1016/B978-1-55860-353-0.50019-7

Shiban, Y., Pauli, P., & Mühlberger, A. (2013). Effect of Multiple Context Exposure on Renewal in Spider Phobia. *Behaviour Research and Therapy*, *51*, 68–74.

Shirk, J. D. (2020). RE: 3D Printing, Augmented Reality, and Virtual Reality for the Assessment and Management of Kidney and Prostate Cancer: A Systematic Review. *Urology*, *145*, 301. doi:10.1016/j.urology.2020.07.061 PMID:32916192

Shu, L., Xie, J., Yang, M., Li, Z., Li, Z., Liao, D., Xu, X., & Yang, X. (2018). A review of emotion recognition using physiological signals. *Sensors (Basel)*, *18*(7), 2074. doi:10.339018072074 PMID:29958457

Siess, A., & Wölfel, M. (2018). User color temperature preferences in immersive virtual realities. *Computers & Graphics*, *81*, 20–31. doi:10.1016/j.cag.2019.03.018

Siff, L. N., & Mehta, N. (2018). An Interactive Holographic Curriculum for Urogynecologic Surgery. *Obstetrics and Gynecology*, *132*(Suppl 1), 27S–32S. doi:10.1097/AOG.0000000000002860 PMID:30247304

Silén, C., Wirell, S., Kvist, J., Nylander, E., & Smedby, Ö. (2008). Advanced 3D visualization in student-centred medical education. *Medical Teacher*, *30*(5), e115–e124. doi:10.1080/01421590801932228 PMID:18576181

Simpfendörfer, T., Baumhauer, M., Müller, M., Gutt, C. N., Meinzer, H. P., Rassweiler, J. J., Guven, S., & Teber, D. (2011). Augmented reality visualization during laparoscopic radical prostatectomy. *Journal of Endourology*, *25*(12), 1841–1845. doi:10.1089/end.2010.0724 PMID:21970336

Sinkin, J., Rahman, O., & Nahabedian, M. (2016). Google Glass in the operating room: The plastic surgeon's perspective. *Plastic and Reconstructive Surgery*, *138*(1), 298–302. doi:10.1097/PRS.0000000000002307 PMID:27348661

Skalicky, S. E., & Kong, G. Y. (2019, December). Novel Means of Clinical Visual Function Testing among Glaucoma Patients, Including Virtual Reality. *Journal of Current Glaucoma Practice*, *13*(3), 83–87. https://doi.org/10.5005/jp-journals-10078-1265

Skiada, R., Soroniati, E., Gardeli, A., & Zissis, D. (2014). EasyLexia: A mobile application for children with learning difficulties. *Procedia Computer Science*, *27*(2), 218–228. doi:10.1016/j.procs.2014.02.025

Slater, M. (2020, May 11). Transforming the Self Through Virtual Reality. *Frontiers Science News*. https://blog.frontiersin.org/2020/05/05/frontiers-in-virtual-reality-online-seminar-series/

Slater, M., Khanna, P., Mortensen, J., & Yu, I. (2009). Visual Realism Enhances Realistic Response in an Immersive Virtual Environment. *IEEE Computer Graphics and Applications*, *29*(3), 76–84. doi:10.1109/MCG.2009.55 PMID:19642617

Slater, M., Spanlang, B., Sanchez-Vives, M. V., & Blanke, O. (2010). First person experience of body transfer in virtual reality. *PLoS One*, *5*(5), e10564. doi:10.1371/journal.pone.0010564 PMID:20485681

Slater, M., & Wilbur, S. (1997). framework for immersive virtual environments (FIVE): Speculations on the role of presence in virtual environments. *Presence (Cambridge, Mass.)*, *6*(6), 603–616. doi:10.1162/pres.1997.6.6.603

Smallwood, J., Davies, J. B., Heim, D., Finnigan, F., Sudberry, M., O'Connor, R., & Obonsawin, M. (2004). Subjective experience and the attentional lapse: Task engagement and disengagement during sustained attention. *Consciousness and Cognition*, *13*(4), 657–690. doi:10.1016/j.concog.2004.06.003 PMID:15522626

Smigelski, M., Movassaghi, M., & Small, A. (2020). Urology Virtual Education Programs During the COVID-19 Pandemic. *Current Urology Reports*, *21*(12), 50. doi:10.100711934-020-01004-y PMID:33090272

Smith, A. M., & Czyz, C. N. (2021). Neuroanatomy, Cranial Nerve 2 (Optic). In *StatPearls*. StatPearls Publishing. https://www.ncbi.nlm.nih.gov/books/NBK507907/

Sohlberg, M. M., & Mateer, C. A. (1989). *Introduction to cognitive rehabilitation: Theory and practice*. The Guilford Press.

Sohlberg, M. M., & Mateer, C. A. (Eds.). (2001). *Cognitive rehabilitation: An integrative neuropsychological approach*. Guilford Press.

Solbiati, L., Gennaro, N., & Muglia, R. (2020). Augmented Reality: From Video Games to Medical Clinical Practice. *Cardiovascular and Interventional Radiology*, *43*(10), 1427–1429. doi:10.100700270-020-02575-6 PMID:32632853

Soleymani, M., Lichtenauer, J., Pun, T., & Pantic, M. (2011). A multimodal database for affect recognition and implicit tagging. *IEEE Transactions on Affective Computing*, *3*(1), 42–55. doi:10.1109/T-AFFC.2011.25

Speare, J. (2018). El retiro del cirujano: ¿Por qué, cuándo y cómo debe retirarse un cirujano? *Anales Médicos de la Asociación Médica del Centro Médico ABC*, *63*(1), 73–79. https://bit.ly/3kI4RqH

Speicher, M., Hall, B. D., & Nebeling, M. (2019). What is Mixed Reality? In *Proceedings of the 2019 CHI Conference on Human Factors in Computing Systems*. Association for Computing Machinery.

Speicher, M., Hall, B., & Nebeling, M. (2019, May). What is mixed reality? In *Proceedings of the 2019 CHI Conference on Human Factors in Computing Systems* (pp. 1-15). 10.1145/3290605.3300767

Spiegel, J. S. (2018). The Ethics of Virtual Reality Technology: Social Hazards and Public Policy Recommendations. *Science and Engineering Ethics*, *24*(5), 1537–1550. doi:10.100711948-017-9979-y PMID:28942536

Spinhoven, P., Penninx, B. W., Van Hemert, A. M., De Rooij, M., & Elzinga, B. M. (2014). Comorbidity of PTSD in anxiety and depressive disorders: Prevalence and shared risk factors. *Child Abuse & Neglect*, *38*(8), 1320–1330. doi:10.1016/j.chiabu.2014.01.017 PMID:24629482

Stanney, K. M., Kennedy, R. S., & Drexler, J. M. (1997). Cybersickness is Not Simulator Sickness. *Proceedings of the Human Factors and Ergonomics Society Annual Meeting*, *41*(2), 1138–1142. doi:10.1177/107118139704100292

Stanton, D., Foreman, N., & Wilson, P. N. (1998, January 1). Uses of virtual reality in clinical training: Developing the spatial skills of children with mobility impairments. *Studies in Health Technology and Informatics*, 219–232. PMID:10350923

Steinberger, J., & Qureshi, S. (2020). The Role of Augmented Reality and Virtual Reality in Contemporary Spine Surgery. *Contemporary Spine Surgery*, *21*(8), 1–5. doi:10.1097/01.CSS.0000689552.57650.21

Sternberg, S. (1967). Two operations in character recognition: Some evidence from reaction time measurements. *Perception & Psychophysics*, *2*(2), 45–53. doi:10.3758/BF03212460

Sternberg, S. (1969). Memory scanning: Mental processes revealed by reaction-time experiments. *American Scientist*, *57*, 421–457. PMID:5360276

Stevens, J. A., & Kincaid, J. P. (2015). The relationship between presence and performance in virtual simulation training. *Open Journal of Modelling and Simulation*, *3*(02), 41–48. doi:10.4236/ojmsi.2015.32005

Strauss, E., Sherman, E. M. S., & Spreen, O. (2006). *A compendium of neuropsychological tests: Administration, norms, and commentary* (3rd ed.). Oxford University Press.

Stroop, J. R. (1935). Studies of interference in serial verbal reactions. *Journal of Experimental Psychology*, *18*(6), 643–662. doi:10.1037/h0054651

Suárez, A. I., Pérez, C. Y., Vergara, M. M., & Alférez, V. H. (2015). Desarrollo de la lectoescritura mediante TIC y recursos educativos abiertos. *Apertura (Guadalajara, Jal.)*, *7*(1), 38–49.

Suenaga, H., Tran, H., & Liao, H. (2013). Real-time in situ three dimensional integral videography and surgical navigation using augmented reality: a pilot study. *Int J Oral Sci.*, *5*, 98–102.

Suryanti, S., Sutaji, D., Arifani, Y., Muyasaroh, M., & Zamzamy, M. (2020). Improved learning accessibility and professionalism of teachers in remote areas through mentoring development of teaching materials based on Augmented Reality. *Kontribusia*, *3*(1), 224–232. doi:10.30587/kontribusia.v3i1.1032

Susi, T., Johannesson, M., & Backlund, P. (2007). *Serious Games : An Overview*. Academic Press.

Sutherland, J., Belec, J., Sheikh, A., Chepelev, L., Althobaity, W., Chow, B., Mitsouras, D., Christensen, A., Rybicki, F. J., & La Russa, D. J. (2019). Applying Modern Virtual and Augmented Reality Technologies to Medical Images and Models. *Journal of Digital Imaging*, *32*(1), 38–53. doi:10.100710278-018-0122-7 PMID:30215180

Sveinsson, B., Koonjoo, N., & Rosen, M. S. (2021). ARmedViewer, an augmented-reality-based fast 3D reslicer for medical image data on mobile devices: A feasibility study. *Computer Methods and Programs in Biomedicine*, *200*, 105836. doi:10.1016/j.cmpb.2020.105836 PMID:33250281

Swacha, J., Queirós, R., & Paiva, J. C. (2019). Towards a Framework for Gamified Programming Education. *2019 International Symposium on Educational Technology (ISET)*, 144–149. 10.1109/ISET.2019.00038

Sweller, J. (1994). Cognitive load theory, learning difficulty, and instructional design. *Learning and Instruction*, *4*(4), 295–312. doi:10.1016/0959-4752(94)90003-5

Sweller, J. (2011). Chapter two – cognitive load theory. *Psychology of Learning and Motivation*, *55*, 37–76. doi:10.1016/B978-0-12-387691-1.00002-8

Sweller, J., Ayres, P., & Kalyuga, S. (2011). Measuring cognitive load. In *Cognitive Load Theory. Explorations in the Learning Sciences, Instructional Systems and Performance Technologies* (Vol. 1, pp. 71–85). Springer., doi:10.1007/978-1-4419-8126-4_6

Sweller, J., Chandler, P., Tierney, P., & Cooper, M. (1990). Cognitive load as a factor in the structuring of technical material. *Journal of Experimental Psychology, 119*(2), 176–192. doi:10.1037/0096-3445.119.2.176

Szpak, A., Michalski, S. C., Saredakis, D., Chen, C. S., & Loetscher, T. (2019). Beyond feeling sick: The visual and cognitive aftereffects of virtual reality. *IEEE Access: Practical Innovations, Open Solutions, 7*, 130883–130892. doi:10.1109/ACCESS.2019.2940073

Tabatabai, S. (2020). COVID-19 impact and virtual medical education. *Journal of Advances in Medical Education & Professionalism, 8*(3), 140–143. PMID:32802908

Tagaya, N., Yamazaki, R., Nakagawa, A., Abe, A., Hamada, K., Kubota, K., & Oyama, T. (2008). Intraoperative identification of sentinel lymph nodes by near-infrared fluorescence imaging in patients with breast cancer. *American Journal of Surgery, 195*(6), 850–853. doi:10.1016/j.amjsurg.2007.02.032 PMID:18353274

Tang, K. S., Cheng, D. L., Mi, E., & Greenberg, P. B. (2020). Augmented reality in medical education: A systematic review. *Canadian Medical Education Journal, 11*(1), e81. PMID:32215146

Tao, H. S., Lin, J. Y., Luo, W., Chen, R., Zhu, W., Fang, C. H., & Yang, J. (2021). Application of Real-Time Augmented Reality Laparoscopic Navigation in Splenectomy for Massive Splenomegaly. *World Journal of Surgery, 45*(7), 2108–2115. doi:10.100700268-021-06082-8 PMID:33770240

Tarassoli, S. (2019). Artificial intelligence, regenerative surgery, robotics? What is realistic for the future of surgery? *Annals of Medicine and Surgery (London), 41*, 53–55. doi:10.1016/j.amsu.2019.04.001 PMID:31049197

Tardif, N., Therrien, C.-É., & Bouchard, S. (2019). Re-Examining Psychological Mechanisms Underlying Virtual Reality-Based Exposure for Spider Phobia. *Cyberpsychology, Behavior, and Social Networking, 22*(1), 29–35. doi:10.1089/cyber.2017.0711 PMID:30256675

Taylor, J. E., Sullman, M. J., & Stephens, A. N. (2018). Measuring anxiety-related avoidance with the Driving and Riding Avoidance Scale (DRAS). *European Journal of Psychological Assessment*.

Taylor, J., Deane, F., & Podd, J. (2002). Driving-related fear: A review. *Clinical Psychology Review, 22*(5), 631–645. doi:10.1016/S0272-7358(01)00114-3 PMID:12113199

Teel, E., Gay, M., Johnson, B., & Slobounov, S. (2016). Determining sensitivity/specificity of virtual reality- based neuropsychological tool for detecting residual abnormalities following sport-related concussion. *Neuropsychology, 30*(4), 474–483. doi:10.1037/neu0000261 PMID:27045961

Ten Cate, O., & Billett, S. (2014). Competency-based medical education: Origins, perspectives and potentialities. *Medical Education, 48*(3), 325–332. doi:10.1111/medu.12355 PMID:24528467

Tepper, O. M., Rudy, H. L., Lefkowitz, A., Weimer, K. A., Marks, S. M., Stern, C. S., & Garfein, E. S. (2017). Mixed Reality with HoloLens: Where Virtual Reality Meets Augmented Reality in the Operating Room. *Plastic and Reconstructive Surgery, 140*(5), 1066–1070. doi:10.1097/PRS.0000000000003802 PMID:29068946

Topçu, Ç., Uysal, H., Özkan, Ö., Özkan, Ö., Polat, Ö., Bedeloğlu, M., Akgül, A., Naz Döğer, E., Sever, R., & Çolak, Ö. H. (2018). Recovery of Facial Expressions Using Functional Electrical Stimulation After Full-face Transplantation. *Journal of Neuroengineering and Rehabilitation, 15*(15).

Torpil, B., Sahin, S., Pekçetin, S., & Uyanik, M. (2021). The effectiveness of a virtual reality-based intervention on cognitive functions in older adults with mild cognitive impairment: A single-blind, randomized controlled trial. *Games for Health Journal, 10*(2), 109–115. doi:10.1089/g4h.2020.0086 PMID:33058735

Torres, J. C., Torres, P. V., & Infante, M. A. (2015). Aprendizajemóvil:perspectivas.RUSC. *Universities and Knowledge Society Journal, 12*, 38–49. https://www.redalyc.org/articulo.oa?id=78033494005

Touati, R., Richert, R., Millet, C., Farges, J.C., Sailer, I., & Ducret, M. (2019). Comparison of two innovative strategies using augmented reality for communication in aesthetic dentistry: A pilot study. *Journal of Healthcare Engineering, 6*(24), 5139.

Towers-Clark, C. (2021). Medicine and Mindfulness: How VR is Helping Healthcare Through the Pandemic. *Forbes.* https://www.forbes.com/sites/charlestowersclark/2021/02/19/medicine--mindfulness-how-vr-training-is-helping-health-care-through-the-pandemic/?sh=36ce916558b9

Trappey, A. J. C., Trappey, C. V., Chang, C. M., Kuo, R. R. T., & Lin, A. P. C. (2021). Virtual reality exposure therapy for driving phobia disorder (2): System refinement and verification. *Applied Sciences (Basel, Switzerland), 11*(1), 347. doi:10.3390/app11010347

Trappey, A. J. C., Trappey, C. V., Chang, C. M., Kuo, R. R. T., Lin, A. P. C., & Nieh, C. H. (2020). Virtual reality exposure therapy for driving phobia disorder: System design and development. *Applied Sciences (Basel, Switzerland), 10*(14), 4860. doi:10.3390/app10144860

Triepels, C., Smeets, C., Notten, K., Kruitwagen, R., Futterer, J. J., Vergeldt, T., & Van Kuijk, S. (2020). Does three-dimensional anatomy improve student understanding? *Clinical Anatomy (New York, N.Y.), 33*(1), 25–33. doi:10.1002/ca.23405 PMID:31087400

Triscari, M. T., Faraci, P., Catalisano, D., D'Angelo, V., & Urso, V. (2015). Effectiveness of cognitive behavioral therapy integrated with systematic desensitization, cognitive behavioral therapy combined with eye movement desensitization and reprocessing therapy, and cognitive behavioral therapy combined with virtual reality expo. *Neuropsychiatric Disease and Treatment, 11*, 2591–2598. doi:10.2147/NDT.S93401 PMID:26504391

Trivedi, P. G. (2018). *Human Emotion Recognition from Physiological Biosignals*. Academic Press.

Trost, Z., France, C., Anam, M., & Shum, C. (2021). Virtual reality approaches to pain: Toward a state of the science. *Pain, 162*(2), 325–331. doi:10.1097/j.pain.0000000000002060 PMID:32868750

Tsapakis, S., Papaconstantinou, D., Diagourtas, A., Droutsas, K., Andreanos, K., Moschos, M. M., & Brouzas, D. (2017). Visual Field Examination Method Using Virtual Reality Glasses Compared with the Humphrey Perimeter. *Clinical Ophthalmology (Auckland, N.Z.), 11*, 1431–1443. https://doi.org/10.2147/OPTH.S131160

Tsutsumi, M., Nogaki, H., Shimizu, Y., Stone, T. E., & Kobayashi, T. (2017, May). Individual reactions to viewing preferred video representations of the natural environment: A comparison of mental and physical reactions. *Japan Journal of Nursing Science, 14*(1), 3–12. doi:10.1111/jjns.12131 PMID:27160351

Tulving, E., & Craik, F. I. M. (Eds.). (2000). *The Oxford handbook of memory*. Oxford University Press.

Tursi, M. F., Baes, C., Camacho, F. R., Tofoli, S. M., & Juruena, M. F. (2013). Effectiveness of psychoeducation for depression: A systematic review. *The Australian and New Zealand Journal of Psychiatry, 47*(11), 1019–1031. doi:10.1177/0004867413491154 PMID:23739312

UNESCO. (2016). *Global Education Monitoring Report: Education for People and Planet*. UNESCO.

UNESCO. (2020). *Embracing Dyslexia - Crossing the chasm and saving lives*. https://bit.ly/2Vzyey2

UNICEF. (2013). *Children with Disabilities*. UNICEF.

Uppot, R. N., Laguna, B., McCarthy, C. J., De Novi, G., Phelps, A., Siegel, E., & Courtier, J. (2019). Implementing Virtual and Augmented Reality Tools for Radiology Education and Training, Communication, and Clinical Care. *Radiology, 291*(3), 570–580. doi:10.1148/radiol.2019182210 PMID:30990383

Urbina, S. (2014). *Essentials of psychological testing* (2nd ed.). John Wiley & Sons Inc.

Vadalà, G., De Salvatore, S., Ambrosio, L., Russo, F., Papalia, R., & Denaro, V. (2020). Robotic spine surgery and augmented reality systems: A state of the art. *Neurospine, 17*(1), 88–100. doi:10.14245/ns.2040060.030 PMID:32252158

Valdés Olmos, R. A., Vidal-Sicart, S., Giammarile, F., Zaknun, J. J., Van Leeuwen, F. W., & Mariani, G. (2014). The GOSTT concept and hybrid mixed/virtual/augmented reality environment radioguided surgery. *The Quarterly Journal of Nuclear Medicine and Molecular Imaging, 58*(2), 207–215.

Valmaggia, L. R., Latif, L., Kempton, M. J., & Rus-Calafell, M. (2016). Virtual reality in the psychological treatment for mental health problems: An systematic review of recent evidence. *Psychiatry Research, 236*, 189–195. doi:10.1016/j.psychres.2016.01.015 PMID:26795129

van der Niet, A. G., & Bleakley, A. (2021). Where medical education meets artificial intelligence:'Does technology care?'. *Medical Education, 55*(1), 30–36. doi:10.1111/medu.14131 PMID:32078175

Van der Schans, E., Hiep, M., Consten, E., & Broeders, I. A. (2020). From Da Vinci Si to Da Vinci Xi: Realistic times in draping and docking the robot. *Journal of Robotic Surgery, 14*(6), 835–839. doi:10.100711701-020-01057-8 PMID:32078114

Van Gog, T., Paas, F., Marcus, N., Ayres, P., & Sweller, J. (2008). The mirror neuron system and observational learning: Implications for the effectiveness of dynamic visualizations. *Educational Psychology Review, 21*(1), 21–30. doi:10.100710648-008-9094-3

Van Merriënboer, J. J. G., & Sweller, J. (2005). Cognitive load theory and complex learning: Recent developments and future directions. *Educational Psychology Review, 17*(2), 147–177. doi:10.100710648-005-3951-0

Van Merriënboer, J. J. G., & Sweller, J. (2010). Cognitive load theory in health professional education: Design principles and strategies. *Medical Education, 44*, 85–93. doi:10.1111/j.1365-2923.2009.03498.x PMID:20078759

van Rijsbergen, M. W., Mark, R. E., de Kort, P. L., & Sitskoorn, M. M. (2014). Subjective cognitive complaints after stroke: A systematic review. *Journal of Stroke and Cerebrovascular Diseases, 23*(3), 408–420. doi:10.1016/j.jstroke-cerebrovasdis.2013.05.003 PMID:23800498

Vankipuram, A., Khanal, P., Ashby, A., Vankipuram, M., Gupta, A., Drumm Gurnee, D., Josey, K., & Smith, M. (2014). Design and Development of a Virtual Reality Simulator for Advanced Cardiac Life Support Training. *IEEE Journal of Biomedical and Health Informatics, 18*(4), 1478–1484.

Vávra, P., Roman, J., Zonča, P., Ihnát, P., Němec, M., Kumar, J., Habib, N., & El-Gendi, A. (2017). Recent Development of Augmented Reality in Surgery: A Review. *Journal of Healthcare Engineering, 4574172*, 1–9. Advance online publication. doi:10.1155/2017/4574172 PMID:29065604

Verhey, J. T., Haglin, J. M., Verhey, E. M., & Hartigan, D. E. (2020). Virtual, augmented, and mixed reality applications in orthopedic surgery. *The International Journal of Medical Robotics + Computer Assisted Surgery, 16*(2), e2067. PMID:31867864

Viehöfer, A. F., Wirth, S. H., Zimmermann, S. M., Jaberg, L., Dennler, C., Fürnstahl, P., & Farshad, M. (2020). Augmented reality guided osteotomy in hallux Valgus correction. *BMC Musculoskeletal Disorders*, *21*(1), 438. doi:10.118612891-020-03373-4 PMID:32631342

Viglialoro, R. M., Condino, S., Turini, G., Carbone, M., Ferrari, V., & Gesi, M. (2021). Augmented Reality, Mixed Reality, and Hybrid Approach in Healthcare Simulation: A Systematic Review. *Applied Sciences (Basel, Switzerland)*, *11*(5), 2338. doi:10.3390/app11052338

Vos, T., Lim, S. S., Abbafati, C., Abbas, K. M., Abbasi, M., Abbasifard, M., Abbasi-Kangevari, M., Abbastabar, H., Abd-Allah, F., Abdelalim, A., Abdollahi, M., Abdollahpour, I., Abolhassani, H., Aboyans, V., Abrams, E. M., Abreu, L. G., Abrigo, M. R. M., Abu-Raddad, L. J., Abushouk, A. I., ... Murray, C. J. (2020). Global burden of 369 diseases and injuries in 204 countries and territories, 1990–2019: A systematic analysis for the Global Burden of Disease Study 2019. *Lancet*, *396*(10258), 1204–1222. doi:10.1016/S0140-6736(20)30925-9 PMID:33069326

Voštinár, P., Horváthová, D., Mitter, M., & Bako, M. (2021). The look at the various uses of VR. *Open Computer Science*, *11*(1), 241–250. doi:10.1515/comp-2020-0123

Vygotsky, L. S. (1978). Zone of proximal development: A new approach. *Mind in society: The development of higher psychological processes*, 84-91.

Wagner, A., Rasse, M., Millesi, W., & Ewers, R. (1997). Virtual reality for orthognathic surgery: The augmented reality environment concept. *Journal of Oral and Maxillofacial Surgery*, *55*(5), 456–462. doi:10.1016/S0278-2391(97)90689-3 PMID:9146514

Wake, N., Nussbaum, J. E., Elias, M. I., Nikas, C. V., & Bjurlin, M. A. (2020). 3D Printing, Augmented Reality, and Virtual Reality for the Assessment and Management of Kidney and Prostate Cancer: A Systematic Review. *Urology*, *143*, 20–32. doi:10.1016/j.urology.2020.03.066 PMID:32535076

Wald, J., & Taylor, S. (2000). Efficacy of virtual reality exposure therapy to treat driving phobia: A case report. *Journal of Behavior Therapy and Experimental Psychiatry*, *31*(3-4), 249–257. doi:10.1016/S0005-7916(01)00009-X PMID:11494960

Waldrop, M. M. (2017). News feature: Virtual reality therapy set for a real renaissance. *Proceedings of the National Academy of Sciences of the United States of America*, *114*(39), 10295–10299. doi:10.1073/pnas.1715133114 PMID:28951492

Walliczek, U., Förtsch, A., Dworschak, P., Teymoortash, A., Mandapathil, M., Werner, J., & Güldner, C. (2016). Effect of training frequency on the learning curve on the da Vinci Skills Simulator. *Head & Neck*, *38*(S1), E1762–E1769. doi:10.1002/hed.24312 PMID:26681572

Wall, K., Stark, J., Schillaci, A., Saulnier, E. T., McLaren, E., Striegnitz, K., Cohen, B., Arciero, P., Kramer, A., & Anderson-Hanley, C. (2018). The Enhanced Interactive Physical and Cognitive Exercise System (iPACES™ v2.0): Pilot Clinical Trial of an In-Home iPad-Based Neuro-Exergame for Mild Cognitive Impairment (MCI). *Journal of Clinical Medicine*, *7*(9), 249. doi:10.3390/jcm7090249 PMID:30200183

Wang, F., Liu, Y., Tian, M., Zhang, Y., Zhang, S., & Chen, J. (2016). Application of a 3d Haptic Virtual Reality Simulation System for Dental Crown Preparation Training. *8th International Conference on Information Technology in Medicine and Education (ITME)*, 424–427.

Wang, J., Suenaga, H., & Hoshi, K. (2014). Augmented reality navigation with automatic marker-free image registration using 3-D image overlay for dental surgery. *IEEE Transactions on Biomedical Engineering*, *61*(4), 1295–1304. doi:10.1109/TBME.2014.2301191 PMID:24658253

Wang, J., Suenaga, H., Liao, H., Hoshi, K., Yang, L., Kobayashi, E., & Sakuma, I. (2015). Real-time computer-generated integral imaging and 3D image calibration for augmented reality surgical navigation. *Computerized Medical Imaging and Graphics*, *40*, 147–159. doi:10.1016/j.compmedimag.2014.11.003 PMID:25465067

Wang, M., Shen, L. Q., Pasquale, L. R., Petrakos, P., Formica, S., Boland, M. V., Wellik, S. R., & ... (2019, January 25). An Artificial Intelligence Approach to Detect Visual Field Progression in Glaucoma Based on Spatial Pattern Analysis. *Investigative Ophthalmology & Visual Science*, *60*(1), 365–375. https://doi.org/10.1167/iovs.18-25568

Wasserman, J. D., & Bracken, B. A. (2003). Psychometric characteristics of assessment procedures. In J. R. Graham & J. A. Naglieri (Eds.), Handbook of psychology: Vol. 10. *Assessment psychology* (pp. 43–66). John Wiley & Sons Inc.

Wechsler, T. F., Kümpers, F., & Mühlberger, A. (2019). Inferiority or Even Superiority of Virtual Reality Exposure Therapy in Phobias? A Systematic Review and Quantitative Meta-Analysis on Randomized Controlled Trials Specifically Comparing the Efficacy of Virtual Reality Exposure to Gold Standard in vivo Exp. *Frontiers in Psychology*, *10*, 1758. Advance online publication. doi:10.3389/fpsyg.2019.01758 PMID:31551840

Weech, S., Kenny, S., & Barnett-Cowan, M. (2019). Presence and Cybersickness in Virtual Reality Are Negatively Related: A Review. *Frontiers in Psychology*, *10*, 158. Advance online publication. doi:10.3389/fpsyg.2019.00158 PMID:30778320

Wei, N., Dougherty, B., Myers, A., & Badawy, S. (2018). Using Google Glass in surgical settings: Systematic review. *JMIR mHealth and uHealth*, *6*(3), e9409. doi:10.2196/mhealth.9409 PMID:29510969

Welie, J. V. (2004). Is dentistry a profession? Part 3. Future challenges. *Journal - Canadian Dental Association*, *70*(10), 675–678. PMID:15530264

Wen, J. C., Lee, C. S., Keane, P. A., & Sa Xiao, A. S. (2019, April 5). Forecasting Future Humphrey Visual Fields Using Deep Learning. *PLoS One*, *14*(4), e0214875. https://doi.org/10.1371/journal.pone.0214875

Werbach, K. (2014). ReDefining Gamification: A Process Approach. In *Proceedings of the 9th International Conference on Persuasive Technology* - Volume 8462. Springer-Verlag. 10.1007/978-3-319-07127-5_23

Whittaker, G., Aydin, A., Raison, N., Kum, F., Challacombe, B., Khan, M. S., Dasgupta, P., & Ahmed, K. (2016). Validation of the RobotiX mentor robotic surgery simulator. *Journal of Endourology*, *30*(3), 338–346. doi:10.1089/end.2015.0620 PMID:26576836

Whittaker, G., Aydin, A., Raveendran, S., Dar, F., Dasgupta, P., & Ahmed, K. (2019). Validity assessment of a simulation module for robot-assisted thoracic lobectomy. *Asian Cardiovascular & Thoracic Annals*, *27*(1), 23–29. doi:10.1177/0218492318813457 PMID:30417680

WHO. (2011). *World report on disability 2011*. World Health Organization.

Wiederhold, B. K., Jang, D. P., Kim, S. I., & Wiederhold, M. D. (2002). Physiological monitoring as an objective tool in virtual reality therapy. *Cyberpsychology & Behavior*, *5*(1), 77–82. doi:10.1089/109493102753685908 PMID:11990977

Wiedermann, J. (2003). Mirror neurons, embodied cognitive agents and imitation learning. *Computer Information*, *22*, 545–559.

Wiles, A.D., Thompson, D.G., & Frantz, D.D. (2004). Accuracy assessment and interpretation for optical tracking systems. *Visual Image Guid Proced Displ, 5367*, 421-32.

Williams, P., Jamali, H. R., & Nicholas, D. (2006). Using ICT with people with special education needs: What the literature tells us. *Aslib Proceedings*, *58*(4), 330–345. doi:10.1108/00012530610687704

Wilson, B. A. (2002). Towards a comprehensive model of cognitive rehabilitation. *Neuropsychological Rehabilitation*, *12*(2), 97–110. doi:10.1080/09602010244000020

Wilson, B. A., & Evans, J. (2020). Does cognitive rehabilitation work? Clinical and economic considerations and outcomes. In *Clinical neuropsychology and cost outcome research* (pp. 329–349). Psychology Press. doi:10.4324/9781315787039-23

Wilson, I., & Shankar, P. R. (2021). The COVID-19 pandemic and undergraduate medical student teaching/learning and assessment. *MedEdPublish*, 10.

Windman, V. (2012). iPad Apps for Students with Autism. *Tech & Learning*, *32*(7), 28.

Winkler, S. L., Kairalla, J. A., Cooper, R., Gaunaurd, I., Schlesinger, M., Krueger, A., & Ludwig, A. (2016). Comparison of Functional Benefits of Self-management Training for Amputees Under Virtual World and E-learning Conditions. *11th International Conference on Disability, Virtual Reality&Associated Technologies*.

Wohlgenannt, I., Simons, A., & Stieglitz, S. (2020). Virtual reality. *Business & Information Systems Engineering*, *62*(5), 455–461. doi:10.100712599-020-00658-9

Wong, A., Leahy, W., Marcus, N., & Sweller, J. (2012). Cognitive load theory, the transient information effect and e-learning. *Learning and Instruction*, *22*(6), 449–457. doi:10.1016/j.learninstruc.2012.05.004

World Health Organisation. (2021). *International Data Online Updates*. https://www.who.int/data

Wouters, P., Paas, F. G. W. C., & Van Merriënboer, J. J. G. (2017). How to optimize learning from animated models: A review of guidelines based on cognitive load. *Review of Educational Research*, *78*(3), 645–675. doi:10.3102/0034654308320320

Wu, J., Sun, Y., Zhang, G., Zhou, Z., & Ren, Z. (2021). Virtual Reality-Assisted Cognitive Behavioral Therapy for Anxiety Disorders: A Systematic Review and Meta-Analysis. *Frontiers in Psychiatry*, *12*, 575094. doi:10.3389/fpsyt.2021.575094 PMID:34366904

Yang, Y., Allen, T., Abdullahi, S. M., Pelphrey, K. A., Volkmar, F. R., & Chapman, S. B. (2018). Neural mechanisms of behavioral change in young adults with high-functioning autism receiving virtual reality social cognition training: A pilot study. *Autism Research*, *11*(5), 713–725. https://doi-org.ezproxy2.umc.edu/10.1002/aur.1941

Yang, X., Yeh, S.-C., Niu, J., Gong, Y., & Yang, G. (2017). Hand Rehabilitation Using Virtual Reality and Electromyography Signals. *5th International Conference on Enterprise Systems*.

Yee, N., & Bailenson, J. (2007). The proteus effect. The effect of transformed self-representation on behavior. *Human Communication Research*, *33*(3), 271–290. doi:10.1111/j.1468-2958.2007.00299.x

Yigitcanlar, T., Butler, L., Windle, E., Desouza, K. C., Mehmood, R., & Corchado, J. M. (2020). Can building "artificially intelligent cities" safeguard humanity from natural disasters, pandemics, and other catastrophes? An urban scholar's perspective. *Sensors (Basel)*, *20*(10), 2988. doi:10.339020102988 PMID:32466175

Yildirim, C. (2020). Don't make me sick: Investigating the incidence of cybersickness in commercial virtual reality headsets. *Virtual Reality (Waltham Cross)*, *24*(2), 231–239. doi:10.100710055-019-00401-0

Yin, Z., Zhao, M., Wang, Y., Yang, J., & Zhang, J. (2017). Recognition of emotions using multimodal physiological signals and an ensemble deep learning model. *Computer Methods and Programs in Biomedicine*, *140*, 93–110. doi:10.1016/j.cmpb.2016.12.005 PMID:28254094

Yu, F., Song, E., Liu, H., Li, Y., Zhu, J., & Hung, C. C. (2018). An Augmented Reality Endoscope System for Ureter Position Detection. *Journal of Medical Systems*, *42*(8), 138. doi:10.100710916-018-0992-8 PMID:29938379

Yuk, F. J., Maragkos, G. A., Sato, K., & Steinberger, J. (2020). Current innovation in virtual and augmented reality in spine surgery. *Annals of Translational Medicine*, *9*(1), 94. Advance online publication. doi:10.21037/atm-20-1132 PMID:33553387

Yung, H. I., & Paas, F. (2015). Effects of computer-based visual representation on mathematics learning and cognitive load. *Journal of Educational Technology & Society*, *18*(4), 70–77.

Zadik, Y., & Levin, L. (2006). Decision making of Hebrew University and Tel Aviv University Dental Schools graduates in every day dentistry-is there a difference? *J Isr Dent Assoc, 4*, 19-23.

Zadik, Y., & Levin, L. (2008). Clinical decision making in restorative dentistry, endodontics, and antibiotic prescription. *J Dent Educ, 72*, 81-6.

Zeng, N., Pope, Z., Lee, J. E., & Gao, Z. (2018). Virtual Reality Exercise for Anxiety and Depression: A Preliminary Review of Current Research in an Emerging Field. *Journal of Clinical Medicine*, *7*(3), 42. doi:10.3390/jcm7030042 PMID:29510528

Zhang, B., & Robb, N. (2020). A comparison of the effects of augmented reality N-back training and traditional two-dimensional N-back training for working memory. *SAGE Open*, 1–14.

Zhao, J., Xu, X., Jiang, H., & Ding, Y. (2020). The effectiveness of virtual reality-based technology on anatomy teaching: A meta-analysis of randomized controlled studies. *BMC Medical Education*, *20*(1), 127. doi:10.118612909-020-1994-z PMID:32334594

Zikl, P., Bartošová, I. K., Víšková, K. J., Havlíčková, K., Kučírková, A., Navrátilová, J., & Zetková, B. (2015). The possibilities of ICT use for compensation of difficulties with reading in pupils with dyslexia. *Procedia: Social and Behavioral Sciences*, *176*(1), 915–922. doi:10.1016/j.sbspro.2015.01.558

Zinzow, H. M., Brooks, J. O., Rosopa, P. J., Jeffirs, S., Jenkins, C., Seeanner, J., McKeeman, A., & Hodges, L. F. (2018). Virtual reality and cognitive-behavioral therapy for driving anxiety and aggression in veterans: A pilot study. *Cognitive and Behavioral Practice*, *25*(2), 296–309. doi:10.1016/j.cbpra.2017.09.002

Zorzal, E. R., Campos Gomes, J. M., Sousa, M., Belchior, P., da Silva, P. G., Figueiredo, N., Lopes, D. S., & Jorge, J. (2020). Laparoscopy with augmented reality adaptations. *Journal of Biomedical Informatics*, *107*, 103463. doi:10.1016/j.jbi.2020.103463 PMID:32562897

Zulkifli, A. F. (2019). Student-centered approach and alternative assessments to improve students' learning domains during health education sessions. *Biomedical Human Kinetics*, *11*(1), 80–86. doi:10.2478/bhk-2019-0010

About the Contributors

Luis Pinto Coelho is an adjunct professor at the Engineering School of Polytechnic Institute of Porto. He is a PhD in Telecommunications and Signal Processing since 2012, and a MsC in Electronics Engineering, since 2005. As a researcher he has published several scientific articles in conferences and journals. He actively collaborates with the scientific community as participant, reviewer, organizer of scientific conferences or as journal editor. His main research interests are on image and signal processing, human-machine interaction and management, all topics with a special focus on the healthcare area.

Ricardo Queirós is a Ph.D. in Computer Science at the Faculty of Sciences of the University of Porto. He is currently a lecturer at the Department of Informatics of the Media Arts and Design School (Polytechnic Institute of Porto). He is also a researcher in the field of e-learning standardization and interoperability, systems architectural integration and gamification in the computer programming domain at the Center for Research in Advanced Computing Systems (CRACS) research group of INESC TEC Porto and uniMAD research group. He has participated in several research projects in his main research areas, including technology transfer projects with industrial partners. He has over 100 publications in books, book chapters, conference proceedings, and journals.

Sara Seabra Reis has an MSc in Clinical Process Optimization and PhD in Bioethics/Biomedical Engineering. She is a Polytechnic Higher Education Teacher with the category of Prof. Adjunct. Interests are in the area of Biomedical Engineering, namely in the areas of Innovation and Health Management.

* * *

Anmol Bagaria is Founder and CEO of CynoDent- Global Healthcare for all. Has Completed BDS from Prestigious Bharati Vidyapeeth Deemed to be University's Dental College & Hospital, Navi Mumbai. And has clinical practice Experience of 3 years. Certified BLS, ACLS and PCLS provider by American Heart Association. Done Fellowship in Facial Aesthetics and Cosmetology from USA; Fellow of the Academy of General Education (FAGE), Manipal; NABH Clinical Auditor by National Accreditation Board for Hospitals & Healthcare Providers of Quality Council of India. She is a Researcher, Oral Health Expert and Social Activist. She has lead various esteemed dental societies and also Headed & Organized Various Projects at National as well as International platforms and has been awarded prestigious awards for the same. She had also designed ideas for oral health awareness & education which had made history on international level. She has headed international projects of UNDP, UNICEF, WHO and also organized international conferences and was award committee head in various organisations.

She is extensively involved in community service. She has more than 50 publications in various indexed national and international journals. She has delivered keynote/Guest lectures internationally. She is a Member, Reviewer, Chief Editor & Advisor Nationally and Internationally. She has been honoured with prestigious awards Nationally & Internationally for remarkable work in the Field of Dentistry.

Jagrika Bajaj received her Master's degree in Clinical psychology from Christ University, India and is currently working as a psychologist. She is an Associate American Psychological Association member. Her interest is in exploring the integration between mental health and technology that can be used as a medium to provide mental health services. Core interests: Psychotherapy, Technology, Virtual Reality.

Israel Barrutia Barreto is a Doctor of Administration, graduate of Centrum, Pucp, candidate for a doctorate in education, Universidad Autónoma Benito Juárez, Mexico, master's degree in business administration and management, graduate of master's degree in public management, master's degree in education, degree in administration, collegiate, specialist in cooperatives and logistics, with 25 years of professional experience in public and private entities, university professor, advisor and jury of undergraduate and graduate theses, author of research books, academic books, scientific articles, nominated for the Master of the Year award Unab - Colombia, with excellent grades in teacher evaluation at universities in Colombia and Peru. Lectures on research, production, logistics, entrepreneurship in prestigious companies and universities in Peru and Colombia, consultant to SMEs, cooperatives, public and private companies, diagnostic capacity of productive units. He currently works as General Manager of the Innova Scientific research center.

Ranjit Barua is a Senior Researcher at Centre for Healthcare Science and Technology, IIEST-SHIBPUR. Core research area Bio-Mechanical System, 3D Bioprinting, Tissue Engineering.

Deborah Chen graduated from the University of California, Berkeley with a Bachelors of Science in Molecular Environmental Biology and a minor in Molecular Toxicology.

Nikita Chigullapally graduated from the University of California, Berkeley with a Bachelors of Science in Nutritional Sciences Physiology and Metabolism.

Suzy Chung graduated from the University of California, Santa Cruz with a Bachelors of Arts in Psychology and Bachelors of Science in Molecular Cell and Developmental Biology.

Fabrizio Del Carpio Delgado is a Master Civil Engineer with a major in construction management. Collegiate and titled. Specialized in Management with processes for the identification of seismic vulnerability. He also works as a university professor at the professional school of civil engineering of the National University of Moquegua. It publishes research within the branches of science and technology. It belongs to the Latin American council of the ASTM in the chapter of soils and aggregates. He has been qualified as a Researcher before the National Council of Science, Technology and Technological Innovation (CONCYTEC) of Peru.

Idalina Cunha de Freitas was born in Johannesburg (South Africa) in 1998, having moved to Madeira Island (Portugal) in 2008 where she completed primary school and high school (2018). Recently she graduated from the Instituto Superior de Engenharia do Porto accomplishing a bachelor's degree in biomedical engineering.

Vitor Gonçalves is a professor in the Department of Educational Technology and Information Management in the School of Education (ESE) of the Polytechnic Institute of Bragança (IPB). PhD in Electrical and Computer Engineering and Master in Multimedia Technology from the Faculty of Engineering of the University of Porto. Degree in Management Informatics from the University of Minho. He is currently a Researcher at the IPB Basic Education Research Center. More information: https://www.cienciavitae.pt/A310-FFD6-55A1.

Catherine Hayes, having qualified as a podiatrist in 1992, is now Professor of Health Professions Pedagogy and Scholarship in the Faculty of Applied Sciences at the University of Sunderland, UK. She is also a UK National Teaching Fellow, Principal Fellow of the Higher Education Academy and Visiting Professor in Higher Education at the Universities of Cumbria and Liverpool Hope in the UK. Catherine is Secretary of the International Federation of National Teaching Fellows and works with the UK's Ministry of Defence's Medical Defence Academy in framing military epistemology within a modernised education and training curriculum for tripartite services provision.

Dorota Kamińska graduated in Automatic Control and Robotics and completed postgraduate studies in Biomedical image processing and analysis at Lodz University of Technology. She received her PhD degree from the Faculty of Electrical, Electronic, Computer and Control Engineering at Lodz University of Technology in 2014. She gained experience during the TOP 500 Innovators program at Haas School of Business, University of California in Berkeley. An educator and researcher at the Institute of Mechatronics and Information Systems, a founder and a leader of the Voxel Research Lab, currently focusing her academic pursuits on cutting-edge VR and AR applications. She is an Associate Editor and Guest Lead Editor of several journals and Special Issues such as Electronics, Entropy, Information. She has received a number of national and European Research grants and has been involved in many international industrial projects. She has published over 50 scientific works and has been organizing challenges and workshops in ECML19 and FG20. She is passionate about biomedical signal analysis and practical applications of machine and deep learning. As a participant in many interdisciplinary and international projects, she is constantly looking for new challenges and possibilities of self-development.

Gino Laque Córdova has 14 years of university teaching at the National University of the Altiplano. At present Appointed Teacher of the Professional School of Civil Engineering - National University of the Altiplano. With an academic degree of Master of Science with a mention in Geotechnical Engineering, at the Alas Peruanas University. Completed doctorate studies in Science and technology and the environment. Currently president of the Quality, Licensing and Accreditation committee of the Professional School of Civil Engineering. With more than 15 years of professional experience developing various engineering studies for civil infrastructure projects.

Allan Lu Lee graduated from the University of California, Berkeley with a Bachelors of Science in Bioengineering.

Scott Lee, MD, MPH, FACS, is a board certified orbit, ophthalmic, and oculoplastic surgeon.

Sonal Mahilkar completed her BDS from Government Dental College Raipur, went on to pursue MSc in Dental Public Health from Queen Mary University of London, UK, and MDS in Periodontology and Implantology from Maitri College of Dentistry and Research Centre, Chhattisgarh. An avid reader with a zeal for academics, she is currently practicing as a periodontist and an implantologist.

Dometila Mamani Jilaja is a Doctor in Education, Master in Education Sciences with a mention in sports education, Bachelor of Physical Education, Bachelor of Initial Education, with studies of Second specialty in EIBI Primary Education, Second specialty in Psychomotricity at the National University of Altiplano Puno, Teacher of Undergraduate and graduate from the Professional School of Physical Education, Faculty of Educational Sciences of the National University of the Altiplano Puno. Member of the Inudi Peru University Research Institute and Innova Educación Magazine.

Lorenz S. Neuwirth is an Assistant Professor at the State University of New York (SUNY), College at Old Westbury and the SUNY Neuroscience Research Institute, both in the United States. He earned his Ph.D. from the City University of New York (CUNY), Graduate Center in New York and his postdoctoral training in molecular epigenetics and neurotoxicology at Thomas Jefferson University in Philadelphia in the United States. Dr. Neuwirth's two main areas of research are in developmental behavioral neurotoxicology and in neuroscience education directed towards undergraduate students. He has been recognized by earning the 2018 Carol Ann Paul Educator of the Year Award by the Society for Neuroscience (SfN) and the Faculty for Undergraduate Neuroscience (FUN) Education. Additionally, he has been recognized by the SUNY 64-Campus system with the 2020 SUNY Chancellor's Award for Excellence in Teaching.

Diane Nguyen graduated from the University of California, Berkeley with a Bachelors of Arts in Integrative Biology.

Angelbert Ramos graduated from the University of California, Berkeley with a Bachelors of Arts in Integrative Biology and Psychology.

Trinity Pauline Rico graduated from the University of California, Berkeley with a Bachelors of Arts in Molecular and Cell Biology with an emphasis in neurobiology.

Maxime Ros is a pediatric neurosurgeon that graduated from Toulouse University, France. He also holds University degrees in Microsurgery, in Medical Education, and a Biomechanics Master of Research degree from Arts-et-Métiers Engineers' School of Paris. He is currently working towards the completion of a Ph.D. at the University of Montpellier, in the School of Education. He founded a Virtual Reality-based educational technology company, Revinax®, to promote skills sharing between healthcare professionals. Notably, he has been elected as a member of the French Academy of Surgery for this project.

Renzo Seminario received his master's degree in biodiversity, landscape and sustainable management from the University of Navarra in 2017. In 2020 he was hired as a researcher by the Innova Scientific research center, a position he held until October 2020. He currently works as Manager of Innovation and Development at Innova Scientific. Writes and presents widely on environmental, technology, social science, and education topics.

Varun Shravah graduated from the University of California, Los Angeles with a Bachelors of Science in Biochemistry with a minor in Science Education.

Subash Sonkar is working as Research Scientist-II Multidisciplinary Research Unit (MRU), Maulana Azad Medical College, University of Delhi, New Delhi, India. Dr. Sonkar Ex-Consultant and Technical Advisor implementation in National Mental Health Program at Indian Council of Medical Research. Dr. Sonkar, Ex-Principal Investigator on NIH funded project affiliated with Florida International University in collaboration with Public Health Research Institute of India. He is an internationally renowned translational research professional and academician with more than 10 years of experience in project planning, review, evaluation and technology assessment. He is associated as Editor, Reviewer and Member of many online journals. His work focuses upon diverse themes crossing the interface between laboratory-based research and translational research in valuating diagnostic tests and effective diseases managements. He did extensive research and published several peer-reviewed national and international research articles in high impacts journals like Nature, Elsevier, BMC, PloS etc. He handled many national and international collaborative research projects that have been successfully completed & Patented in India. Dr. Sonkar received various International and National awards for his research like, Young Investigator, Young Scientists, Best Young Scientist, Young Leader Awards, IASSTD Awards, GHES Fellow Awards Etc. His part of research was also nominated for president awards in 2015 by University of Delhi, India.

Emily Tarver is an Assistant Professor of Emergency Medicine at the University of Mississippi Medical Center (UMMC). She completed her residency training at UMMC in 2009 and worked in community practice for 9 years before a return to academic medicine. She is a strong advocate for simulation as a means of immersive, hands-on training for all healthcare professions. She has a particular interest in virtual simulation for both remote and classroom based learning in healthcare education and has been the first simulation fellow at her institution.

Amy J. C. Trappey received her PhD in Industrial Engineering from Purdue University (USA). Prof. Trappey's research interests are in knowledge engineering and intelligent systems, particularly for IP and patent analytics, e-business and e-manufacturing. Prof. Trappey is currently serving as the Associate Editor for World Patent Information, Advanced Engineering Informatics and IEEE Transactions on SMC: Systems. Dr. Trappey is an ASME, ISEAM, and CIIE Fellow.

Charles V. Trappey received his PhD in Consumer Science from Purdue University (USA), MS in Quantitative Business Analysis from Louisiana State University (USA), and LLM in IP Law from Queensland University of Technology (Australia). Prof. Trappey's research interests are in innovation and technology forecasting, patent informatics, and technology marketing. Dr. Trappey is an Australia Trademark Attorney.

Aparna Sahu holds a PhD in Experimental-Cognitive Psychology, from the University of Toledo, Ohio, USA, and has received post-doctoral training from the Cognitive Neuropsychology Centre, Department of Experimental Psychology, University of Oxford, UK. Her research interests are in the areas of creating technology based cognitive tests and retraining modules, and exploring the roles of individual differences in cognitive performance. She has authored publications in areas such as laterality, technology and cognitive testing, and memory processing

Michael Youn graduated from the University of California, Berkeley with a Bachelors of Arts in Psychology.

Grzegorz Zwoliński received the M.Sc. and Electr. Engineer degrees from the Institute of Mechatronics and Information Systems (TUL), in 1992, and the Ph.D. degree from TUL, in 1999. He specializes in electrical machines, computer graphics, and graphics programming. He has been a university teacher of TUL, since 1993, and the University of Computer Sciences and Skills, since 1995. He is a Creator of many IT management systems, computing systems for electrical machines, and 3D graphics. He is currently working in several international projects on virtual and augmented reality.

Index

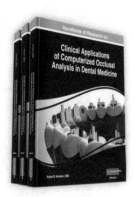
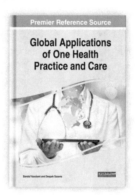
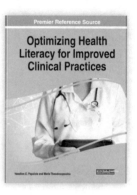
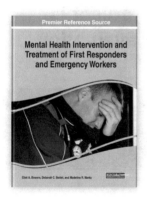
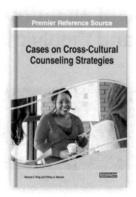
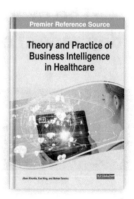
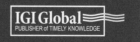

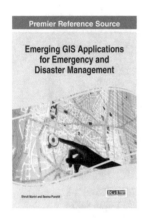
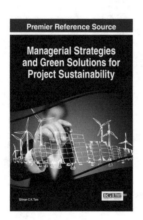
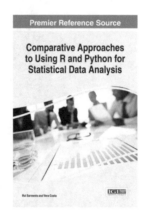
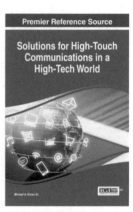

IGI Global Author Services

Providing a high-quality, affordable, and expeditious service, IGI Global's Author Services enable authors to streamline their publishing process, increase chance of acceptance, and adhere to IGI Global's publication standards.

Benefits of Author Services:

- **Professional Service:** All our editors, designers, and translators are experts in their field with years of experience and professional certifications.

- **Quality Guarantee & Certificate:** Each order is returned with a quality guarantee and certificate of professional completion.

- **Timeliness:** All editorial orders have a guaranteed return timeframe of 3-5 business days and translation orders are guaranteed in 7-10 business days.

- **Affordable Pricing:** IGI Global Author Services are competitively priced compared to other industry service providers.

- **APC Reimbursement:** IGI Global authors publishing Open Access (OA) will be able to deduct the cost of editing and other IGI Global author services from their OA APC publishing fee.

Author Services Offered:

 English Language Copy Editing
Professional, native English language copy editors improve your manuscript's grammar, spelling, punctuation, terminology, semantics, consistency, flow, formatting, and more.

 Scientific & Scholarly Editing
A Ph.D. level review for qualities such as originality and significance, interest to researchers, level of methodology and analysis, coverage of literature, organization, quality of writing, and strengths and weaknesses.

 Figure, Table, Chart & Equation Conversions
Work with IGI Global's graphic designers before submission to enhance and design all figures and charts to IGI Global's specific standards for clarity.

 Translation
Providing 70 language options, including Simplified and Traditional Chinese, Spanish, Arabic, German, French, and more.

Hear What the Experts Are Saying About IGI Global's Author Services

"Publishing with IGI Global has been an amazing experience for me for sharing my research. The strong academic production support ensures quality and timely completion." – **Prof. Margaret Niess, Oregon State University, USA**

"The service was very fast, very thorough, and very helpful in ensuring our chapter meets the criteria and requirements of the book's editors. I was quite impressed and happy with your service." – **Prof. Tom Brinthaupt, Middle Tennessee State University, USA**

Learn More or Get Started Here:

For Questions, Contact IGI Global's Customer Service Team at cust@igi-global.com or 717-533-8845

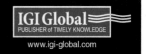
www.igi-global.com

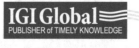

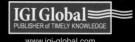

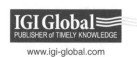
www.igi-global.com

Publisher of Peer-Reviewed, Timely, and Innovative Academic Research Since 1988

IGI Global's Transformative Open Access (OA) Model:
How to Turn Your University Library's Database Acquisitions Into a Source of OA Funding

Well in advance of Plan S, IGI Global unveiled their OA Fee Waiver (Read & Publish) Initiative. Under this initiative, librarians who invest in IGI Global's InfoSci-Books and/or InfoSci-Journals databases will be able to subsidize their patrons' OA article processing charges (APCs) when their work is submitted and accepted (after the peer review process) into an IGI Global journal.

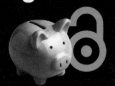

How Does it Work?

Step 1: **Library Invests in the InfoSci-Databases:** A library perpetually purchases or subscribes to the InfoSci-Books, InfoSci-Journals, or discipline/subject databases.

Step 2: **IGI Global Matches the Library Investment with OA Subsidies Fund:** IGI Global provides a fund to go towards subsidizing the OA APCs for the library's patrons.

Step 3: **Patron of the Library is Accepted into IGI Global Journal (After Peer Review):** When a patron's paper is accepted into an IGI Global journal, they option to have their paper published under a traditional publishing model or as OA.

Step 4: **IGI Global Will Deduct APC Cost from OA Subsidies Fund:** If the author decides to publish under OA, the OA APC fee will be deducted from the OA subsidies fund.

Step 5: **Author's Work Becomes Freely Available:** The patron's work will be freely available under CC BY copyright license, enabling them to share it freely with the academic community.

Note: This fund will be offered on an annual basis and will renew as the subscription is renewed for each year thereafter. IGI Global will manage the fund and award the APC waivers unless the librarian has a preference as to how the funds should be managed.

Hear From the Experts on This Initiative:

"I'm very happy to have been able to make one of my recent research contributions *freely available* along with having access to the *valuable resources* found within IGI Global's InfoSci-Journals database."

— **Prof. Stuart Palmer**, Deakin University, Australia

"Receiving the support from IGI Global's OA Fee Waiver Initiative *encourages me to continue my research work without any hesitation*."

— **Prof. Wenlong Liu**, College of Economics and Management at Nanjing University of Aeronautics & Astronautics, China

For More Information, Scan the QR Code or Contact:
IGI Global's Digital Resources Team at eresources@igi-global.com.

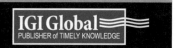
IGI Global
PUBLISHER of TIMELY KNOWLEDGE

Printed in the United States
by Baker & Taylor Publisher Services